The Politically Incorrect Guide® to
Pandemics

"Steven Mosher has a rare capacity to understand and explain big subjects. Fluent in Mandarin, he was among the first to reveal the evils worked by the modern Chinese regime. Now he sets the contemporary Chinese pandemic in historical context. In a disturbing conclusion, he shows what is different about this pandemic and why its costs have been multiplied. It is a fascinating read and should be on every bookshelf."

—**Dr. Larry P. Arnn**, president, Hillsdale College

"If you want to know what was really going on in the Wuhan Institute of Virology in the months and years leading up to the Covid pandemic, read Steven Mosher's book *The Politically Incorrect Guide to Pandemics.* Mosher challenges the narrative propagated on both sides of the Pacific by those who want to obscure the origins of the China Virus and reveals the who, what, when, how, and why of its creation—in the lab."

—**Lawrence Sellin**, Ph.D., colonel, U.S. Army Reserve, retired

"Steven Mosher is an old 'China Hand'—he knows the country, the people, the good and the bad, what's vital and what's irrelevant. In *The Politically Incorrect Guide to Pandemics* you feel that experience and depth as he takes you on a journey of exploration to find out the truth about Covid-19. That truth is unpleasant and uncomfortable—that it's imperative to understand the world of biological weapons. And that we are closer to the beginning than the end of the story of this plague."

—**Stephen K. Bannon**, host, *WarRoom*, and former White House chief strategist

"What do smallpox, bubonic plague, Spanish Flu, and other assorted influenzas have in common? As Steven Mosher's *The Politically Incorrect Guide to Pandemics* tells us, they all came from one country. And in this thoroughly researched and documented work, he also explains how Covid-19 and the world's next global disease differ from all others in history. Mosher gives us a comprehensive and compelling account, essential reading for all."

—**Gordon Chang**, author of *The Coming Collapse of China*

The Politically Incorrect Guide® to Pandemics

Steven W. Mosher

In Life!

REGNERY PUBLISHING
A Division of Salem Media Group

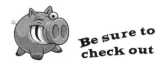
Be sure to check out

The Politically Incorrect Guides® to...

American History
Thomas Woods
9780895260475

The American Revolution
Larry Schweikart
Dave Dougherty
9781621576259

The Bible
Robert J. Hutchinson
9781596985209

The British Empire
H. W. Crocker III
9781596986299

Capitalism
Robert P. Murphy
9781596985049

Catholicism
John Zmirak
9781621575863

Christianity
Michael P. Foley
9781621575207

The Civil War
H. W. Crocker III
9781596985490

Communism
Paul Kengor
9781621575870

The Constitution
Kevin R. C. Gutzman
9781596985056

Darwinism and Intelligent Design
Jonathan Wells
9781596980136

English and American Literature
Elizabeth Kantor
9781596980112

The Founding Fathers
Brion McClanahan
9781596980921

Global Warming
Christopher C. Horner
9781596985018

The Great Depression and the New Deal
Robert Murphy
9781596980969

Hunting
Frank Miniter
9781596985216

Immigration
John Zmirak and Al Perrotta
9781621576730

Islam (And the Crusades)
Robert Spencer
9780895260130

Jihad
William Kilpatrick
9781621575771

The Middle East
Martin Sieff
9781596980518

The Presidents, Part 1
Larry Schweikart
9781621575245

The Presidents, Part 2
Steven F. Hayward
9781621575795

Real American Heroes
Brion McClanahan
9781596983205

Science
Tom Bethell
9780895260314

The Sixties
Jonathan Leaf
9781596985728

Socialism
Kevin D. Williamson
9781596986497

The South (And Why It Will Rise Again)
Clint Johnson
9781596985001

The Vietnam War
Phillip Jennings
9781596985674

Western Civilization
Anthony Esolen
9781596980594

Women, Sex, and Feminism
Carrie L. Lukas
9781596980037

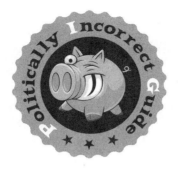

The Politically Incorrect Guide® to
Pandemics

Steven W. Mosher

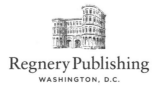

Regnery Publishing
WASHINGTON, D.C.

Politically Incorrect Guide® and Regnery® are registered trademarks of Salem Communications Holding Corporation

Cataloging-in-Publication data on file with the Library of Congress

ISBN: 978-1-68451-261-4
eISBN: 978-1-68451-277-5

Published in the United States by
Regnery Publishing
A Division of Salem Media Group
Washington, D.C.
www.Regnery.com

Manufactured in the United States of America

10 9 8 7 6 5 4 3 2 1

Books are available in quantity for promotional or premium use. For information on discounts and terms, please visit our website: www.Regnery.com.

I dedicate this book to my nine children and twelve grandchildren (and counting), in the hope that they may never again have to endure a man-made pandemic

Contents

The Plague Village of Hamin Mangha, China (circa 3000 BC)

The bodies were piled helter-skelter. Almost a hundred corpses had been hastily thrown into a small house, which was then burned to the ground, and the village itself was abandoned. Fire was the chief purifying agent of primitive man.

The village was located in China's Northeast, a vast area stretching from just north of Beijing all the way to the Amur River, which marks the border with Russia. Hamin Mangha, as it is called today, was excavated in 2011 by a team of Chinese anthropologists, who wrote in the journal *Chinese Archeology* that it was "the largest and best-preserved prehistoric settlement site found to date in northeast China."[1]

Altogether, the researchers discovered the foundations of twenty-nine houses, but one in particular caught their attention. The house, which consisted of a single 14 x 15 foot room, was filled with human bones. The ninety-seven bodies had been stacked two and three high, suggesting that the deaths had taken place so quickly that there was no time for them to be properly buried. Half were children, the others were adults, but not a single one was over thirty.

After considering a number of different scenarios, including warfare and earthquakes, the anthropologists concluded that "the large death toll might have been caused by a plague in the Horqin Sandy Land [in northeast China] 5,000 years ago."

★ ★ ★

"The Great Breeding Ground of Epidemics"

It is perhaps fitting that the earliest known epidemic for which we have archeological evidence swept across northeastern China five thousand years ago. It was a precursor of things to come.

Genomic analyses have shown that smallpox, the bubonic plague, and multiple deadly influenzas, including the "Spanish flu," actually originated in China.

It was for good reason that Francis Gasquet called China "the great breeding ground of epidemics" over a hundred years ago in his book about the bubonic plague, *The Black Death of 1348 and 1349*.[2]

The outbreak does not seem to have been restricted to Hamin Mangha, judging from the existence of another mass burial site dating from the same time. A couple hundred miles away lies Miaozigou, which was excavated some years earlier. The skeletons unearthed there were the same age as the Hamin Mangha victims and had been piled together in similar fashion. As in Hamin Mangha, something had happened in Miaozigou that killed a lot of people in a hurry and led the survivors to abandon the spot as accursed.

Identifying the Cause of the Disaster

"This similarity [between the two sites] may indicate that the cause of the Hamin Mangha site [disaster] was similar to that of the Miaozigou sites," authors Yonggang Zhu and Ping Ji wrote. "That is, they both possibly relate to an outbreak of an acute infectious disease."[3]

But if an epidemic devastated the entire region, what disease caused it?

Chinese scientists are unable to give a clear answer to the question of what killed the residents of Hamin Mangha and other settlements up to hundreds of miles away. It could have been smallpox, which, in one form or another, plagued humanity for at least ten thousand years until it was eradicated a few decades ago.

We know from written records that practitioners of traditional Chinese medicine have been grappling with deadly strains of smallpox since well before the birth of Christ. By 200 BC, as we will see in chapter 1, they had already invented an early form of vaccination, called variolation, to protect people against the disease.[4]

Smallpox is certainly deadly enough to have killed half the population of Hamin Mangha, a death toll so high it may have led the survivors to burn the victims' remains and flee the village in horror.[5]

But there is an invisible killer even deadlier than smallpox that may have struck Hamin Mangha. This would be the same disease that was responsible for three of the greatest pandemics in recorded history—the Plague of Justinian, the Black Death, and the Yunnan Plague (see chapters 2, 3, and 4 below): the bubonic plague.

All three plagues, each of which eventually made its way West, can be traced back to major epidemics in China. But the Chinese empire also endured many other outbreaks over the course of time. The historical record suggests that China, at least from the time of the first Shang Dynasty (1600–1046 BC), has probably never been completely free of the plague.[6] It is the ancestral home of the plague bacillus *Yersinia pestis,* and certain populations of rats and other rodents there serve as natural reservoirs of the disease.

The preliterate people who lived in Hamin Mangha could not leave us a written record of their travails, but the archeological record establishes that they relied on both farming and hunting for food. And among the animals they hunted was a ground-dwelling rodent—something like a prairie dog—called a marmot. Marmots, as it happens, are among the natural reservoirs of the bacillus that causes bubonic plague.

Even today, marmot hunters in northeast China occasionally come down with one or another variety of the plague through contact with infected animals. Hunters can become infected not just through bites from infected fleas, but by direct infection while handling or skinning the carcasses of infected marmots. For this reason, illnesses and even deaths from the bubonic plague bacillus are not uncommon in northeast China, but the disease itself can now be treated with antibiotics if diagnosed early.[7]

The last major epidemic of the plague occurred in China's Northeast from 1910 to 1911. Medical experts trace this epidemic back to marmot hunting as well. This time the outbreak was of the deadly pneumonic variety of the plague. There are three varieties of the disease caused by the bubonic plague bacillus *Yersinia pestis*. The disease known simply as the bubonic plague attacks the lymphatic system, the pneumonic plague infects the lungs, and the septicemic plague infects the circulatory system. One-third of those who come down with the bubonic variety survive; the other two are generally fatal.

Estimates of the death toll range up to sixty thousand, but this approximation may rely too heavily on urban statistics.[8] It is impossible to know how many people in the surrounding countryside or remoter villages succumbed.

The pneumonic plague is among the deadliest diseases on earth, with a fatality rate close to 100 percent. If an outbreak of the pneumonic variety had occurred in Hamin Mangha, few residents would have been left standing.

Aside from the bubonic plague bacillus, there is one other suspect in the murder mystery that is Hamin Mangha. We cannot rule out the possibility that this early epidemic was caused by a novel influenza virus. Many influenzas have crossed the species barrier over the millennia and taken up residence in new host populations of human beings. The disease at Hamin Mangha may have been a true zoonosis, as such infectious diseases are called—a virus new to human beings.

We know such zoonotic transmission has often occurred in China. The Chinese have eaten not just marmots but pretty much everything that flies, walks, crawls, and swims since time immemorial, providing countless opportunities for such infections to occur.[9] And once they do, China's large population provides ample opportunity for such a virus (or a bacteria) to gain a permanent foothold among its new hosts and become an endemic disease. The several viral pandemics that have emerged from China over the past century or so (see chapters 6 and 7) are proof enough of this.

We cannot know at this great remove whether the villagers of Hamin Mangha perished of smallpox, the bubonic plague, or some unknown but deadly flu virus.

The only thing we are sure of is that the residents of Hamin Mangha did not die of Covid-19 or, as I call it, the China Virus. That particular scourge would have to wait until bioweapons experts of the People's Liberation Army had mastered twenty-first-century genomic technology, created an enhanced coronavirus in the lab, and let it out into the world.

Which they did.

Plague Planet

History is largely the story of man's inhumanity to man. From Cain and Abel to Herod's Slaughter of the Innocents, from the Aztecs' cannibalistic slaughter of neighboring tribes to the Chinese Communist Party's elimination of roughly 500 million of its own citizens, born and unborn,[10] since it came to power in 1949, the death toll from the violence that men have wrought upon other men is staggering.

Natural disasters have also taken a heavy toll on humanity. From the eruption of Mount Vesuvius in AD 79 to the 1976 earthquake in Tangshan, China, that killed 240,000, from the Yangtze River flood of 1931 that killed 3.7 million to the famine that took 42.5 million Chinese lives in the wake of the Great Leap Forward, tens of millions of people have been burned, crushed, drowned, and starved to death over the centuries.

But all of these causes of death pale in comparison to the wide swath that a host of tiny killers has cut through humanity. The butcher's bill from these killers, invisible to the naked eye and unknown until the advent of modern science, numbers in the billions. Over the course of

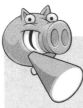

Then and Now: Zoonotic Diseases

Humanity is constantly being bombarded with zoonotic bacteria and viruses that, by reason of random genetic mutations and recombinations, manage to cross the species barrier to infect mankind. If the virus in question is highly lethal but only moderately infectious, it infects a small number of people, kills them quickly, and then dies out with its hosts. If, on the other hand, the virus is highly infectious but, say, causes little more than the sniffles, it may stick around for centuries in the human population. The common cold has been with us since the beginning of time and may well still be around at the end.

Every once in a while, however, a nightmare emerges from nature. Often as a result of a close encounter with a bird or a pig, a novel pathogen arrives on the scene that both spreads quickly and also kills mercilessly. A pandemic follows, and millions, or tens of millions, of people die. The China Virus is different. It did not manage to cross the species barrier on its own. In fact, its precursor did not even exist in nature. It is a man-made virus, the result of laboratory insertions into an existing coronavirus. The goal was to create an "unrestricted bioweapon"—a virus that was highly infectious but only moderately lethal and whose makers could plausibly deny any connection with it. The pandemic that followed the virus's release, like the virus itself, was the first man-made pandemic in the history of the world. But perhaps not the last.

human history, far more people have been felled by microorganisms than by any other cause of death.

Until fairly recently, half of all newborns did not survive to adolescence but were struck down in infancy or childhood by one of a host of waterborne and airborne pathogens. It was largely because of these tiny packets of poison—bacteria and their even smaller cousins, viruses—that human life spans averaged only twenty years or so throughout most of human history.

Many of these pathogens have probably coexisted with humanity from the beginning. We are also constantly being bombarded with zoonotic pathogens—viruses or bacteria that cross over the species barrier and "learn" to infect human beings. The vast majority of these microbes cause mild symptoms; the diseases they cause do not reach epidemic proportions; and the pathogens themselves die out after infecting, sickening, or, in the worst case, killing a small number of people. They are self-limiting.

But a deadly few—smallpox, bubonic plague, and certain respiratory viruses—have proven to be both infectious and deadly to peoples and to empires. These tiny invaders have hollowed out populations, destroyed economies, and left the survivors too weak to resist the barbarians at the gates—or even to bury the dead.

We are living on a plague planet.

PART ONE

THE CHINESE POX

CHAPTER 1

Who Conquered Whom?
The Antonine Plague (165–180)

As we know from the Neolithic plague village of Hamin Mangha,[1] mankind has been plagued with pestilence since the beginning of time. But the first plague we have good records of took place in the Roman Empire.

In AD 165, the Romans were at the height of their power. The Pax Romana—the Roman Peace—had begun in 27 BC. For almost two centuries the empire's economy had flourished, its population had burgeoned, and its well-trained and widely feared legions had maintained order and kept the barbarians at bay.

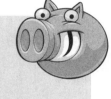

Then and Now: Pandemics

Mankind has probably been plagued with pandemics—from nature, not from bio-labs—since the beginnings of the human race. The first well-recorded one took place in the second century AD.

It would not be the barbarian hordes, though, that brought the Pax Romana to an end, but an invisible enemy against whom the legionaries' weapons were useless.

The die was cast when the Parthians, whose empire occupied the territory that makes up modern-day Iraq and Iran, defeated the Roman forces in Armenia in AD 161 and advanced against the cities of Syria, and Roman co-emperor Lucius Verus was dispatched to deal with the invaders. Over the next couple of years, the tide turned in the direction of Rome. Verus's forces pursued the defeated Parthians along the Euphrates River back to their capital and, according to the Roman historian Dio Cassius, Verus "destroyed Seleucia by fire and razed to the ground the palace of [the Parthian King] Vologases at Ctesiphon. In returning, he lost a great many of his soldiers through famine and disease, yet he got back to Syria with the survivors."[2]

What Dio Cassius left out of his account was that a plague was sweeping through Parthia at the time of the Roman attack on Parthia. Upon entering Parthian cities, the Roman soldiers immediately began to fall ill. In fact, the plague may have led them to make a hasty withdrawal, burning the Parthians' pestilential capital to the ground before they fled.[3] Fire has often been used as a defense against the spread of disease.

Verus's legions, laden with the spoils of plundered Parthian temples and herding droves of slaves and cattle, had meant to return in triumph. But as they marched west back across the desert to the Mediterranean, the deadly disease continued to eat away at their ranks. And the microscopic counter-invader that the cohorts carried back to the Roman Empire did not stop there. It ignited a devastating pandemic that would reach all corners of the Roman world over the next two decades, killing millions.

Depopulation by Plague

The Antonine Plague, as it came to be known, from the family name of the emperors Marcus Aurelius and Lucius Verus, who were both members of the Antonine family,[4] would forever alter the trajectory of the Roman Empire. It seems to have claimed the life of co-emperor Lucius Verus himself in the year 169, and arguably that of Emperor Marcus Aurelius as well, a little over a decade later. The deaths of both emperors left the unstable, even insane, Commodus (later of *Gladiator* movie fame) in charge and had other disastrous consequences as well.

Dio describes a particularly lethal outbreak of the pestilence in AD 189—"the greatest of any of which I have known" he says—in which up to two thousand people a day were dying in Rome alone.[5] Some historians estimate that between 7 and 10 percent of the population of the empire perished over the course of the twenty-three years of the Antonine Plague, although the death rate would have been considerably higher in Rome's densely populated cities and even higher in the Roman legions where it started.[6] But even this may underestimate the severity of the pandemic.

We now know that smallpox—which, it turns out, as we shall see below, was the pestilence in question—may kill up to 40 or even 50

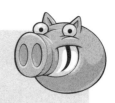

Then and Now: Mortality Rates

Given a death rate around one in three or even higher, the Romans' fear was a rational response to the actual threat level of the Antonine Plague. They personally saw many friends and family members dying. Americans in 2020 and 2021 were terrorized by media reports and official pronouncements that relentlessly exaggerated the danger of the China Virus and stoked irrational panic.

percent of the individuals it afflicts.[7] It has mercilessly devastated numerous populations in the past, including the Native American populations of the New World following their encounter with settlers from the Old. In 1707 Iceland suffered an epidemic of smallpox that swept away eighteen thousand people—a full 36 percent of the total population of fifty thousand—in a single year.[8]

With a death rate of 30 percent or more, smallpox was far more deadly than any viral plague since. Had Covid-19 struck at the time, it would scarcely have been noticed by the Romans, since its mortality rate is scarcely higher than that of a severe flu.

How many deaths would such a fatality rate have meant in Roman times? Estimates of the population of the Roman Empire during the time of Marcus Aurelius run from 60 million upwards, to 100 million or so.[9] At the low end, the Antonine Plague may have killed 5 to 10 million. But

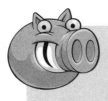

Then and Now: Flight Patterns

Just as the ancient Romans fled their plague-infested cities for the safer and more open environs of the countryside, Americans fled locked-down cities and states in 2020 and 2021 for the freer environs of states such as Florida and Texas. The difference is that there were no lockdowns in the Roman Empire, while Americans had to break quarantine to escape.

easily double this number may well have perished.[10] Those who survived were left scarred, and all too often blind.

An Equal Opportunity Killer

No one, from emperor to slave, was safe from the new disease. The ranks of upper-class Athenians were so ravaged by the outbreak that in the year 174 Marcus Aurelius relaxed the requirements for membership in the city's ruling council, the Areopagus, lest its seats go unfilled.[11] Marcus Aurelius himself lost his co-emperor to the plague, and had to bear the burdens of empire alone until his own death in AD 180, when he, too, succumbed to the disease.

As the plague spread across the empire, many cities experienced significant population decline, both from direct mortality and from the subsequent flight of fearful survivors into the countryside—an ancient but effective form of social distancing. Egyptian tax documents of the time show a sharp decline in tax revenues, much like New York and other American states experienced with the Covid-19 pandemic.[12] Civic building projects ground to a halt as well, as architectural evidence from both Rome and London shows.[13] Internal trade routes were disrupted, both between Mediterranean ports and along the extensive road system that Rome had

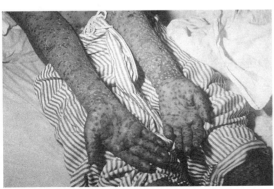

The arms and hands of a smallpox patient, Kosovo, Yugoslavia, 1972. *William Foege*[14]

built into the interior, and the economy fell into a deep recession.

Aside from the economic consequences of the outbreak, think about the fear and helplessness that the Romans must have felt in the face of a virulent disease that left you either dead or disfigured. The psychological impact of seeing friends, neighbors, and family members swept away must have been devastating. With death all around them, and recognizing their own mortality, the ancient Romans not surprisingly turned to the divine.

Some sought to win back the favor of the empire's ancient gods, who they feared had abandoned them. Marcus Aurelius himself put civic architectural projects on hold to set about restoring temples and shrines to placate the old Roman deities.[15]

Romans also turned to Christianity in large numbers. The plague pushed them into churches to petition God for protection. But there were "pull" factors at work as well,

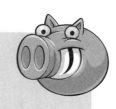

Then and Now: Resorting to Prayer

The natural reaction of people faced with their own mortality is to turn to the divine. Imagine how the Romans would have reacted if Marcus Aurelius, instead of keeping the shrines and temples open, had barred people from their places of worship, as state and local authorities across the world did during the Covid-19 pandemic. At the same time that Dr. Anthony Fauci was warning that millions might perish, he was pushing to close the very places where people might go to seek solace. With a few brave exceptions, most of the religious leaders in the United States—Catholic and Protestant alike—meekly complied.

which proved even more important. Christians were "inoculated" against their fear of death by their belief in the resurrection of the dead. Once Romans accepted this belief, they were able to say, along with St. Paul, "Death, where is thy sting?" Romans were also drawn to Christianity by the example of Christians who put their faith into action. Unlike other people, Christians did not flee from the plague. Instead, defying the disease, they "did unto others" by staying in the cities and tending to the sick and the dying. By the end of the second century—probably, in no small part, because of the plague—Christianity had spread throughout the Roman Empire.

While the Christian church was burgeoning with converts, Rome's legions were having trouble filling their ranks.

At the outbreak of the plague, Rome's military was composed of approximately 165,000 legionaries divided into some 30 legions, bolstered by 224,000 auxiliaries.[16] This professional force was highly trained and well-armed, but neither training nor weapons were able to protect Rome's military from the invisible enemy that the war with Parthia had introduced into its ranks.

Rome's soldiers had been the vectors by which the plague entered the empire, and they not surprisingly bore the brunt of the assault. Barracks life put sick soldiers in close proximity with their fellows, and the disease spread through their close-packed quarters like wildfire. Legions everywhere in the empire were stricken, weakening Rome's ability to defend the empire. Commanders in the Balkans, seeing their shrinking ranks, refused to allow old soldiers to retire from military service. In Egypt the legions replaced the fallen by enlisting the sons of soldiers who had died.[17]

The garrisons along the German frontier to the north were particularly hard hit. Both co-emperors, along with their Greek physician Galen, were present with the legions in the strategic frontier fortress of Aquileia during the winter of 168. As the plague swept through the ranks, the emperors quickly decamped to Rome, leaving their nervous physician behind to attend to the troops. Unfortunately, his humoral theory of disease was useless in dealing with an infectious disease like the plague.[18]

To bolster the depleted ranks, Marcus Aurelius began recruiting every man who could fight, including criminals, freed slaves, Germans, and even gladiators. This meant fewer games in the Colosseum, depriving the Romans of one of their chief entertainments. Still, despite the emperor's efforts, not enough soldiers could be found, and gaps in the ranks remained.

Rome's weakness invited aggression, and the Germanic tribes on the empire's northern frontier, the Marcomanni, did not hesitate. Neither did the Sarmatian tribes farther to the east, who launched their own invasion.[19] Rome's armies, already laid low by the pandemic, were ill-prepared to respond.

Not surprisingly, the hastily recruited troops failed in their duty. In AD 167, for the first time in over two centuries, Germanic tribes crossed over the Rhine. The success of the invasion was a sign that the Pax Romana was coming to an end. The empire would henceforth be beset from within and without, as civil wars at home alternated with incursions along its long northern and eastern frontiers.

Identifying an Invisible Enemy

So how do we know just what was the pestilence that Verus's legions brought back from the Middle East? Was it smallpox or, as some have thought, measles? Later historians have been frustrated by the fact that Galen, the author of *Methodus Medendi* and one of the most influential physicians of all time, treated patients at the time of this plague but did not describe it well enough to allow modern medical historians to choose between the two. His surviving case notes of the initial outbreak in Rome could describe either illness. They describe a disease that was both highly infectious and often fatal. Among the more common symptoms were fever, diarrhea, vomiting, thirstiness, swollen throat, and coughing. He wrote of a rash—he called it an "exanthem," as doctors still do today—that was highly distinctive that erupted all over the bodies of victims. He noted that the illness usually ran its course in about two weeks, and that not all who caught the disease died. Those who survived were immune from further outbreaks.

Measles and smallpox are both deadly viruses that can be said to cause a rash. Modern doctors have no trouble distinguishing between the

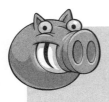

Then and Now: Medical Advice

The Roman physician Galen's best advice when dealing with a plague was to flee. He coined the Latin phrase *Cito, longe, tarde*: "Leave quickly, go far away, and come back slowly." When the Antonine Plague struck the Roman Empire, he acted on his own advice and fled to Pergamon in Asia Minor. America would arguably have been better off if many of our public health officials had done the same thing in 2020—or had simply been fired.

measles and smallpox. The "exanthem" of measles consists of a red, flat rash that starts on the face and then spreads to the rest of the body. Smallpox victims, on the other hand, develop distinctive bumps all over their bodies. The bumps are filled with thick fluid and have a characteristic depression or dimple in the center.

It wasn't until 2010 that a trio of Japanese scientists settled the issue once and for all. Measles turns out to have been a Johnny-come-lately in the plague wars. The scientists pointed out that it was not until the ninth century AD that the first scientific description of measles and smallpox—and the differences between the two—was provided by Abu Bakr, known as Rhazes.[20] And the first epidemics clearly identified as measles were not recorded until the eleventh and twelfth centuries.

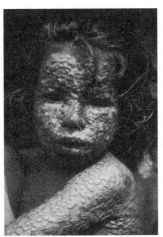

A child with smallpox in Bangladesh in 1973. *James Hicks*[22]

But the icing on the genetic cake came from comparing measles and a cattle disease called Rinderpest Virus, its closest known relative. Assuming standard mutation rates, the authors concluded that the two seem to have diverged around the eleventh or twelfth century. As they pointed out, "The result was unexpected because emergence of MeV [measles] was previously considered to have occurred in the prehistoric age."[21]

Mystery solved. Measles didn't even exist at the time of the Antonine Plague. It didn't jump from cattle to humans until a millennium later.

Smallpox, on the other hand, seems to have been around in one form or another for ten thousand years or so.[23] Its distinctive pustules have been found on three Egyptian mummies dating back to three thousand years ago, including on the mummified head of Pharaoh Rameses V, who died in 1145 BC.[24] Two hundred years earlier, it reportedly helped the Egyptians defeat the Hittites in war. The Hittite king and his son were among those who perished of the disease, after which the surviving Hittites accused the Egyptians of—you guessed it—germ warfare.[25]

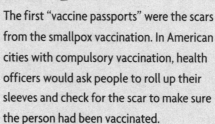

Then and Now: Vaccine Passports

The first "vaccine passports" were the scars from the smallpox vaccination. In American cities with compulsory vaccination, health officers would ask people to roll up their sleeves and check for the scar to make sure the person had been vaccinated.

The Athenian epidemic of 430–426 BC, which coincided with the opening battles of the Peloponnesian War, caused the death of the great statesman Pericles, decimated the population, and contributed significantly to the decline and fall of classical Greece. Recent scholarship suggests that it, too, was smallpox.[26]

The greatest success story in the history of vaccines has been the complete eradication of smallpox from humanity. Mass vaccination campaigns worldwide eliminated the deadly variola virus from the human population, and it has no other natural reservoirs. Many older Americans still carry a scar from the vaccination on their upper arm. The only remaining samples of the virus are confined in P4 high-containment labs.

Could smallpox make a comeback—because of a lab leak or, worse yet, at the hands of some bad actor with a bioweapons program? If a coronavirus can be weaponized and released by China—as we will see it was—then smallpox could be too.

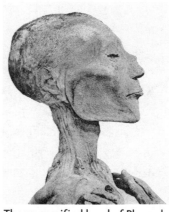

The mummified head of Pharaoh Rameses V, who died in 1145 BC, shows signs of smallpox pustules. *G. Elliott Smith*[27]

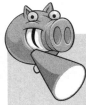

Then and Now: Vaccine Mandates

More than a century ago, a Massachusetts state law allowed cities to compel residents to be vaccinated in order to stop the spread of smallpox. The city of Cambridge mandated smallpox vaccinations, but resident Henning Jacobson refused, arguing that the law violated his Fourteenth Amendment due process rights. In 1905, in *Jacobson vs. Massachusetts*, the Supreme Court held that compulsory vaccination was a legitimate exercise of the state's police power to protect the health and safety of its citizens. At the same time, however, it underlined the importance of allowing local boards of health to make such decisions, which must be grounded in the "necessity of the case." The government could not exercise its power to mandate vaccines in "an arbitrary, unreasonable manner" or exceed "what was reasonably required for the safety of the public."[28]

According to the Congressional Research Service (CRS), the principles laid out in *Jacobson* support modern state and local vaccine mandates. But the CRS analysis notes that there are no federal laws that allow the federal government to issue mandates to the general population. Indeed, a one-size-fits-all federal vaccine mandate for the entire country would seem to be the very definition of the "arbitrary, unreasonable" measure going beyond the "reasonably required for the safety of the public" standard that the Supreme Court set out in *Jacobson*.

And what about the right to privacy that the Supreme Court has found in the Fourteenth Amendment? At what point does the state's interest in protecting health and safety override the right to privacy and bodily integrity? It was one thing to compel vaccinations for smallpox, which had a case fatality rate of 30 percent. It is quite another to impose a similar vaccination mandate for Covid-19, which has an infection fatality rate of 0.17 percent, according to an early but persuasive estimate by John Ioannidis, professor of medicine at Stanford University.[29]

Few people would argue against mandatory vaccinations for a disease as deadly as smallpox. But mandates for influenza-like illnesses are an overreach, especially when there are therapeutic treatments available that greatly reduce the already comparatively small number of fatalities.

Not All Strains of Smallpox Are Created Equal

If the Antonine Plague was a smallpox pandemic, where did it ultimately come from? Did it originate in Seleucia, where Rome's legions contracted it, or farther east? The evidence suggests that it may have started with a particularly vicious strain of the pox that originated in, of all places, China.

All viruses produce variants, and all variants of the variola virus, which causes smallpox, are not created equal. Whereas some of the variants later found in Africa and the Americas were relatively mild, the original virus, which seems to have originated in Asia in the early centuries of the Christian era—variola major— was much more deadly.[30]

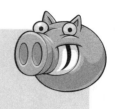

Then and Now: Origins

The Antonine Plague may have started with a particularly vicious strain of smallpox that originated in China. Odds are it did, although it was not deliberately spread from there. At that time, biowarfare was still in its infancy.

This may explain why the ancients overlooked it, as smallpox researcher C. W. Dixon was surprised to note. Dixon wrote, "The most striking thing about smallpox is its absence from the books of the Old and New Testaments, and also from the literature of the Greeks and Romans. Such a serious disease as variola major is very unlikely to have escaped a description by Hippocrates if it existed."[31]

Well, it did exist, but perhaps not yet in its most virulent form. The particular variant that struck down the Roman legions seems to have been incubating in China for some time before it burst forth from the Middle Kingdom during the second century AD. Chinese historical records record a series of plagues that broke out near the end of the Eastern Han Empire. The first occurred in AD 151, during the reign of Emperor Huan of Han (r. 146–168). Another major outbreak occurred ten years later, in AD 161, and then regularly thereafter for the next couple of decades.

China had apparently been grappling with deadly strains of smallpox for centuries by that point.[32] As early as 200 BC, practitioners of traditional Chinese medicine had invented an early form of vaccination, called variolation, which involved grinding up smallpox scabs and blowing the resulting powder, virus and all, up into someone's nostrils.

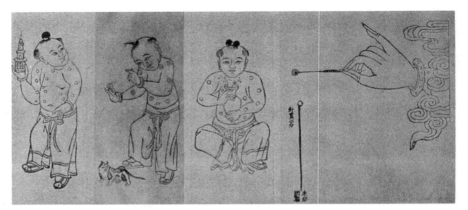

Smallpox symptoms and inoculation. Chinese images presented at the XVIIth International Congress of Medicine, London, 1913. *Wellcome Library*[33]

As you can imagine, this was a pretty risky procedure. You were deliberately infecting yourself with live smallpox. Most people contracted a mild case of the disease. But one in fifty contracted a case of smallpox severe enough to kill him. These odds might seem pretty daunting—until you remembered that you had a one in three chance of dying from the real thing. So . . . variolate me, said many Chinese over the centuries.

This includes Qing dynasty emperor Kangxi (1654–1722), who survived the ravages of smallpox as a child. The disease left his face pockmarked but paradoxically made him a prime candidate for the Dragon Throne on the grounds that he was now immune from the deadly disease. Kangxi had the most children of any emperor—the official number is twenty-four sons and twelve daughters—and had them all inoculated. It is not known if any of them died from the procedure.

Another fact that suggests that the Middle Kingdom was the original epicenter of the Antonine Plague is that the earliest accurate description of the symptoms of smallpox comes from China. A practitioner of traditional Chinese medicine by the name of Ge Hong (AD 284–364) anticipated later (seventh- and tenth-century) descriptions by Indian and Persian physicians by several centuries. Apparently the Chinese suffered an especially virulent variant of the disease.

Australian sinologist and historian Rafe de Crespigny is among those who believe that the Antonine Plague was born in China. He points to a plague that, according to the records of the Eastern Han dynasty, broke out in China before AD 166.[34]

If smallpox was originally confined to the Han Empire, how did it spread outside the country? Undoubtedly in the same way that later diseases, such as the Wuhan Virus, spread in 2019 and 2020: along trade and travel routes. In the second century AD this meant the Silk Road, which linked Han China to the Roman Empire by land and by sea.

The route of the Silk Road varied over time, but the twin cities of Seleucia and Ctesiphon lay on the main route used in Roman times. Roman legions advancing against the Parthians reached those cities some time in late AD 165, but the invisible enemy—which had gotten there before them, traveling along the Silk Road from China—met them there.[35]

The plague could also have reached Rome on trading ships that plied the Indian Ocean—not to mention the fact, which Rafe de Crespigny notes, that there was direct contact between Rome and China. "It may be only chance" writes de Crespigny, "that the outbreak of the Antonine plague

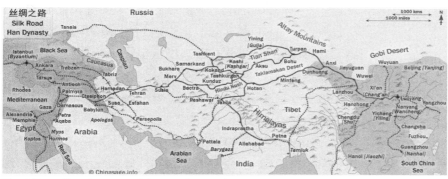

The Silk Road at the time of the Han Dynasty. *Courtesy of China Sage*[36]

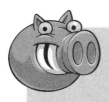

Then and Now: Natural Immunity

Natural immunity has been known in the West at least since the Plague of Athens, which raged on and off in the city from 430 to 426 BC. The Greek historian Thucydides describes in gruesome detail how tens of thousands of his fellow Athenians fell ill and died, with "men dying like sheep, through having caught the infection from nursing each other."

But he also noted that "it was with those who had recovered from the disease that the sick and the dying found most compassion. These [survivors] knew what it was from experience, and had now no fear for themselves; for the same man was never attacked twice—never at least fatally."[38]

in 166 AD coincides with the Roman embassy of 'Daqin' (the Roman Empire) landing in Jiaozhi (northern Vietnam) and visiting the Han court of Emperor Huan."[37] The returning Roman embassy is another possible vector by which the Han plague may have reached Roman territory.

Every pandemic in history has been ended by natural immunity. And so it was with the Antonine Plague. The survivors found they had not suffered in vain, but were henceforth immune to the disease. When the numbers of the newly immune grew large enough, herd immunity was reached, and the pandemic vanished for want of new victims.

How to Kill an Empire

By the time the plague had run its course, the Pax Romana was over. The population of the empire had been greatly reduced, the economy had been devastated, the imperial coffers had been emptied, and the army was a hollow shell of its former self, unable to fend off increasingly aggressive incursions from foreign invaders.

But the plague did more than end the Pax Romana. It precipitated the long decline and fall of the Roman Empire. The third century AD saw a series of upheavals—crises in which emperors came and went as if through a revolving door. The empire was besieged from all sides and came near to collapse, mostly because the plague had deprived it of the one resource a great empire cannot do without: people.

And a similar drama was playing at the other end of the Eurasian continent. In the latter half of the second century AD, a series of plagues also hollowed out the population of China and crushed its economy. De Crespigny believes that the repeated outbreaks of the plague, and the terror they generated among the population, led directly to the rise of a millenarian movement led by Zhang Jue (d. 184). This was not a peaceful movement that promoted selfless love of neighbor like Christianity. Zhang and his followers engaged in faith healing, but his cult also instigated the disastrous Yellow Turban Rebellion (184–205).[39] This rebellion was eventually suppressed, but not before the Eastern Han dynasty was fatally weakened. A state of turmoil obtained in China until the dynasty finally collapsed in AD 220.

Pandemics, it turns out, often mark the beginning of the end for empires.

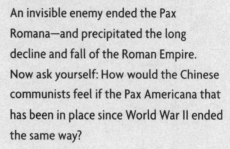

Then and Now: Geopolitical Implications

An invisible enemy ended the Pax Romana—and precipitated the long decline and fall of the Roman Empire. Now ask yourself: How would the Chinese communists feel if the Pax Americana that has been in place since World War II ended the same way?

PART TWO

THE CHINESE PLAGUES

CHAPTER 2

The Rats and the Roman Empire: The Plague of Justinian (541–750)

"During these times, there was a pestilence, by which the whole human race came near to being annihilated. Now in the case of all other scourges sent from Heaven some explanation of a cause might be given. . . . But for this calamity, it is quite impossible either to express in words or to conceive in thought any explanation except indeed to refer it to God. . . . It started from the Egyptians who dwell in Pelusium."

—Procopius, *History of the Wars*

By AD 541 the Roman emperor Justinian was well on his way to cobbling back together the greatest empire the Western world had ever known—when another microscopic invader from the East began ravaging his dominions. Justinian had inherited a rump Roman Empire shorn of its western provinces, but had energetically set in motion plans for recovery.

Victory followed victory as he subjugated the Vandals in North Africa, won victories over the Ostrogoths in Italy, and began making inroads into Spain. The population of the empire was growing, the economy was strong, and tax revenues were increasing. Morale in the increasingly numerous legions was excellent, and the recovery of the remaining lost provinces seemed just a matter of time. No enemies formidable enough to stop him stood in the way.

At the same time, the last Roman emperor who deserves to be called Great was creating legal and architectural edifices that stand to the present day. Chief among these were the Code of Justinian and the Hagia Sophia—whose name means "Holy Wisdom"—the greatest cathedral the world had ever seen. With these and other accomplishments, Justinian was on a trajectory not only to reassemble the Roman Empire but to restore its greatness.

Then came the Plague of Justinian, as it is called. Starting in the year 541, the first truly global pandemic spread across the empire, emptying out its cities and destroying its economy.

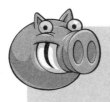

Then and Now: Bubonic Plague

The Black Death in the Middle Ages was actually the bubonic plague's second invasion of Europe. The first had occurred seven hundred years before, in the Plague of Justinian. As in the first—and in many a pandemic that came after—the invading pathogen came from China. Unlike smallpox, the bubonic plague has not been eradicated. The CDC estimates there have been an average of between five and six cases of bubonic plague per year in the United States in recent decades.[1]

For the rest of Justinian's long rule—he reigned until AD 565—he accomplished little beyond dealing with the problems caused by the disease. The plague that not only killed millions of his subjects but also ended his dream of a restored Roman Empire bears his name. Who said history was fair?

"It Started from the Egyptians Who Dwell in Pelusium"

It was the year AD 541, Justinian's court historian Procopius recalled, when a plague "started among the Egyptians who dwell in Pelusium." This small port city, located on the east side of the Nile Delta, was a propitious entry point for the plague—at least from the plague's point of view. Alexandria, one of the Roman Empire's largest cities, was situated on the western side of the same delta—only 160 miles away, well within striking distance.

The city founded by and named after the great conqueror boasted the busiest harbor in the empire. Egyptian grain fed the great cities of the empire, and massive grain ships regularly left from Alexandria for Constantinople and Rome. Smaller coastal traders carried grain and other goods up and down the coasts of Africa and Syria. And no ship in those days, whatever its size or cargo, was without a pack of hungry rats as supercargo. While rats, like humans, will eat almost anything, their favorite food is grain.

By the following year, the plague was raging in Alexandria and throughout Egypt. Besides grain and rats, each ship leaving the harbor now carried something else as well: a microscopic demon hidden away in the guts of the tiny fleas that the rats always carried. When the ships arrived at their destination and offloaded their grain, the rats scurried ashore as well, carrying their deadly supercargo with them. This is why, as Procopius notes, the plague always started in the empire's coastal cities, and then spread inland from there to cities along the Roman roads.[2]

No place was spared. As Lester K. Little, the author of *Plague and the End of Antiquity*, writes, "From Alexandria it spread all over the Mediterranean, to Libya, Africa, Italy, Sicily, Gaul, and Spain. It also spread from Alexandria to Palestine via the ports of Gaza and Ashkelon, going from the coast inland to the region around Jerusalem."[3] But it was in Constantinople, the very heart of the empire, that the plague was to exact the highest price.

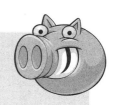

Then and Now: Modes of Transport

The bubonic plague was spread via ships carrying it to ports all around the Mediterranean, by a bacterium hitching a ride on fleas on rats. The Covid-19 pandemic was spread via airplanes carrying it to cities all over the world, by a virus hitching a ride on people from Wuhan. Except that, as we shall see, was done deliberately.

The Circle of Death: Bacteria, Fleas, Rats, Humans—We All Fall Down

Procopius can be forgiven for thinking of the plague as divine punishment. Not only did it kill with a vengeance, it seemed to have no natural explanation. It would take the advent of modern medicine to discover the complex life cycle of the Black Plague: the rats that carried the flea that carried the deadly bacteria that caused a pandemic that would nearly destroy the empire.

Most bacteria rely on human or animal droppings to make their way from one host to another. The bacterium that causes the plague, *Yersinia pestis*, however, is not content to simply wait around for someone to step in it. Instead it has hijacked the flea. It takes up residence in the flea's foregut and waits for its ride to find a host for both of them. The tiny insect is able to jump two feet high and, upon landing on a host animal, to latch onto it with built-in grappling hooks. The flea's preferred host is a rat, but a ravenous flea will bite just about anything warm-blooded, and the clever passenger riding inside it has found a way to make the flea very, very hungry.

The flea, like the mosquito, is a bloodsucker. It has two hollow lancets—one on either side of its mouth—that penetrate the rat's skin and connect its two pumping systems directly to its host's bloodstream. In this way it creates a pathway for the bacteria to get from inside its foregut to inside the rat. But to complete its journey from flea to rat, the bacteria has to somehow "swim against the tide" of incoming blood.

Y. pestis does this in an ingenious way. The bacteria glue themselves together in the flea's foregut, thus blocking the blood from flowing into the flea's stomach. As the hungry flea begins to frantically bite its host over and over again in an effort to get nourishment, this bacterial plug acts in reverse, forcing out the blood and bacteria from inside the flea into the rat and infecting it.[4]

Yersinia pestis is fatal for rats. And when the rat dies, the now ravenous fleas abandon the corpse in a frantic search for food, biting any warm-blooded creatures they happen upon. This includes any humans who might happen to be in the vicinity. And there were many humans within their reach in Roman times, when rats were a fixture in and around Roman dwellings. The fleabites that followed generally proved fatal for the person on the receiving end of the flea's lancets.

Of course, none of this was known at the time. People simply had no idea where the pestilence came from or how it was being spread. As Procopius, watching in fearful confusion as people of all ages and walks of life were cut down, observed,

But for this calamity it is quite impossible either to express in words or to conceive in thought any explanation, except indeed to refer it to God. For it did not come in a part of the world, nor upon certain men, nor did it confine itself to any season of the year, so that from such circumstances it might be possible to find subtle explanations of a cause. But it embraced the entire world, and blighted the lives of all men, though differing from one another in the most marked degree, respecting neither sex nor age. For much as men differ with regard to places in which they live, or in the law of their daily life, or in natural bent, or in active pursuits, or in whatever else man differs from man, in the case of this disease alone the difference availed naught.[5]

Then and Now: Methods of Transmission

Bubonic plague, the deadliest disease in mankind's history, is not directly contagious between people; it has to hitch a ride on a flea. The China Virus, on the other hand, was engineered to be highly infectious and can easily spread through the air from person to person—a fact that the CCP initially tried to hide, in order to jump-start the pandemic.

The best advice of the medical practitioners of the time remained the prescription that Galen had written out four hundred years before: *Cito, longe, tarde.* "Leave quickly, go far away, and come back slowly." Or as Denethor, Steward of Gondor in the *Lord of the Rings* movies, put it even more succinctly when Sauron's forces attacked his city: "Flee, flee for your lives!"

"Lord of Demons"

The residents of Constantinople, the densely populated imperial capital, were especially hard-hit. Many of the city's residents had no permanent lodging—they slept in homeless shelters run by the city's monasteries and churches.

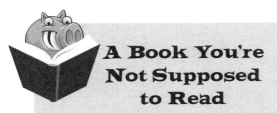

A Book You're Not Supposed to Read

If you want to know what a real pandemic is like, read Procopius's *History of the Wars*. As Justinian's court historian, Procopius was at the emperor's right hand throughout the plague. He wrote the best eyewitness account we have of the devastation that it wrought.

The crowded conditions of their lodgings made them vulnerable to infection and contributed mightily to the spread of the disease.

To make matters worse, those who lived in the city were soon facing a food shortage. Justinian, continuing a practice from Rome's heyday, had long offered a free bread ration to many of his citizens, something that required almost daily shipments of grain from Alexandria. And every ship tying up to the city's docks brought new packs of flea-bitten rats to the capital.

Once the pandemic took off in earnest the shipments slowed down, and then all but stopped. The emperor found it impossible to continue feeding his people. The grain mills stopped milling, the bakers stopped baking, and the bread ration stopped. Widespread hunger quickly turned into starvation, lowering people's resistance to the plague and greatly increasing the mortality rate.

The survivors began blaming the emperor for their misery and death, cursing him, Procopius says, as the "Lord of Demons." It's probably a good thing that Justinian, unlike President Donald Trump in 2020, did not have an election coming up.

Constantinople came to resemble a ghost town, even without the imposition of Covid-like lockdowns. As Procopius writes:

> During that time it seemed no easy thing to see any man in the streets of Byzantium, but all who had the good fortune to be in health were sitting in their houses, either attending the sick or mourning the dead. And if one did succeed in meeting a man going out, he was carrying one of the dead. And work of every

description ceased, and all the trades were abandoned by the artisans, and all other work as well, such as each had in hand.[6]

Before long, thousands of the city's residents were becoming infected every day—and two-thirds of the infected would be dead within the span of two weeks. It proved impossible to bury all the dead, and with the corpses piling up at an alarming rate, Justinian turned to the city walls to dispose of the bodies. He decided to use the hollow towers that dotted the walls as crude mausoleums and ordered the bodies of the dead to be flung into them. This got the bodies off the streets and out of sight but not, unfortunately, out of mind. "As a result of this an evil stench pervaded the city," Procopius noted. "[This] distressed the inhabitants still more, especially when the wind blew fresh from that quarter."[7]

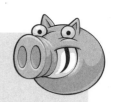

Then and Now: Bodies in the Streets

From the if-you-thought-Covid-was-bad annals: When the plague hit Constantinople in earnest, people began wearing identification tags so that if they should die in the street their families could be notified and their corpses collected for burial. The only place people "died in the streets" from Covid was China—and many of them revived as soon as the CCP propaganda teams were done filming.

As the Plague of Justinian killed off the agricultural workforce, the economy went into free fall. Even people living in the smaller cities found it difficult to feed themselves and their families. Some cities attempted to control the spread of the disease by shutting themselves off from the outside world. Quarantining, however, created—as always—a new set of problems. Bishop Nicholas of Sion banned farmers from entering his city on market days, trying to stop the plague, but he had to withdraw his edict after local authorities unfairly accused him of trying to drive up food prices.

Even those who escaped being infected by the plague were often "infected" by hysterical rumors. As the death toll mounted, panic began to spread among the survivors, many of whom thought that the end of the world was upon them. In September 541, as the plague broke out in

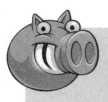

Then and Now: Superstitious Beliefs

We moderns may be tempted to mock the citizens of sixth-century Constantinople for their superstitions, but their beliefs were not all that different from the modern hysteria surrounding masks, driven by the debunked notion that wearing a piece of paper over one's mouth and nose protects against a virus tiny enough to pass right through it.

Constantinople, a woman attracted a large following by prophesying that "in three days' time the sea would rise and swallow everything."[8] Another rumor that spread throughout the city was that breaking pottery would drive the plague out. The streets filled with shards—and the dead.[9]

Justinian's officials did everything they could to calm the public and reduce panic, but the death toll even in smaller Roman cities was horrific. Bishop Gregory of Tours, writing a half century later, described the situation in the city of Arvernis in Gaul (modern-day Clermont, France): "Since soon no coffins or biers were left, six and even more persons were buried together in the same grave. One Sunday, 300 corpses were counted in Saint Peter's Basilica alone."[10]

Procopius, in his *Anekdota*, says that some people viewed the plague as retribution for sin. This Old Testament view of the matter conflicts with the New, however, in which Christ makes clear that disease and disability are not punishments for sin.[11] Others set about caring for the sick. Christians were in fact responsible for the one great medical innovation of late antiquity: the hospital. These centers for caring for the sick and dying spread from Judea in the late fourth century to cities throughout the empire. Victims of the Plague of Justinian in cities including Rome, Ephesus, and Constantinople sought and received care in these Christian-run hospices, and often themselves became Christian as a result.[12]

As to how many died in the Plague of Justinian, we can only speculate. Most authorities suggest that Europe as a whole lost something between one-third to one-half of its people to the sixth-century plague. Even if we take the lower estimate, this would have been a devastating blow to Justinian's empire, reducing its population from 26 million to 17 million or less by the time the plague had run its course.[13]

The capital itself was particularly hard-hit, losing half its population. At the height of the plague, Procopius says, 10,000 people a day were dying in Constantinople.[14] Historian T. H. Hollingsworth suggests that out of an initial population of 508,000 almost half, or some 244,000 people, succumbed to the pandemic.[15] No wonder Justinian ran out of room to bury the dead.

As the plague raged all across the Eurasian continent and even into Africa, the global death toll must have been horrific. Given the high mortality rate of the disease, 10 percent or even more of the world's population may have died.

"God Bless You"

The first symptom of bubonic plague is a mild fever and a headache. By the second day many of the infected are already in delirium—confused, fatigued, and slurring their speech. By the third day the lymph glands in the neck, armpits, and groin begin to swell painfully into the characteristic "buboes"—sometimes as small as a pea, other times to the size of goose eggs. Purplish blotches show up on the skin as the tiny capillaries underneath rupture, while the fleabites—the original source of the infection—grow from dark-ringed red spots to open putrid lesions. As if this isn't enough, the disease also attacks the victim's nervous system, causing excruciating pain, wild anxiety, and bizarre behavior.

Some plague victims will develop infections in their blood or their lungs—the septicemic or pneumonic plague. Both are almost invariably

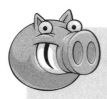

Then and Now: Episcopal Blessings

Sixth-century pope Gregory the Great did not order the churches shut down and Masses suspended. He did not suggest that everyone, sick or not, needed to quarantine themselves, or that everyone, indoors and outdoors, needed to wear masks. That particular brand of episcopal madness—or cowardice—would have to wait for the twenty-first century.

fatal. The pneumonic plague is also highly infectious, since the sufferer often has uncontrolled bouts of coughing and sneezing, which aerosolize the bacillus, allowing it to spread directly from person to person.

Pope Gregory the Great (r. 590–604), noting that coughing and sneezing were early warning signs of infection, suggested that everyone respond with a blessing. We've been blessing each other when we sneeze ever since.

There was nothing that Roman doctors could do to alter the course of the disease; the only care they could offer was palliative. To alleviate the pain, doctors administered the "juice of the opium poppy," which was in common use in the Roman cities of the time, to those who could afford it.[16] Of those infected with the bubonic plague, seven out of ten would die an agonizing death.[17] How painful? Thousands of the citizens of Constantinople threw themselves into the sea in order to end their agony. It was said that those who did not die envied the dead.

The epidemic initially lasted for just over three years, from 541 to 543, but then it recurred periodically for the next two centuries. Between 541 and 750 there were no fewer than eighteen outbreaks. Those who survived the plague, including Justinian himself, developed robust and long-lasting natural immunity to the subsequent episodes of the disease—similar to the robust natural immunity enjoyed by those who have had Covid-19 in our time—but each new generation had to run the plague gantlet, and a large percentage of them would die.[18]

Another Plague That Brought Down Another Empire

The Plague of Justinian was a pandemic the likes of which would not be seen again in Christendom until the Black Death in the fourteenth century. The drastic reduction of the population caused a near collapse of the economic base of the late Roman Empire. The great depression that followed greatly reduced the tax revenue that the imperial state could collect. Among other things, it forced Justinian to cut his once strong army in half, so that he no longer had the military strength he needed to continue his efforts to reconstitute the Roman Empire.[19] From that point forward he was simply trying to hold things together.

None of Justinian's successors was ever again in a position to attempt—as he had—the restoration of the empire's lost provinces. They continued to be hamstrung by outbreaks of the plague every ten years or so, and the empire went into a long, slow decline. With the treasury often running at a deficit, no more basilicas arose, no more public baths were built, and no more city walls were constructed to protect the empire's cities. The construction of new housing by private citizens ceased as well, since the recurrent plagues regularly produced a plentiful and regular supply of vacant residences.[20]

The emperors of what came to be known as the Byzantine Empire were hard-pressed to maintain their current borders. They were often unsuccessful. The Roman-Sasanian War that raged from 602 to 628 ended in a stalemate, but not so the war that followed. The forces of Islam erupted out of Arabia in 629, swiftly overrunning the entire Sasanian Empire and also Roman provinces in Syria, the Caucasus, Egypt, and North Africa. Constantinople's holdings were reduced to Anatolia (modern-day Turkey), Greece, and a few enclaves in Italy and the Balkans. But for the plague, that conflict might well have ended differently.

The Plague of Justinian laid the groundwork for the medieval world. Labor shortages and an abundance of available land led to the end of slavery, as landowners raised slaves to serfs and offered them protection in return for their loyalty. With the disintegration of the empire and its civil institutions, the only remaining institution that spanned the entire Latin Christian world was the Catholic Church. Catholic bishops were looked to for guidance not just in ecclesiastical matters but in other issues of public concern as well. Almost by default, the Church became the dominant power in medieval Europe, with both peasants and feudal lords submitting to its authority for centuries to come.

Tracing "Patient Zero"

Procopius pointed to "the Egyptians who dwell in Pelusium" as the source of the plague, but this was merely the point at which the disease had entered the empire. The actual origin of this particular plague, like that of many others, was much farther east. It was, as historian John Barker remarks, "an unexpected bonus, perhaps, of Justinian's southern trade route to the Far East."[21] As in later bubonic plagues (as we shall see in the next chapters) the original patient was not from the Mediterranean, but in far-away China along the Silk Road.

The Silk Road of the time had both land and sea routes. While Constantinople was a hub of the northern overland routes, the initial outbreak in Egypt suggests that the rats carrying the fleas carrying the deadly bacillus came from China by boat via the southern route.

The demon had come from the East and did not spare the East, though it had only a minor impact on China as a whole. Major cities and some provinces experienced breakouts, but the plague advanced only a few miles per day and could not easily spread throughout the whole of China's huge land-based empire. Each of China's provinces constituted a self-contained agricultural economy, and most were separated by mountains and rivers. The fact that trade between the different provinces was limited helped to contain the spread of disease-laden rats.

Still, like the Roman Empire, the Chinese, going through a period of disunion after the fall of the Han dynasty in the third century, suffered repeated outbreaks of the plague. It was not until the year 689 that the emperor Yang Jian successfully reunited the country, founding the Sui dynasty. China may be the source of most pandemics, but historically it has been better able to cope with them than those it infects.

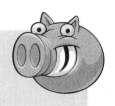

Then and Now: Patient Zero

In plague after plague, pandemic after pandemic, the original "patient zero" turns out to have been in China. The Covid-19 pandemic is not the exception but the rule. With, as we shall see, one important difference—this one was on purpose.

The Roman Empire, as we have seen, was not nearly so fortunate. Rome's provinces ringed the Mediterranean, and the ships that fueled its economic life also carried the plague with a speed and deadliness unmatched in any other part of the world.

The Plague of Justinian permanently shattered the Roman world, ushering in the medieval European world, which would last for another eight centuries or so, until it was—ironically enough—brought down in turn by the next bubonic plague, the Black Death of the fourteenth century.

And "patient zero" would once again be in the Far East.

The Greatest Public Health Disaster in History: The Black Death (1347–1351)

On the eve of the Black Death, Europe was populated and prosperous. The European population had tripled in the previous three centuries, and additional land had been brought under cultivation.[1] Cities were growing even faster, as craftsmen set up shops and organized guilds, and merchants took advantage of expanding local markets to set up trading networks. The cathedrals, fortifications, abbeys, and private homes constructed during this period—many built of expensive stone rather than cheaper wood—testify to the aggregate wealth of the early-fourteenth-century economy.

At the same time, the lot of ordinary peasants did not seem to be improving, as rents were high and the soil was becoming exhausted. To make matters worse, the "Little Ice Age," which began in 1300, was shortening the growing season and causing crop failures.[2] Those peasants who made their way to the cities were no better off than their country cousins, since as unskilled laborers they had difficulty earning their daily bread.

Gunpowder had been invented by the Chinese and made its way westward, rendering castle walls easier to breach. Still, the feudal lords remained in control.

The citizens of both the crowded, unsanitary cities and the largely destitute countryside fell to the Black Death like wheat before the scythe. Over the five years from 1347 to 1352, perhaps half the population of Europe contracted the plague. In the words of the old "Ring around the Rosie" nursery rhyme, many were to "fall down," never to rise again.

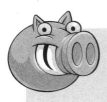

Then and Now: Naming Rights

The word "Black" in the Black Death does not refer to the color or a symptom of the disease—it's just a synonym for "terrible" or "dreadful."[4] Similarly, the term China Virus is not a reference to a people or a culture, but rather to the country controlled by the Chinese Communist Party, whose military bioengineered the coronavirus and released it upon the world. President Donald Trump was once asked why he insisted upon calling the coronavirus the "China Virus." His answer? "Because it comes from China." Enough said.

Breaching the Portals of Europe

The earliest known episode of biological warfare in human history involved weaponizing the Black Death against Europe. The year was AD 1346, and the Tatar Mongols were besieging the Genoese port of Caffa on the Black Sea.[3] The Mongols had brought the plague with them, and when their ranks began to thin from the disease, they thought to use the diseased corpses of their fallen comrades against their walled enemies.

As Mark Wheelis has written, the Mongols "ordered corpses to be placed in catapults and lobbed into the city in the hope that the intolerable stench would kill everyone inside. What seemed like mountains of dead were thrown into the city, and the Christians could not hide or flee or escape from them."[5]

The city did not fall, but as conditions grew worse, some of the Genoese fled in their ships, unwittingly carrying the plague with them. By the following year the Black Death had entered Europe. History records that four Genoese ships from Caffa landed in Messina, Sicily, in the fall of 1347. These were carrying grain, and each of them—like the Alexandrian grain ships of centuries before—carried a full complement of flea-infested rats and sick crewmembers. Within a few days, the city was in the grip of a full-blown epidemic.[6]

The plague reached a number of other ports, including Constantinople and Marseilles, by ship that same year. But the disease was so virulent that some vessels became ghost ships "whose whole crews had been carried off by the plague, and which drifted about as derelicts until cast upon some coast where they brought death and destruction to those who hastened to the rescue."[7]

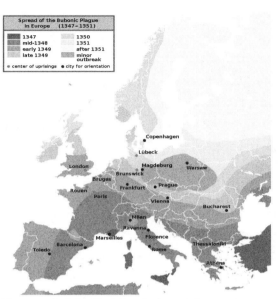

The spread of the Black Death through Europe (map shows modern borders), 1347–1351. *Original by Robert Zenner, enlarged, translated, and edited by Jaybear*[8]

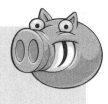

Then and Now: Biowarfare

Biological warfare isn't new, but it has been considerably refined since the Mongol army hurled plague-infected dead into the besieged Crimean city of Caffa. The Chinese Communist Party has advanced to using the infected bodies of the people they control while they are still alive, as we shall see. These disease vectors, as we might call them, were allowed to travel all around the world, shedding the deadly coronavirus as they went on their way to their unsuspecting targets.

The Black Death spread inland from the coast, reaching Rome and Paris in the summer of 1348. The first wave of the pestilence would not die out until it reached Scandinavia and the Russian wilderness in 1351. The plague continued to return periodically for the next century or more. It continued to pop up in England until 1665, while for France the horror did not end until 1720. The demographic effect was equivalent to Europe's major population centers being periodically nuked.

A Civilizational Apocalypse

Had the Black Death been a one-and-done affair, it would have been bad enough. But for five long years after the initial pandemic, the plague would retreat during the winter, when infected fleas would die before they could

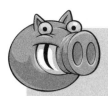

Then and Now: Panic

In the midst of a deadly plague that killed more than half the population, unbridled fear and mass panic naturally reigned. The authorities tried—and largely failed—to prevent a complete breakdown of society. In the face of the China Virus that kills only a fraction of 1 percent of the population, many politicians deliberately stoked fear and panic so as "not to let a crisis go to waste"—as they took the opportunity to remake society along their preferred lines.

latch onto human beings, only to return in the spring with a vengeance. And each year it spread more widely.

Knowing that cities were centers of infection, people fled to the country as they had during the Plague of Justinian. Trade and commerce ground to a halt, and the price of food and other goods skyrocketed. The peasants, for as long as they stayed healthy, continued to plow their fields—they and their families had to eat—but tradesmen closed their shops, schools closed their doors, and municipal governments ceased functioning, as officials and common people alike abandoned their posts. Everything from government and science to arts and religion was negatively affected. It was a civilizational apocalypse.

Those who fled to the countryside found the villages as blighted as the cities, perhaps even more so. As in all pandemics, the poor suffered most, and no wonder. The peasants died in droves, as Francis Gasquet wrote, "living as [they] . . . did in close, unclean huts, with no rooms above ground, without windows, artificial light, soap, linen; ignorant of certain vegetables, constrained to live half the year on salt meat; [afflicted by] scurvy, leprosy, and other diseases, which are engendered by hard living and the neglect of every sanitary precaution."[9] As we have learned during the Covid pandemic, comorbidities kill.

The plague was omnipresent; nowhere was safe. As Marchionne de Coppo di Stefano Buonaiuti, who lived through the Black Death, wrote, "Some fled to the country, and some to provincial towns, to get a change of air; where there was no plague they brought it, and where it already existed they added to it."[10] As the death toll mounted, the mood of the people darkened. The abbot of Tournai, Gilles li Muisis, recorded in his diary how some people sought release from the fear in free love, while others engaged in intense devotions and ritualistic purging.[11]

As fast as the disease spread, a fatalistic sense of utter hopelessness and despair spread even faster. "'Ha, ha,' quoth Death, 'that ye may know that no fortress can resist me and even if it had bastions . . . and if it were surrounded by a moat which could supply water to the mighty ocean, in spite of all this I will take the town.'"[13]

★ ★ ★

An Image So Vivid It May Put You Off Italian Food for a While

Buonaiuti famously compared the mass graves, in which the corpses were sandwiched between thin layers of soil, to lasagna, with its layers of sauce, noodles, and cheese.[12]

As the plague took its toll on the population, the survivors became suspicious of everyone outside of their rapidly shrinking immediate circles. Travelers, beggars, and strangers were all looked upon with jaundiced eyes, if not outright hostility. The authority and respect once enjoyed by governors, priests, and physicians ebbed away, as they all, in their own different ways, proved unable to cope with the spread of the disease.[14] Society was riven by the same kinds of division that we saw during the Covid pandemic, when the fearful are maddened by the sight of a maskless face, and Karens are quick to report on people not keeping the proper "social distance"— though with considerably more justification, since mortality rates were running at 70 percent.

The fear gnawing away at people's very souls ran so deep that it often fractured families, the very bedrock of society. According to Marchionne de Coppo di Stefano Buonaiuti, people would often abandon members of their own families if they showed signs of the disease: "When evening came, the relatives said to the patient: 'So that you don't have to wake up the people looking after you at night, asking for things, because this is going

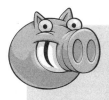

Then and Now: Rhyming Epitaphs

The only mass deaths that occurred in the Covid-19 pandemic of 2020–2021 took place in nursing homes, chiefly in New York and New Jersey. Andrew Cuomo, the governor of New York at the time, forced these homes to accept patients who were already infected. These superspreaders promptly infected the other elderly residents within, who died in droves in the days and weeks following. Their gravestones could read: "Is it not sad and painful to relate, that Cuomo's decision sent fifteen thousand to their fate."

on day and night, you yourself can reach for cakes and wine or water, here they are on the shelf above your bed, you can get the stuff when you want.' And when the patient fell asleep, they went away and did not return."[15]

Gravestones from the time of the Black Death and the subsequent plagues that continued to break out in Europe over the next centuries tell the sad tale of how the bubonic plague felled entire families and devastated communities:

- St. John's churchyard at Nuremberg, 1437: "Was that not sad and painful to relate, I died with thirteen of my house on the same date?"
- And from the same churchyard in Nuremberg, 1533: "Is it not sad and moving to relate, I, Hans Tuchmacher, died with fourteen children on the same date?"
- St. Leonard's graveyard in Swabian Gmuend: "Is that not a painful sight, seventy-seven in the same night, Died of the plague in the year 1637."[16]

The last major outbreak of the Black Death in Great Britain was not until the middle of the seventeenth century. The Great Plague of London caused a mass exodus from London, led by King Charles II. The plague started in April 1665 and spread rapidly through the hot summer months. By the time the plague ended, about 100,000 people, including 15 percent of the population of London, had died.

There were so many dead that open pits were dug, *Robinson Crusoe* author Daniel Defoe wrote. "There was a strict order to prevent people coming to those pits, and that was only to prevent infection. But after some time that order was more necessary, for people that were infected and near their end, and delirious also, would run to those pits, wrapt in blankets or rugs, and throw themselves in, and, as they said, bury themselves."[17]

Mass casualty events throughout history have driven people to their knees to plead for divine assistance. Churches and hospitals were the only institutions that did not close during the plague, and worship services continued throughout. Defoe noted that in the Great Plague of London, from 1665 to 1666, "People showed an extraordinary zeal in these religious exercises, and as the church-doors were always open, people would go in single at all times, whether the minister was officiating or no, and locking themselves into separate pews, would be praying to God with great fervency and devotion."[18] As he noted, "The Government encouraged their devotion, and appointed public prayers and days of fasting and humiliation. . . . The people . . . flocked to the churches and meetings, and they were all so thronged that there was often no coming near, no, not to the very doors of the largest churches."[19]

Putting faith into action, believers cared for the sick and the dying as well, risking—and often losing—their own lives in the process. The clergy were especially hard-hit, "as they stayed at the side of their suffering parishioners and probably nursed them or delivered the last unction at the most dangerous time in pneumonic or septicemic plague."[20] But lay believers

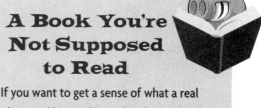

A Book You're Not Supposed to Read

If you want to get a sense of what a real plague is like, read Daniel Defoe's *A Journal of the Plague Year* about the 1665–1666 Great Plague of London. Defoe published this account of the 1664–65 London plague in 1772, probably based on notes left him by his uncle, Henry Foe. Defoe, who is best known as the author of *Robinson Crusoe*, obviously thought being marooned on a desert island would be a preferable fate.

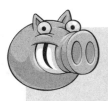

Then and Now: Religion and Politics

The government of Defoe's time may have encouraged people to go to church, but the reaction of the authorities in many Western countries to the Covid-19 pandemic was the complete opposite. They locked churches down, and even had some pastors and congregants arrested for holding worship services—even if they were "locked in separate pews," in Defoe's words for social distancing. Politics, rather than religion, was the order of the day.

stepped up as well. When the Italian city of Siena was struck by the plague, the city's officials fled. But many Christians followed the example of St. Catherine of Siena, who stayed behind and helped to create and run the hospitals that were needed.[21]

The Black Death devastated the economy of Europe for a generation. As James Westfall Thompson wrote, "Those who survived found themselves personally richer than before; but Europe was immeasurably poorer, for production absolutely ceased for months, even a whole year, and when it was renewed the productive capacity of Europe was found to be much impaired, while the waste had been terrific."[22]

Like all plagues, the Black Death resulted in an enormous redistribution of wealth. Those who did not perish returned to their homes and belongings, but many houses remained empty, their former residents having died. Distant heirs often went from rags to riches overnight and felt guilty about profiting off of the misfortune of their deceased kinsmen. The poor, however, got poorer—they had barely been scraping by before the plague brought the economy to a halt, and they didn't have wealthy relatives with assets to inherit.

The continent-wide epidemic had burned itself out by 1353, but the pestilence never really went away. Outbreaks continued to occur for the next four hundred years here and there in Europe in country after country—Italy in 1630, Germany in 1709 and 1713, France in 1720, and so on. London experienced recurring epidemics—outbreaks were recorded in 1563, 1593, 1603, 1625, 1636, 1665—which reduced the population of the city by 30 percent over the course of a century.

The last recorded plague occurred in Marseille in 1720, when an estimated four out of every ten people died.

Among the few jurisdictions to respond effectively to the Black Death was Venice, where public health may be said to have been born. As reports of the advancing pandemic reached the city, Andrea Dandolo, the Doge of Venice,

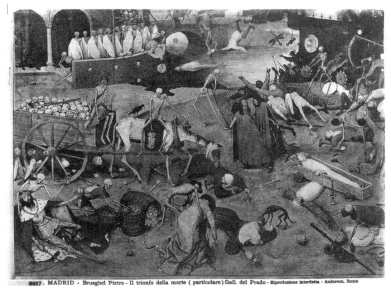

Detail of *The Triumph of Death* by Pieter Brueghel the Elder, c. 1562, inspired by the waves of bubonic plague that swept Europe for centuries, beginning with the Black Death in 1347–1351. *Wellcome Library*[23]

convened the Great Council. A committee of leading nobles was formed to make recommendations on how to protect the city and its citizens from the pestilence while continuing the commerce that was Venice's lifeblood. They came up with a sensible set of measures that constituted what was perhaps the first coherent public health policy in history.

- Every ship entering Venetian waters was boarded and searched. Vessels with dead bodies or foreigners on board were "sanitized" by being set on fire and sunk.
- Ships carrying only Venetians and showing no signs of plague were quarantined off a nearby island for forty days—from the biblical account of the life of Christ, who had prayed and fasted alone—self-quarantined—in the desert for forty days.

Then and Now: Profiting from the Plague

Massive transfers of wealth accompany every plague. But few people have ever profited to the extent that Amazon's Jeff Bezos did in 2020–2021. When state governments locked down his brick-and-mortar competitors—many never to reopen—millions of customers were forced onto his website. From March 2020 to March 2021, Bezos made $65 *billion*.

Forty in Italian is *quaranta*, from which we get the world quarantine.

- All taverns and inns were shut down. Anyone caught selling wine was fined, and had his stock confiscated and poured into the canals. There would be no wild bacchanalias—superspreader events—in Venice.

- The city hired gondolas to go up and down the canals collecting the dead. The gondoliers accomplished their grisly task by shouting "Dead bodies! Dead bodies!" (*Corpi morti! Corpi morti!*) In this way corpses, which were themselves sources of infection, were quickly collected, carried to an outer island, and buried there.

- Venetians sick with the plague were confined to an island called Lazaretto Vecchio—"Old Lazaretto." Thus in Italian "lazaretto" has come to mean a hospital treating infectious diseases.

These commonsense public health policies did not prevent the plague from reaching Venice—the worst recorded episode, which occurred in 1630, cost the lives of an estimated one-third of the population—but they may have limited the frequency of the outbreaks. And they did allow the economy of this thriving port city to continue to function, which in its own way was just as important to the health of its citizens. Equally important, the Venetian Grand Council's policies allayed the fears of the public and helped to avert panic.[24]

"Lunch with Your Friends, and Dinner with Your Ancestors in Paradise"

At the time of the Black Death, eight hundred years had passed since the Plague of Justinian, and at first people didn't connect the two. And yet both plagues were caused by a strain of the bacterium *Yersinia pestis* that was spread by infected fleas riding on rodents. And both were really three plagues in one, depending upon what part of the body was infected—the bubonic plague attacked the lymphatic system, the pneumonic plague the lungs, and the septicemic plague the circulatory system.

The Italian author Giovanni Boccaccio, who lived through the plague and used it as the setting for his classic *The Decameron*, described the characteristic buboes that

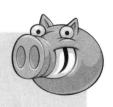

Then and Now: Panic

The fourteenth-century Doge and Grand Council of Venice, with their prudent public health policies, stand in sharp contrast to the Anthony Faucis of our day who seemed determined to spread panic with their nonstop warnings about endless variants, looming lockdowns, mandatory vaccines, and repeated boosters. Public health is not only about keeping people safe, it is also about making people *feel* safe. The actions of official Washington during the Covid-19 pandemic often had the opposite effect, perhaps because a panicked people are easier to regiment and control.

began in both men and women with certain swellings in the groin or under the armpit. They grew in size to a small apple or an egg, more or less, and were vulgarly called tumors. In a short space of time the tumors spread from the two parts named all over the body. Soon after this the symptoms changed and black and purple spots appeared on the arms or thighs or other parts of the body, sometimes a few large ones, sometimes many little ones. These spots were a certain sign of death, just as the original tumor had been and remained. . . . In any case very few recovered, most people died within about three days of the

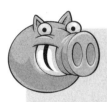

Then and Now: Infected by Fear

As in Defoe's day, some people at the present time have been "frightened into despair and lunacy" or "melancholy madness." But today it is the vast majority, rather than just "some" who have succumbed to "mere fright and surprise without any infection at all." Millions of people who have not contracted Covid-19 have been frightened out of their wits by media hyperbole, unscientific projections, and self-serving politicians who, in order to "never let a crisis go to waste," have portrayed the coronavirus as the second coming of the Black Death.

Dr. Robert Malone, the inventor of the mRNA vaccine technology, has described this phenomenon as "mass formation psychosis," which seems an accurate description of the hysteria that held so many people in its grip in 2020 and 2021.[28]

appearance of the tumors described above, most of them without fever or any other symptoms.[25]

Actually, about one-third of those who came down with the bubonic variety of the plague did manage to survive; it was the other two varieties that were almost invariably fatal. The septicemic plague in particular killed with a suddenness and a ferocity that shocked people. The average survival time from the onset of symptoms to death was only 14.5 hours.[26] Boccaccio, who lost both his father and his stepmother to the plague, wrote that "its victims ate lunch with their friends and dinner with their ancestors in paradise."[27]

Overall, of those who contracted any form of the Black Plague, an estimated 70 percent died.

As during the Plague of Justinian, the suffering of those who had the misfortune to contract the disease was almost beyond description. "It is scarce credible what dreadful cases happened in particular families every day," Defoe wrote. "People in the rage of the distemper, or in the torment of their swellings, which was indeed intolerable, running out of their own government, raging and distracted, and oftentimes laying violent hands upon themselves, throwing themselves out at their windows, shooting themselves, mothers murdering their own children in their lunacy, some dying of mere grief as a passion, some of mere fright and surprise without any infection at all, others frightened into idiotism and foolish distractions, some into despair and lunacy, others into melancholy madness."[29]

The horror of the Black Death was amplified by the fact that the physicians of the time had no idea how the disease was contracted or spread. In fact, some doctors were convinced that looks could kill—the plague spread so quickly. "Instantaneous death occurs," wrote a Montpellier physician, "when the aerial spirit escaping from the eyes of the sick man strikes the healthy person standing near and looking at the sick."'[30]

Plague victims could not expect anything in the way of help from the medical science of the day. Dr. Guy de Chauliac, celebrated as the father of French surgery, wrote, "The disease was most humiliating for the physicians, who were unable to render any assistance, all the more as, for fear of infection, they did not venture to visit patients, and if they did could do no good and consequently earn no fees, for all infected died with the exception of some towards the end of the epidemic, who escaped, as the boils had been able to mature." Physician Chalin de Vinario put it more succinctly: "Every pronounced case of plague is incurable."[31]

The famous "beak doctors" practiced an early form of masking. They believed that the "air was . . . stiff in times of plague" and that wearing masks with long beaks filled with herbs and flowers would cleanse the air they breathed.[32] Like modern-day cloth and paper masks, such beaks were largely useless in stopping the disease, although they probably did serve to mask the

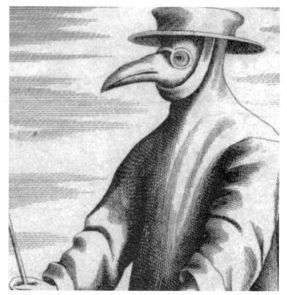

Depiction of a Black Death doctor wearing a beak-shaped mask in a vain effort to protect against the plague. *Gerhart Alzenbach*

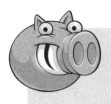

Then and Now: Treatments

There were no therapeutic drugs available to treat the Black Death. In the Covid-19 plague, we had antiviral medications available but were, in many cases, forbidden from using them. It's almost as if someone wanted to profit by making expensive experimental vaccines the only option. And it is true that in 2021 Big Pharma took in $100 billion selling shots under liability-free guaranteed contracts with governments around the world.[34]

horrendous stench that accompanied the Black Death. Of course, not everyone wore them, and no one was ordered to.

Physicians had nothing more to offer the suffering than palliative care, and no explanation for their illness other than vague references to God, the stars, or other remote causes. "The art of Hippocrates was lost," Montpellier doctor Simon de Couvain lamented in 1350.[33] The Black Death completely flummoxed the medical professionals of the time.

"Leave Quickly"

If the art of Hippocrates was lost, the advice of Galen was still useful. The Roman physician had been dead for a thousand years, but when the Black Death swept over much of Asia, Europe, and parts of Africa in the mid-1300s, his *Cito, longe, tarde* ("Leave quickly, go far away, and come back slowly") was still the best medical advice around. In England, it even inspired a nursery rhyme:

> Three things by which each simple man, from plague escape and sickness can.
> Start soon, flee far from town or land, on which the plague has laid its hand.
> Return but late to such a place, where pestilence has stayed its pace.[35]

The Black Death not only brought death, it sowed mass panic and, over time, a popular obsession with death. Each time that the pestilence returned over the following decades, the people grew more terrified. It was not only its lethality but its sheer unpredictability that kept Europeans in constant fear, which found expression in the writers and artists whose works, one historian noted, "reflected a loss of optimism and a preoccupation with death. A common theme was the danse macabre, or 'dance of death,' and murals on church walls showed death as the Grim Reaper."[36]

While it took years and even decades for the Black Death to create the fear-obsessed culture of the late Middle Ages, it only took a few short months to recreate this culture following the outbreak of the Covid-19 pandemic in China. The hysteria over the China Virus was based not on reality but on warnings of impending doom—including grossly exaggerated projections that millions would die. The mass graves never materialized, but the specter remained, engraved on the minds of millions of frightened Americans. Unlike pandemics in past history, it wasn't the actual disease that sowed fear and mass panic, but scientific "experts" and public figures manipulating the flow of information about the disease.

Most scholars agree that the first wave of the Black Plague, which raged from 1347 to 1351, cost Europe some 25,000,000 dead, one-third or more of its population.[37] But the death toll continued to climb throughout the on-again, off-again pandemic for the next four centuries. By the time the Black Death's reign of terror in Europe was finally over, the butcher's bill was up to an estimated 137 million people. The number of deaths worldwide during this period from bubonic plague would be much higher, especially if the death toll at plague central—which, as we shall see, was China—is counted. But the true number is unknowable.

Once Again, a Plague Changes the Course of History

In the absence of the Black Death, the feudal civilization of the Middle Ages might have continued indefinitely. But by killing off a majority of the serfs, the plague sounded the death knell of feudalism.

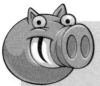

Then and Now: "Overpopulation"

Thomas Malthus, the inventor of the theory of "overpopulation," wrongly blamed people in their numbers for the Black Death.[38] Today, many of our elites believe that the world is overpopulated. The World Economic Forum (WEF), whose yearly conference at Davos is attended by the leaders of some of the most powerful nations on earth, frequently publishes articles warning that "overpopulation remains a global challenge." Were they hoping to see a depopulation silver lining in the pandemic cloud?[39]

With so many dead, it was no longer land but labor that was in short supply. The surviving workers could and did command a higher price for their labor, and as a result gained more control over their lives. As John Kelly notes in *The Great Mortality*, "In the fifty years after the Black Death, the medieval world's traditional economic winners and losers exchanged places. The new losers, the landed gentry, began to see their wealth shredded by the scissors of low food prices and high labor costs; the new winners, the people at the bottom, saw their one marketable asset—labor—increase dramatically in value."[40] Workers and their families saw their diets improve. Higher-quality bread and even meat appeared on their tables, and lifespans lengthened as a result.[41]

The Origin of the Black Death

The Mongols brought the Black Death to Caffa, but where did they contract it? Ibn al-Wardi, an Arab historian who lived in the Syrian town of Aleppo, believed that the plague originated in the East, where, he says, it had raged unchecked for fifteen years before arriving in the West.[42] Situated on the boundary between east and west, he was in a position to know.

Other records suggest that the Mongols had been suffering from the plague for some time. Kelly recounts that the chronicles of the Great Mongol Khanate of Mongolia and Northern China state that in 1332, "The twenty-eight-year-old Mongol Great Khan Jijaghatu Toq-Temur and his sons died suddenly of a mysterious illness."

What illness, and where did it come from? The year before the Great Khan's death, Kelly writes, "Chinese records also make reference to a mysterious illness; this one, a treacherous epidemic, that swept through Hopei province in the northeast region of the country and killed nine-tenths of the population."[43]

And the bubonic plague bacillus that caused both the Black Death and the Plague of Justinian has now been traced back by modern genomic analysis to an earlier outbreak in China. Even the particular strain of *Yersinia pestis* that we know caused the Black Death has been traced back there. The original patient zero was from China. China was the point of origin—and the original killing grounds—of the bubonic plague bacillus itself.[44]

Then and Now: Made in China

Given that the both the smallpox virus—which caused the Antonine Plague—and *Y. pestis* bacillus—which caused the Black Death, and before it the Plague of Justinian—have now been positively identified as coming from China, it is hardly racist to ask: *Why is it always China?*

The Black Death was devastating on both ends of the Eurasian continent. While Europe lost perhaps a third of its people, some of China's provinces may have lost a full half—while China was recorded as having a population of more than 120 million in AD 1200, a 1393 census counted only 65 million. Admittedly, the dynastic transition from Mongol to Ming rule was accompanied by upheaval and famine, and the borders of the new dynasty were somewhat reduced, but tens of millions may have died of the bubonic plague.

It is possible that the bubonic plague may have traveled from China to Europe even before the Mongols' act of biological warfare. Pasta may not have been the only thing that Marco Polo brought back along the Silk Road from China in 1295.

CHAPTER 4

Shipping Routes: The Yunnan Plague (1772–1960)

It was the fifty-sixth year of the reign of the emperor Kangxi of the Qing dynasty. From his Dragon Throne in the Forbidden City, the emperor ruled a vast domain, which stretched far beyond China proper to include Tibet in the south, Turkestan in the west, Mongolia in the northwest, and his own ancestral homeland in the northeast, the original homeland of the Manchus before they conquered the land south of the Great Wall. "All under Heaven"—in the phrase the imperial court often used to refer to its rule—was at peace.

British emissaries paid a visit to the imperial court that year—the year Europeans called AD 1792—in the hope of setting up a trading relationship. They were haughtily dismissed by the emperor, who instructed them to tell "the King of England . . . that the Celestial Empire, ruling all with the four seas . . . has not the slightest need of his country's manufactures." Instead, King George III was merely commanded to "swear perpetual obedience" to the Chinese emperor.

The British nevertheless remained hungry for Chinese silk, tea, and ceramics—and they didn't realize that China would be exporting something else as well. Far in the south, in the province that the Chinese call "South of the Clouds," or Yunnan, another bubonic plague was brewing. Or, more likely, it had never really gone away.

Riding on Rodents

There is always a reservoir of the plague bacillus circulating through the wild rodent population of China, occasionally infecting humans through the handling of infected animals or bites from their fleas. But the plague only reaches epidemic proportions in large towns and cities, which support not only dense populations of humans but also, in years past, large populations of rats.

Over the course of the eighteenth century, immigrants from other parts of China poured into Yunnan province. "It should not surprise us that the first recorded incidence of what can confidently be identified as bubonic plague occurred in the 1790s, precisely the time when Yunnan's urban population was growing most rapidly," explains Carol Benedict in *Bubonic Plague in Nineteenth-Century China*.[1]

Chinese dietary practices may also have played a role. Adding rat to your chow mein greatly increases your chances of contracting the plague. Killing and eating a rat infected with the plague bacillus exposes you to infection in two ways. The first danger comes from the fleas that, as soon as their luncheon host is butchered, start frantically hopping about to find a dinner companion. The second danger comes from exposure to the flesh and bodily fluids of the infected rat itself.

The population—both of rats and of humans—in Yunnan continued to increase in the nineteenth century, and by 1855 a major epidemic of bubonic plague had erupted in the province. From county records, which document the advance of the "rat plague," we know that it reached the provincial capital of Kunming in 1866 and the provincial border a few years later. From Yunnan, the plague continued spreading eastward through the even more densely populated provinces of Guangxi and Guangdong. The advancing front of the epidemic moved relatively slowly. Kelly estimates that "*Y. pestis* traveled at an average of eight miles per year."[2]

★ ★ ★

The Death of Rats

Rats die in the East, rats die in the West!

Men fear dead rats, as if they were tigers.

The rats die, and before long, men are dying like falling walls!

Countless men die each day, the sun grows dim, the clouds are grey.

Three men set out upon a walk, two fall dead while they talk!

Men are dying in the night, but no one dares to cry out.

The lamplight grows dim, as the Plague demon comes into the room.

The light then dies, leaving ghost and corpse in the darkness of the tomb.

Crows sound their raucous cry, while the dogs howl bitterly.

The living resemble the dead, while the ghosts of the dead fool the living.

The dead litter the ground, the homes of Men fall into ruin.

The wind blows for a time, the bones of Men are scattered.

The crops are ready for the harvest, but there is no one in the fields.

This year the officials will find no one to tax.

I hope to ride on a fiery dragon, to see God in heaven.

Begging him to spread heavenly milk, so that the dead will come back to life.

—eighteenth-century Chinese poet Shi Daonan (translation by the author)

Shi succumbed to the Yunnan Plague a short time after writing this melancholy poem.[3]

Moving eastward at this leisurely pace, the bacillus reached Guangzhou (Canton), the provincial capital of Guangdong, in 1888. From there it made its way to the coast eighty miles away, with the first cases in the British Crown colony of Hong Kong being reported in 1894. Now the bacillus was able to find its way aboard ships, as it had in the ports of Pelusium and Caffa in earlier times. But this time around, thanks to steam power, it would be carried much faster, and much, much farther.

The bacillus was spreading much more quickly now. Within the year, traveling along the Chinese coast, it had ignited epidemics in Macau and

Fuzhou. By the following year, 1896, it had reached Singapore and Bombay, from whence it spread quickly throughout the Indian subcontinent. At the time there was no question about its point of origin. As Francis Gasquet, whose book on the Black Death was published in 1908, affirmed, "The origin of the Indian plague, as indeed that of the great pestilence of 1348–9, is China, the great breeding ground of epidemics."[4]

Over the next few years, British steamships carried infected crew members, rats, and their insect passengers throughout the empire. By the turn of the twentieth century, the Yunnan Plague was a pandemic by anyone's reckoning: it had reached every continent.[5] "From the perspective of the microorganism, the bacterium *Yersinia pestis*, the third pandemic was a great success," Myron Echenberg writes. "Before the arrival of modern shipping technology, the pathogen had been confined to [China]. By the middle of the twentieth century, however, *Yersinia pestis* was permanently established in wild rodent reservoirs the world over."[6]

The plague burned through South China, killing countless millions. How many millions, we simply don't know. By way of comparison, British sources estimate that India, which is roughly comparable in size and population density to China proper, lost 10 million people to the plague over the course of a couple decades. It seems certain that China, where the pandemic began, and where outbreaks continued for more than a century, lost many more.

The reason the bubonic plague was almost endemic in China was not just because it had natural reservoirs in local rodent populations. It was also because of dietary habits, dense human settlement patterns, and a burgeoning population, which provided multiple opportunities for both zoonotic and human-to-human transmission over time. Samuel Cohn suggested that the reason for the repeated outbreaks was that humans are not able to acquire permanent natural immunity to all variants of *Yersinia pestis*. If true, this would mean that, after a period of time, people who have recovered from the plague would once again become vulnerable to infection.[7] But this view is contradicted by the historical record, which consistently shows that survivors are unlikely to contract the infection again. This is why they were often recruited—or volunteered—to take care of plague victims.[8]

Not everyone agrees that China suffered worse losses than India. One Chinese researcher, Xu Lei, has produced detailed maps showing that over the course of a century or more the Yunnan Plague "spread to 541 counties in 21 provinces in China"—which is to say across half the country—but claims that this wide-ranging epidemic only "infect[ed] 2.5 million people and caus[ed] 2.2 million deaths."[9]

Given the high mortality rate of the bubonic plague, which is well established, such low numbers make no epidemiological sense. Nor are they based on accurate demographic data;

> ★ ★ ★
> ## P.C. Today:
> Did Xu Lei lowball his numbers? He claims that in all of China only 2.2 million died of the Yunnan Plague from 1772 to 1964. But in Yunnan province alone the registered population—many were not registered—fell by over 4.5 million from 1855 to 1884. The plague, along with a local Muslim rebellion and famine, helped to depopulate the province.[10]
>
> Xu's claim is no more credible than the CCP's absurd insistence that only 14,742 people have died from Covid from January 2020 to April 2022. We know that in Wuhan alone the bodies of over 50,000 Covid victims were incinerated in the city crematoria in just the first few months of the pandemic.[11]

imperial China did not carry out reliable censuses. In fact, local Qing dynasty officials did not keep detailed statistics of any kind even in the best of times—especially ones that might make them look bad. And China was in the throes of turmoil from the mid-nineteenth to the mid-twentieth centuries, from the Taiping Rebellion through the Sino-Japanese War of 1895 and the Boxer Rebellion to World War II and Mao's Communist Revolution.

And today, statistics out of CCP-controlled China are *always* massaged for political purposes, in order to show not just the Chinese Communist Party but also China's entire history in the best possible light. I suspect that Xu may have lowballed his numbers to save China's "face."

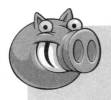

Then and Now: Crossing the Pacific

The Covid-19 pandemic is not the first time that a plague from China has reached America's shores. The Yunnan Plague arrived in San Francisco harbor on board a Japanese ship, the SS *Nippon Maru*, in 1899.

Certainly Westerners living in China at the time thought that the death tolls were significantly greater. A French doctor suggested that the total number of deaths in Guangzhou over the course of the plague was 174,000, or more than a third of the city's population of 400,000. A British doctor living in that same city estimated that 10,400 people had died in the first four months of the 1894 pandemic alone.[12]

Unlike Qing officials, the British authorities in Hong Kong did keep detailed records of births and deaths. Or at least they attempted to—they were handicapped by the reluctance of Chinese residents to self-report illness, or even deaths. The records in Hong Kong report only 2,500 cases of the plague in 1894, dropping to only 44 cases the year following, which cannot possibly be correct. Local Western doctors put the numbers of dead much, much higher, with one French doctor estimating the 1895 total alone at closer to 12,000.[13]

Coming to America

By the 1890s, the world was aware that the bubonic plague had once again broken out in China, and the passengers and crews of ships arriving in American or European ports from the Far East were carefully screened to see if anyone was ill. The first cases were discovered in summer of 1899, when a ship arrived in San Francisco harbor from Hong Kong. The captain first reported that everyone on board was healthy, although he admitted that two passengers had fallen ill during transit.

But when the ship was quarantined and searched, eleven Chinese stowaways were found. Two disappeared that same night. They were probably tossed overboard by the frightened crew—when their bodies were later recovered from the bay they were found to have been suffering from the plague. The news sent shock waves through the city, although no other cases were immediately discovered. Nine months later, however, the plague struck Chinatown. It is likely that infected stowaways and rats from this and other ships had made it ashore while the authorities were looking for sick passengers.

What followed was a frantic effort to contain the spread of the plague, whose complicated germ–flea–rat–human cycle was still not well understood. The first measure taken by the city board of health was, quite naturally, to quarantine the area where the outbreak had occurred. The twelve blocks of Chinatown were cordoned off. But that measure was met with bitter criticism from business owners, who argued that if word got out that the plague was loose in the city it would be very bad for business.

The board retreated after two days, and instead instructed its officials to go door-to-door to identify any who might be infected. The Chinese refused to open their doors and went to great lengths to hide their dead and dying. Still, two more cases of the plague were discovered, and the board was forced to admit publicly that plague had been found in the city.

At one point the U.S surgeon general instructed local health officials to inoculate everyone in Chinatown against the plague using an experimental vaccine developed by microbiologist Waldemar Haffkine in India. Similar to the Chinese practice of variolation, it used a small amount of the plague bacillus to generate an immune reaction. As you might expect, this "formulation had nasty side effects, and did not provide complete protection, though it was said to have reduced risk by up to 50 percent."[14] The Chinese community, up in arms, refused to submit to what they called mass experimentation, and the idea was dropped.[15]

Cases of the plague continued to occur sporadically among the Chinese population, and in April 1901 a massive clean-up campaign was launched

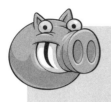

Then and Now: One Man's Anti-Vaxxer Is Another Man's Freedom Fighter

When the Chinese in San Francisco's China-town refused to take an experimental vaccine that "had nasty side effects, and did not provide complete protection, though it was said to have reduced risk by up to 50 percent," the idea was dropped.[16] During the Covid pandemic a number of nations, U.S. states, and companies attempted to impose a similar mandate for an experimental vaccine on their citizens or employees, enforcing it by restricting the liberties or even terminating the employment of those who refused. Many objected, and eventually the mandates were rescinded nearly everywhere except in the China Virus's country of origin.

in Chinatown. Over 1,200 houses and 14,000 rooms were cleaned and disinfected. By 1904, the plague was over. There had been 122 deaths, all but a couple of them in San Francisco's Chinatown.

The San Francisco earthquake of 1906 led to another small outbreak of the plague the following year, but it was quickly quelled by a new kind of public health measure. Officials, who at that point understood the key role that rats played in spreading the disease, put a bounty on their furry little heads. The rat population was hunted to near extinction, and the plague died out. Mild outbreaks in Los Angeles and New Orleans were quickly quelled the same way.

Chinese herbal doctors didn't understand the germ theory of disease, but they did grasp that the plague had something to do with rats—they called it *shuyi*, or rat plague. And in Yunnan, where the plague was endemic, people kept a wary eye out for sick rats. As the eighteenth-century Chinese poet Shi Daonan noted, "Men fear dead rats, as if they were tigers."[17]

A French visitor to Yunnan during the pandemic noted that when sick rats started staggering out of their burrows, people who lived in the vicinity immediately "purified their houses by lighting a fire in every room and in some districts stopped eating meat."[18] Did burning infected fleas out of their houses and keeping rodent meat out of their woks help to protect them? Perhaps.

All told, five hundred deaths in the United States were attributed to the plague between 1899 and 1950. European fatalities over the same time period were seven thousand, while the Central and South American death toll is estimated at thirty thousand. In both India and China, however, the death toll was in the millions. Together, the two countries accounted for the vast majority of deaths.

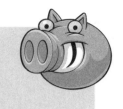

Then and Now: The Golden State

The last rat-borne epidemic in the United States occurred in Los Angeles in 1924–1925. Given the large and growing homeless encampments in Los Angeles and other California cities today, each with its complement of rats, some have warned that another outbreak may be on the horizon there.[19]

That Western countries were largely spared is a reflection not only of the effective quarantine and public health measures that were put in place, but also of the relatively sophisticated medical services available in the West. At the time, China and India were premodern societies where the method of dealing with the plague was little improved over that of Galen so many centuries before. India was under British rule, of course, but few Indians had access to the relatively sophisticated colonial medical service.

Even where such medical service was active and available, as in Hong Kong, the fears and anti-foreign sentiments of ordinary Chinese largely kept them from benefiting from it. Xenophobia ran high in China. When the British governor of Hong Kong made it clear that he was determined to take strong public health measures to curb the spread of the disease, an anti-government poster campaign was launched in the port city. Rumors began circulating that English doctors "were cutting open pregnant women and scooping out the eyes of children to make medicines for the treatment of plague-stricken patients."[20] Few Chinese would seek medical care from such purported monsters.

At least 15 million people would die before the plague burned itself out, making it one of the deadliest pandemics in the history of the world.

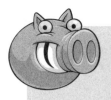

Then and Now: Coming to America

The Yunnan Plague was largely, though not entirely, contained within China. While India did suffer greatly as well, America did not. Americans wouldn't be so fortunate with later viral epidemics that originated in China.

Solving the Plague Mystery

It was not easy for nineteenth-century science to unravel the mystery of the plague. It simply had too many moving parts—bacteria, fleas, rats, and humans—all performing an intricate dance of death. Until the 1890s physicians were still flailing about for an explanation, with some pointing to dirt and garbage and others blaming the mysterious "miasma"—noxious fumes that supposedly rose from the ground from decaying organic materials and sickened those they enveloped. That's why rats caught it first, they said—they live underground.

It wasn't until 1894 that a student of Louis Pasteur by the name of Alexander Yersin reported a breakthrough. Yersin, who was working in Hong Kong, found rod-shaped bacteria in the swollen lymph nodes—the buboes—and other organs of patients who had died of the plague. To confirm that this bacterium was actually the cause of death, he injected it into a number of different animals. All of the animals died within days, their organs riddled with the same bacteria.[21] Today the bacillus that causes the bubonic plague bears its discoverer's name—Yersin. *Yersinia Pestis* means "Yersinia the Pestilence," which the invisible killer of the bubonic plagues surely is.

A French researcher working in India solved another part of the mystery a few years later. Paul-Louis Simond had learned that residents of the island of Taiwan (then called Formosa) avoided handling dead rats because they were fearful of contracting the plague. Suspecting that fleas might be serving as the vector, Simond set up an ingenious experiment to test his hypothesis. Two cages were put side by side, the first containing a newly dead, plague-infected rat and the second a healthy rat. After fleas from the infected rat hopped onto the healthy rat it, too, contracted the bubonic plague and died. Hypothesis proved.

Now, for the first time, we knew the life cycle of the plague bacillus. It goes like this:

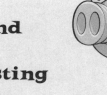

Then and Now: Contrasting Causes

Human beings were simply collateral damage in the three worst plagues in recorded history. The plague bacteria had blindly evolved to hunt rats, not man.

The China Virus, on the other hand, was deliberately engineered—by men—to target man himself.

1. A flea bites a rat infected with the plague bacterium;
2. Plague bacteria multiply in the flea's gut;
3. The infected rat dies, and the bacteria-laden flea hops off;
4. The flea looks for another rat, but will bite anything warm-blooded;
5. The flea bites its new host, transmitting the plague bacterium.

It is sobering to note that, in the three worst plagues in recorded history, which collectively killed well over 100 million people, the actual target of *Yersinia pestis* was not man, but the lowly rat. Humans were simply collateral damage.

Yersinia Pestis as a Bioweapon

Now that the bacterium responsible for the Yunnan Plague had been identified, it was perhaps inevitable that military minds would begin thinking about how to weaponize it. It was to forestall such an eventuality that the 1925 Geneva Protocol included a prohibition on the use of biological weapons in war.[22]

But the horror and dread with which the world regarded the prospect of germ warfare seems only to have encouraged the chief medical officer of the Imperial Japanese Army, Shiro Ishii, to envision waging just that. Ishii was able to convince his superiors that spreading lethal diseases would be an effective way of defeating Japan's enemies.[23] When Japan seized control of Manchuria from the Chinese in the early 1930s, Ishii set about creating a network of bioweapons research and development facilities there, which at one point employed over ten thousand personnel. Its central hub was called Unit 731.

After Japan went back to war with China again in 1937, Unit 731 began feverishly weaponizing the pathogens it had been researching. It provided the Japanese army with vials of cholera and typhoid germs that could be dumped into wells and marshes and spread in homes to cause local outbreaks. It infused germs into snacks and clothing that could be handed out or airdropped to the unsuspecting enemy.

But the Japanese army wanted a weapon that would devastate entire cities, and so Ishii turned to the bubonic plague. He knew that the pneumonic plague, which is both highly infectious and almost invariably fatal, would be the ideal biological weapon to incapacitate the enemy. Its victims die quickly—remember Boccaccio's description of having lunch with your friends and dinner with your ancestors in paradise—and in horrific fashion, suffering from high fevers and coughing up blood.

Ishii ordered Unit 731 to breed swarms of plague-infected fleas and devised a way that they could be spread by low-flying planes over Chinese cities. The World Health Organization later calculated that fifty kilograms of the deadly pneumonic plague, if it were widely dispersed over a major city, would be capable of infecting and killing virtually the entire population. From the point of release, the bacteria would remain viable within a radius of about nineteen kilometers for about one hour.[24]

Ishii was working with grams, rather than kilograms, of the bacteria, but was still able to inflict considerable damage on the civilian population. The first aerial attack occurred on October 27, 1940, when Japanese warplanes dropped plague-contaminated fleas and rice into the cities of Ningbo and Quzhou, China. This led to an outbreak of pneumonic plague that reportedly killed tens of thousands and was judged a great success.[25] Other attacks followed, such as the November 4, 1941, bombing of the Hunan city of Changde. A single plane sowed infected fleas, along with some other plague-infused items, over the city, causing almost eight thousand fatalities over the next few weeks.[26]

Japan surrendered in 1945, but the plague bacteria did not. The plagues unleashed by the Japanese went on to kill tens of thousands more before dying down in 1948. Even today, rats with antibodies to the specific *Yersinia pestis* strain used in Japan's biowarfare attacks are still being found in China. In all, historian Sheldon H. Harris estimates that over two hundred thousand people were killed by the Imperial Japanese Army's germ warfare program and other human experiments.[27]

Estimates of the death toll made by the Chinese authorities run much higher. An "International Symposium on the Crimes of Bacteriological Warfare" was held in Changde—the city that was "bombed" with plague fleas—in 2002. The Chinese presenters claimed that 580,000 people had died at the hands of Unit 731, most from the Japanese biological warfare attacks.[28]

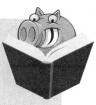

A Book You're Not Supposed to Read

The definitive account of how the Japanese military used the bubonic plague and other pathogens in China in World War II has been told by Sheldon H. Harris in *Factories of Death: Japanese Biological Warfare 1932–45 and the American Cover-Up* (New York: Routledge, 1994). Harris also tells the story of how Ishii and others escaped being put on trial for war crimes following the war: they received immunity from prosecution in return for handing over their research to the United States.

Plague Central?

The Plague of Justinian, the Black Death, and, of course, the Yunnan Plague can all be traced back to major epidemics in China. But these are only the three occasions when the plague impacted the West in a significant way. The historical record suggests that China, at least from the time of the first Shang dynasty (1600–1046 BC), has probably never been completely free of the plague.[29]

Indeed, it is not unreasonable to think that the people of the plague village of Hamin Mangha in Neolithic China may have died from eating marmots infected with the bubonic plague. People living in Inner Mongolia today still hunt marmots, and as a result are still—even today—dying of the plague.[30]

It is not hard to see why the plague might have been endemic in China for thousands of years. China has a number of natural animal reservoirs for the plague throughout the country, from rats in Yunnan in the south to marmots in Manchuria and Mongolia in the north, so the plague is always just a burrow away. Chinese cuisine, as everyone knows, has always included almost everything that walks, flies, crawls, or . . . burrows.[31] The combination of a diet that includes rats and rodents and a high population density ensured that there were always pockets of plague percolating in different parts of China. In fact, the bubonic plague was so common that it was often simply called *yi*, or "plague," or *dayi*, "large plague," instead of being separately identified in Chinese medicine as was, for example, smallpox.

Epidemics that affected large parts of China—such as the devastating series of epidemics that hit China during the Manchu conquest in the mid-seventeenth century—were noted in official dynastic records. But smaller, localized outbreaks were frequently mentioned only in the pages of local county gazetteers, such as the one from Shunde county, Guangdong province, in my possession. That the outbreaks in question are sometimes referred to as *shuyi*, or "rat plague," is further evidence that the "plague" in question was of the bubonic variety.[32]

Of course, none of this evidence proves that *Yersinia pestis* originated in China rather than, say, India or Africa, although it certainly points in that direction. But, thanks to modern genomic science, the matter is no longer in doubt. It is now clear that *Yersinia pestis*, which so cleverly hijacks the flea to infect the rat, originally evolved in China long ago.

The first piece of genetic evidence came from French biologist R. Devignat, who identified three major variants of *Yersinia pestis*. Thinking that these corresponded to the three bubonic plagues, he named the first Antigua after the Plague of Justinian in the ancient world, the second Medievalis after the Black Death of the Middle Ages, and the third Orientalis after the Yunnan Plague, which was largely confined to Asia.[33]

The French microbiologist Michel Drancourt was able take the investigation one step further. A sixth-century mass grave had been found in southern France in which sixty victims of the Plague of Justinian had been hastily buried. From their skeletons he was able to extract enough genetic material from the original infection to conclude that they had died not from the Antigua or Medievalis variants, but from the Orientalis strain. The demon that had come to Pelusium in AD 540 had started its journey in China.[34] The other two variants were later spin-offs.

Modern science has confirmed what the historical record suggests, that the proximate cause of the bubonic plagues was a *Yersinia pestis* variant from China. But the question of ultimate origin remains. When and, more important, where did the plague bacterium itself mutate into its present deadly form?

Here again, modern genetics has provided the answer. A team of medical geneticists collected data on all the known strains of *Yersinia pestis* and constructed a family tree of the bacteria. The major branches of the tree—corresponding to the three great waves of plague—can all be traced back to China, where the root of their phylogenetic tree is located. They concluded that "*Y. pestis* evolved in or near China, and has been transmitted via multiple epidemics that followed various routes, probably including transmissions to West Asia via the Silk Road and to Africa by Chinese marine voyages."[35] Or as Gasquet put it somewhat more succinctly in his 1908 book, "China [is] the great breeding ground of epidemics."[36]

Aside from the three major plagues, the researchers were also able to trace other outbreaks back to their point of origin in China. They showed that repeated epidemics in Mongolia, Siberia, and Russia over the centuries were caused by Chinese variants, for instance. And they concluded from the genetic evidence that it was the Chinese admiral Zheng He's several voyages of exploration to the East African coast from 1417 to 1431 that brought the plague to sub-Saharan Africa.[37]

Since mutations tick off at a fairly constant rate over time, the team was even able to estimate that the bacteria evolved into its present lethal state at least 2,600 years ago, and perhaps as long as 28,000 years ago. In other words, long before it reached the Roman Empire in the second century AD, it had been plaguing the people of China.

The Bubonic Plague Is Never Going Away

Setting aside Japan's biowarfare attacks, the last major outbreak of the Yunnan Plague—the last "natural" outbreak, that is—occurred in Manchuria in 1909–1910. While it may have started as the bubonic variety, it quickly morphed into the even more infectious and deadly pneumonic version. People themselves become disease vectors, passing it along by coughing, sneezing, or even by exchanging a friendly hello. And, as everyone who lived through the pandemic of 2020–2021 knows, it's almost impossible to stop the spread of an airborne virus. It claimed at least sixty-three thousand lives.

The last recorded rat-borne epidemic in the United States occurred in Los Angeles in 1924–1925. A century later, some have warned that another outbreak may not be too far off. The City of the Angels is dotted with large and growing homeless encampments, each with its complement of rats.[38]

A number of efforts have been made to develop a vaccine to the bubonic plague, but their efficacy is unproven.[39] The chief breakthrough in treatment came in 1945 with the discovery of Streptomycin, which has proven so effective against *Yersinia pestis* infections that it is still the antibiotic of choice today seventy-five years later.[41] But what really ended the plague's reign of terror was the discovery of DDT, a potent new insecticide that, by eradicating flea populations, literally cut the plague's legs out from under it. The cycle of death had been broken.

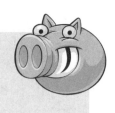

Then and Now: Big Budget

It may not always be possible to create a vaccine to protect people from a dangerous pathogen, but it is certainly easy to spend billions of dollars in the effort. From 2000 to 2019, an estimated $15.3 billion was spent in the effort, unsuccessful to this day, to develop a vaccine against HIV/AIDS.[40] Useful therapeutic drugs, however, have been developed and deployed over that same time period—and at a fraction of the cost.

The World Health Organization declared victory over the Yunnan Plague in 1960, when the number of deaths worldwide fell to around two hundred. And in 2003 it stopped requiring the routine reporting of plague cases.

It seems a little premature to declare victory. The Yunnan Plague has never really ended, nor is it likely to. *Yersinia pestis* is no longer limited to a few rodent reservoirs in China but is found among rodent populations around the world. Indeed, from the perspective of the bubonic plague bacteria, the Yunnan Plague was a great success. And human beings continue to be collateral damage, as *Yersinia pestis*–carrying fleas

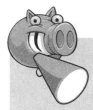

Then and Now: The Hunter Becomes the Hunted

As CNN reported in 2020,

Authorities in the Chinese region of Inner Mongolia have sealed off a village after a resident there died from bubonic plague, a centuries-old disease responsible for the most deadly pandemic in human history. . . . Authorities also urged people to reduce contact with wild animals while traveling and avoid hunting, skinning or eating animals that could cause infection.

Last month, two cases of bubonic plague were confirmed in Mongolia—brothers who had both eaten marmot meat, according to China's state-run news agency Xinhua. In May 2019, another couple in Mongolia died from the plague after eating the raw kidney of a marmot, thought to be a folk remedy for good health.

Marmots [are] a type of large ground squirrel that is eaten in some parts of China and the neighboring country Mongolia, and which have historically caused plague outbreaks in the region.

The marmot is believed to have caused the 1911 pneumonic plague epidemic, which killed about 63,000 people in northeast China. It was hunted for its fur, which soared in popularity among international traders. The diseased fur products were traded and transported around the country—infecting thousands along the way.[42]

bite them in densely populated cities and towns and people in the countryside continue to recklessly expose themselves to the bacteria by killing and eating infected wild rodents.

This is why there have been repeated outbreaks of plague in such places as China and Tanzania (1983), Zaire (1992), and India, Mozambique, and Zimbabwe (1994). During the 15-year period from 1989 to 2003, 25 countries reported a total of 38,359 cases of the plague and 2,845 deaths to the World Health Organization, which works out to about 2,500 cases and almost 200 deaths a year. The vast majority of the cases are reported from Africa[43] but, not surprisingly, China remains an epicenter as well. Yunnan was hit by another outbreak between 1986 and 2005, and another case was diagnosed there in 2016.[44] As we have seen, marmot hunters in northeastern China also continue to come down with the disease.[45]

Meanwhile the bacillus continues to evolve. In the mid-1990s a multi-drug resistant strain of the plague arose in Madagascar.[46] Unlike smallpox, which has been totally eradicated, *Yersinia pestis* seems to be capable of surviving any and all human efforts to eradicate it.

Then and Now: Rat's Back on the Menu, Boys

How does a nice bowl of rattail soup sound? Rats and other rodents have been part of Chinese cuisine since ancient times. In recent times, in order to keep the rat population down, Communist officials have encouraged their consumption, and many restaurants have rats on the menu.[47]

Geostrategic Effects

Unlike the first two bubonic plagues, the West escaped the third largely unscathed. But the effect of the Yunnan Plague in the East was profound. The sickness and death it visited upon the Chinese empire's most populous and prosperous provinces in the last few decades of the nineteenth century undermined the Qing dynasty at a time when it was already struggling to cope with an increasingly restive Han Chinese majority at home and increasingly aggressive great powers abroad.

But the greatest geostrategic consequence of the Yunnan Plague lies elsewhere.

Despite the example of the Mongol assault on the Black Sea port of Caffa, biological warfare had not generally been a part of the arsenal that nations deployed against their enemies. The decision of the Japanese to weaponize natural pathogens and use them in repeated attacks on the civilian population of China changed warfare forever. It persuaded the Chinese Communist

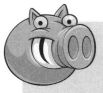

Then and Now: Germ Warfare (and Projection)

Communist Party leader Mao Zedong accused the United States of carrying out germ warfare against Chinese and North Korean troops during the Korean War. Premier Zhou Enlai was even more specific, claiming that U.S. troops had sown the smallpox virus in Pyongyang and other North Korean provinces to cover their retreat southward to the 38th parallel, from December 1950 to January 1951.[48] The charge was false, and perhaps it was a case of projection. Mao longed to unleash biological weapons on his enemies. And in 2019 Xi Jinping, who emulates Mao in all things, actually did.

Party that biological warfare was the wave of the future.

After the war, China took over the Japanese biowarfare facilities in Manchuria, and it has been operating them, with increasing sophistication, ever since.

The CCP was eager to go from being the victim of germ warfare to the victimizer. In 2019, as we will see in a later chapter, it succeeded.

PART THREE

THE CHINESE INFLUENZAS

CHAPTER 5

The First (and Worst) Truly Global Pandemic: The Spanish Flu (1918–1920)

*"Before and after 1918, most influenza pandemics developed in Asia
and spread from there to the rest of the world."*

—Jeffery K. Taubenberger and David M. Morens

The year was 1918, and the world had been at war for four years.

What came to be known as the Great War had begun on June 28, 1914, when Archduke Franz Ferdinand, heir to the throne of the Austro-Hungarian Empire, was assassinated in Sarajevo. On the western front, it had quickly bogged down into trench warfare. When the Germans' advance stalled in late 1914, they dug in along a line running from Alsace-Lorraine to the North Sea coast. The British and French armies likewise entrenched themselves, a few hundred yards away.

Both sides built ever more elaborate systems of trenches as the war ground on. Defended by barbed wire and machine gun emplacements and with batteries of artillery in the rear providing precision strikes, such entrenched positions could only be breached at tremendous human cost. The ground between the trenches was not called "no-man's land" for nothing. No man could long survive the storm of steel that would greet him if he tried to cross.

The war proved deadly—to both soldiers and civilians. By the time it ended, on November 11, 1918, an estimated 8.5 million combatants had died, and an even greater number of civilians.

But as bad as the carnage of trench warfare was, something worse was on the way. By 1918 another deadly threat was stalking humanity. It would, in the end, rack up a far higher casualty total than the war itself. The battle lines in World War I were drawn in Europe, but the new influenza virus was no respecter of human borders. The Armistice stopped human beings from killing one another, but the virus was not a signatory. It continued its relentless campaign of devastation, going everywhere and infecting seemingly everybody for two more years.

As the virus raged, new trenches had to be dug—not to protect the bodies of the living, but to serve as graves for the corpses of the dead. By the time the disease had run its course, some 500 million people were estimated to have contracted it—nearly 30 percent of the world's population of 1.8 billion in 1918. And of those who fell ill, 50 million may have died. Perhaps more. No one knows for sure.

The soldiers called it "the Spanish Flu."

Spain Wasn't to Blame

It was not unusual for the soldiers in the trenches in France to complain of headaches, fevers, sore throats, and aches and pains. Large numbers of soldiers came down with flu-like illnesses such as trench fever from the bites of the omnipresent body lice. They suffered other maladies as well, including trench foot and dysentery, because of the unhealthy conditions in the muddy ditches they were forced to live in.

In the spring of 1918, large numbers of them were complaining of symptoms typical of the flu. A few deaths were noted, but this was also not unusual. This spring outbreak, however, turned out to be a prelude to something much worse—the most deadly influenza epidemic in the history of the world.

What is now understood to be the first wave of the Spanish Flu was quickly followed by a second. The new variant—if that's what it was—was much more deadly. This time large numbers of soldiers began dying. Within a couple of weeks some seventy thousand American soldiers had fallen so ill they had to be hospitalized, and roughly one in three of these never left their hospital beds alive. The other armies on the front lines—British, French, and German—suffered a similar fate.

The highly infectious influenza spread through the trenches like wildfire, sped on its way by the cramped and miserable conditions in those muddy ditches, the generally weakened physical condition of the soldiers, and the other maladies they were already suffering from. Soon more soldiers were falling to the flu than were being felled in combat.

Wartime censorship kept reports of how the deadly disease was ravaging the ranks of their armies out of the newspapers in France, Great Britain, Germany, and the United States. No country wanted to reveal its own weakness, or the weakness of its allies, to the enemy; nor did any country want to demoralize citizens back home with the news that their sons were dying from a stealth attack by an invisible enemy.

But the press in neutral Spain was not subject to the same restrictions. With the flu also running rampant there, the Spanish newspapers were full of reports about its spread on the Iberian Peninsula, where it reportedly killed at least 150,000 people. Because Spain was not involved in the war, the censors in Allied countries allowed stories of this catastrophe to run freely in their own newspapers. Thus Spain became indelibly identified with the flu in the mind of the public, especially after King Alfonso XIII himself came down with the disease. The king survived, but the name Spanish Flu stuck.

Fewer soldiers would have died, perhaps, if the Allied leaders had not been readying a final push to defeat the Central powers, relying heavily on the fresh troops of the American Expeditionary Force. "The European allies ignored the disease as much as they could in the last months of the war," writes Milorad Radusin in his account of the Spanish Flu. "The Central Powers were being given the final blow and there was no room for drastic prophylactic and hygienic measures, which would stop or at least slow down the spread of the pandemic. The war logic was also against health

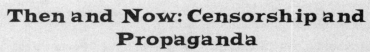

Then and Now: Censorship and Propaganda

During the Spanish Flu, countries with troops in the field engaged in strict wartime censorship to keep news of the epidemic from undermining military and civilian morale. As long as the war was in progress, the sharing of news, research, and data on the influenza was limited, even among the Allies.

A century later we have the ability to communicate instantaneously with all corners of the globe, but the sharing of data, research, and news about the China Virus is still limited. In the United States, the Biden administration encouraged Big Tech to censor criticism of its ever shifting Covid policies on masks, vaccines, therapeutics, closures, and lockdowns.[1]

China went even further, engaging in full-blown wartime censorship and propaganda.[2] The Chinese Communist Party suppressed information about the origins and early spread of the China Virus in part because, like Germany in World War I, it was in a contest with the United States and its allies for global dominance.

But there was another, even more important, reason for the CCP's disinformation campaign. While the deadly influenza virus of 1918 had been an accident of nature, the China Virus of 2019—SARS-CoV-2—was created in the Wuhan Institute of Virology.

None of the warring parties of World War I were responsible for the pandemic that followed the arrival of the Spanish Flu, but the 2020–2021 pandemic does have a progenitor: the CCP, which deliberately—with malice aforethought—unleashed a bioweapon on the world.

interests in the countries faced with a foreboding of defeat. . . . The flu was ignored to the greatest possible extent."[3]

But they should have been paying attention, because the flu left the armies prostrate. Statistics from the American Expeditionary Force show that while 227,000 soldiers were hospitalized with battle wounds in 1918, 340,000—half again as many—had to be hospitalized for influenza over that same period.[4] It was the flu, rather than the bullets and bombardments of the enemy, that caused the greatest loss of life among American soldiers and sailors during the war.

Nor was the epidemic confined to the military—it almost simultaneously ripped through civilian populations in Europe, Asia, and North America. The infection reached Glasgow in May 1918, and over 228,000 British died in the months following. By the end of the summer, an epidemic was raging in Germany, claiming an estimated 400,000 victims in a country already prostrate from the war. The French suffered an equal number of civilian deaths.

Following the shipping lanes, as always, the epidemic quickly became a pandemic, spreading to Asia, Australia, and throughout the Americas. The worst-hit country seems to have been India. The influenza arrived in the port of Bombay in June 1918, and cases were soon being reported in other major port cities such as Karachi and Chennai (Madras). With few hospitals and scarce medical personnel—many of India's doctors had been drafted into the British army—the influenza was to claim its biggest death toll ever in the Indian subcontinent. An estimated 16 million Indians died over the following twelve months.

The influenza reached the United States in September, and within the next three months some 20 million people fell ill. By the end of 1918, 450,000 Americans had died, a number that would increase to an estimated 675,000 by the time the epidemic had run its course in 1920.

The signing of the Armistice in November 1918 only made things worse, since with the end of the war millions of soldiers were demobilized. As they returned home to their cities and towns, they brought the influenza with them. A third wave of the pandemic ensued.

Before the pandemic ended a little over a year later, the Spanish Flu had reached almost every corner of the globe. The world was much less well-connected in those days, but the highly infectious virus even managed to make its way up to remote Inuit villages in the Alaskan wilderness and to isolated islands in the South Pacific, which suffered some of the highest mortality rates in the world. Some 22 percent of Western Samoa's population died.[5]

The Spanish Flu was the first truly global pandemic. Few places on earth were spared.

Pandemic, What Pandemic?

For those who lived through the Covid-19 pandemic of 2020–2021, with the endless panic over case numbers, hospitalizations, and deaths, it's surprising to learn of the unruffled demeanor of officials and the muted reaction of the press in the United States in the late summer of 1918. After all, the second wave of the Spanish Flu was rapidly spreading across the country at that very moment, and it was at least as infectious—and far, far more deadly—than the China Virus at its worst.

President Woodrow Wilson, whose sole focus was winning the war, brushed off concerns about the Spanish Flu. He released no public statements and insisted that the troop transports keep ferrying American soldiers to Europe, even as many on board were falling ill and dying along the way.[6]

His officials took their cues from their boss. Surgeon General Rupert Blue insisted, "There is no cause for alarm if proper precautions are observed." Another official dismissed the pandemic as "ordinary influenza by another name." It most definitely was not, but local health officials followed the same line. Chicago's director of public health, for instance, decided that it was not his job to "interfere with the morale of the community," maintaining rather that "it is our job to keep people from fear. Worry kills more than the disease."[7] In New York City, home of the best-respected of local health departments, "the initial reaction appeared aimed at calming, rather than alerting, the public about the possible dangers from the approaching epidemic."[8]

John Barry, author of *The Great Influenza*, accuses both the Wilson administration and the press of behaving irresponsibly in failing to immediately sound the alarm when the second wave of the Spanish Flu arrived. "[T]here was outright censorship" in Europe, Barry noted.[9] "In the United States, they didn't quite do that, but there was intense pressure not to say anything negative."

The Committee on Public Information, as it was called, was an independent federal agency set up to create a positive narrative about the war. It churned out thousands of feel-good stories about the conflict, which newspapers often republished word for word. News about the spread of the Spanish Flu in the trenches in France would have been devastating for morale at home, so it was deliberately suppressed. And even when the influenza was ripping across the United States itself, most newspapers downplayed its severity so as not to undermine the war effort.

While his officials were damping down concerns about the influenza so as not to undermine the war effort, Wilson himself had an additional motivation. He saw the war as an opportunity to create a new international order based on his idea for a League of Nations—a kind of proto–New World Order—and in pursuit of his grand scheme appears to have been simply indifferent to an influenza pandemic that was killing hundreds of thousands of his fellow Americans.

As the death count in the United States rose in the fall of 2018, city and county authorities responded to local outbreaks by instituting public health measures such as masks and restrictions on gatherings. This worked better than imposing a one-size-fits-all solution on a continent-sized country in which rates of illness varied not only state by state but also city by city, and even town by town.

As the Spanish Flu continued to spread, the media's reluctance to report the truth began to break down. Stories about the rising death toll and the new health measures being instituted in response began to appear in local

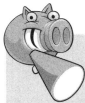

Then and Now: Pandemic Panic

John Barry has furiously criticized what he calls the "lies and silence" of Woodrow Wilson and his administration during the Spanish Flu pandemic, which "cost authority figures credibility and trust." Even worse, he writes, was that "with no public official to believe in, people believed rumors and their most horrific imaginings. A man living in Washington described the result: 'People were afraid to kiss one another, people were afraid to eat with one another. . . . It destroyed those contacts and destroyed the intimacy that existed amongst people. . . . There was an aura of a constant fear that you lived through from getting up in the morning to going to bed at night.'"[10]
To anyone who lived through the Covid pandemic, these behaviors sound drearily familiar. The only difference was that in 2020–2021, "the intimacy that existed amongst people" was deliberately discouraged by government orders to socially distance, wear masks, and avoid touching one another, even to shake hands. (Of course, New York City's board of health, aware that some people might violate the "no touching" rule, did suggest, "If you must have sex with strangers, be sure and mask up first.")
If in 1918 Wilson's silence *allowed* the rise of a pandemic of fear, in 2020 health officials deliberately *created* the pandemic of fear surrounding Covid. You can decide for yourself which is worse: for officials to remain silent in the face of the worst pandemic in human history, or for officials to endlessly warn of a coming Covid apocalypse that, for all of their efforts to magnify it, turned out in the end to be more akin to a couple of severe flu seasons. And, as we shall see, by "distancing" people from needed medical treatments and panicking them into taking an experimental vaccine, the climate of fear that they created may ultimately kill more people than it saved.

newspapers. At the same time, however, no one had much to offer about the nature of the disease that was causing the carnage. The result was mass panic. In rural Kentucky, the Red Cross reported, "people were starving to death not from lack of food but because the [healthy] were panic stricken and would not go near the sick."[11] If this sounds like a scene straight out of the Black Death, it's because it was. History was rhyming—and not in a good way.

Masks, Closures, and Travel Bans—but No Lockdowns

If there was any single public health measure that became emblematic of the Spanish Flu, it was the pervasive masking. The advice of the time was generally to wear masks when in rooms where people were sick. But what started with nurses and doctors covering their faces with gauze masks quickly spread to other municipal employees, such as policemen and firemen, and soon panicked citizens were following suit.

Some jurisdictions mandated masks on public transportation, and some even attempted a universal mask mandate. The city of San Francisco, for example, passed a city-wide mask ordinance that required everyone to wear a cotton or gauze mask when going out in public. There was immediate pushback from the public—including a group calling themselves the San

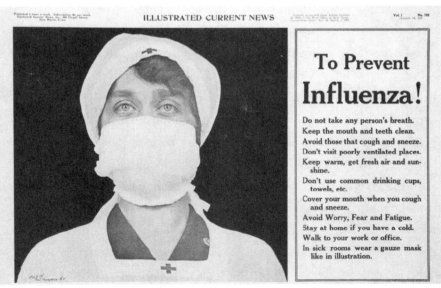

Public health advice in 1918. *Paul Thompson for the* Illustrated Current News, *New Haven, Connecticut*

Francisco Anti-Mask League. Other groups around the country organized to fight some of the new restrictions as well, primarily because they were affecting businesses and livelihoods.[12]

Those who resisted wearing masks argued that mandating mask-wearing was a restriction on their liberties and that there was no scientific evidence that masking helped to stop the spread of the Spanish Flu. They were proven right by later studies showing "that the . . . impact [of masks] on the spread of the disease was very low or nonexistent."[13] A cotton mask would have stopped bacteria, but this was a virus which was a thousand times smaller than a bacterium—and several thousand times smaller than the gaps in a cotton cloth mask.

In dealing with a pandemic of unknown origin, it is only common sense to try and keep people from communicating the disease to one another. Besides mask mandates, some local public health agencies took actions that actually did slow the spread of disease, such as forbidding handshakes and spitting. They even attempted—with, one imagines, somewhat less success—to ban coughing and sneezing. Physicians everywhere encouraged social distancing. "Don't take anyone's breath," was a slogan of the day.

Local jurisdictions took the lead in adopting public health policies—shuttering theaters, shutting down saloons, and even closing sidewalks—in response to outbreaks. State governments, on the other hand, did little, and the federal government did even less. Americans in those days still confidently governed themselves through locally elected officials.

Countries with different political traditions, on the other hand, took a very different approach. Mexican officials, for example, attempted to contain the influenza by issuing national regulations which "targeted urban public spaces in which large numbers of people congregated, closing theaters, cinemas, schools, nightclubs, churches, cantinas, and *pulquerías* [Mexican taverns]. Curfews were established, and violation of them carried a modest but not insignificant fine, especially for the poorest citizens."[14]

In other Western countries there were no centrally imposed lockdowns, although to slow down the spread of the infection many did shut down their cinemas, theaters, dance halls, and churches for anywhere from a few weeks to several months. But exceptions were made. In the United Kingdom, the BBC reports, "pubs, which were already subject to wartime restrictions on opening hours, mostly stayed open. The Football League and the FA Cup had been cancelled for the war, but there was no effort to cancel other matches or limit crowds, with men's teams playing in regional competitions, and women's football, which attracted large crowds, continuing throughout the pandemic. . . . Some people wore anti-germ masks, as they went about their daily lives." But no mask mandate was imposed, and people were not shut up in their homes for days or weeks on end.[16]

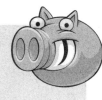

Then and Now: The Sanitary Dictatorship

The phrase "sanitary dictatorship," which was frequently applied to the 2020–2021 Covid-19 lockdowns, was coined in Mexico during the Spanish Flu pandemic of 1918 in Mexico City's attempt to impose nationwide restrictions on the country.[15]

Most localities suspended public gatherings for a time. Paris postponed a sporting event in which ten thousand young people had been invited to participate. "[S]ome churches in Italy suspended confessions and funeral ceremonies," reports Eugenia Tognotti.[17] But, in general, European countries, perhaps because they were already devastated by the war, put little effort into widespread public health measures.

If there was any country that anticipated the travel bans, quarantines, and lockdowns of today, it was Australia. The influenza arrived in Sydney in late January 1919, and the state government of New South Wales (NSW) immediately sprang into action. "The day after NSW was proclaimed to be 'infected,'" writes James Bishop, "all libraries, schools, churches, theatres, halls and indoor entertainment venues were shut down. Six days later, racecourses and hotels were closed and people on public transport and in public places were

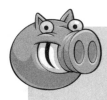

Then and Now: Once a Prison Colony, Always a Prison Colony

In 1919 the Australian state of New South Wales became the first state or province in the world to institute an across-the-board travel ban, quarantine, and lockdown. A century later, when Covid-19 hit, it imposed an even more stringent lockdown on its population.

One is tempted to say that Australia overreacts in this way because it began its national life as a tyranny—a prison colony—whereas the United States began its national life by revolting *against* a tyranny. Once a prison colony, always a prison colony, one might say.

required to wear masks. NSW schools remained closed throughout February."[18]

As other Australian states adopted similar measures to contain the virus, state borders were closed and movement by public and private transport was restricted. Urban streets were sprayed with the disinfectant phenyl. The public were told to open their windows, disinfect their homes, frequently wash their hands, and never, ever cough or sneeze on anyone else. Above all, they were urged to stay home.

While some countries attempted to keep the Spanish Flu at arm's length by means of travel bans, few succeeded. Take the case of Mexico, for example.

As the Spanish Flu raged through northern Mexico in the fall of 1918, President Rodriguez ordered municipal officials to shut down local rail lines to stop it from spreading farther south. Not everyone complied. "The mayor of Torreón, Coahuila, Celso Castro, told Rodríguez that some train travel had stopped, but that shipments to Saltillo, the state's capital, continued with vigor. . . . Ultimately, economic pressure and the realization that the disease was too widespread to be affected by restricting train travel led officials to back off from shutting down the trains."[19] The influenza was so infectious that it generally outran the ban.

There was only one place where travel bans were an unequivocal success. As soon as the governor of American Samoa heard about the Spanish Flu, he immediately barred ships from docking on the islands. He also requisitioned vessels from the U.S. Navy on which to quarantine anyone suspected of having the disease. The result of his aggressive actions was that not a single life was lost to the influenza on American Samoa during the entire pandemic.

Western Samoa, some forty miles away, was not nearly so fortunate. Its New Zealand governor took a hands-off approach—at one point he even rejected an offer of medical assistance from his American counterpart—and the flu raged out of control. By the time herd immunity had been achieved, ending the outbreak, twenty-two out of every one hundred people had died. Western Samoa suffered one of the highest death rates in the world.

Did any of the standard public health measures adopted markedly reduce the number of people who died of the Spanish Flu? Martin Bootsma and Neil Ferguson looked at data from twenty-three different American cities to see the effect of local mask requirements and restrictions on movement and gatherings. These measures, they concluded, "reduced total mortality only moderately (perhaps 10–30%)," and "the impact was often very limited because of interventions being introduced too late and lifted too early."[20]

In the face of a devastating pandemic, even a moderate reduction in mortality sounds pretty good. That is, until you reach the end of the "Results" section and read what sounds like an afterthought: "These figures . . . do not allow for the mortality that may then have resulted when controls were finally lifted."

In other words, the authors are saying, the public health measures that these cities took—masking, closures, and quarantines—"flattened the curve," but once they were lifted, a second wave of the Spanish Flu occurred, and many of the lives that the measures had "saved" in the first wave were then lost in the second.

Like every other pandemic in human history, it was not public health measures that ended the Spanish Flu, but herd immunity.

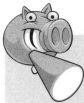

Then and Now: Progressives and Totalitarians

But even at the height of the disease, when ten thousand people were dying each day, there was no thought of a national lockdown in the United States. Wilson wasn't interested, and the states deferred to the cities. Dozens of cities closed theaters and saloons and—in a few cases—tried to enforce mask mandates. It was a textbook case of federalism and subsidiarity. Herd immunity was achieved in a hurry, though not without great loss of life, and the Spanish Flu subsided as quickly as it had arisen.

Of course, in 1918 we didn't have the example of China locking down entire provinces and welding people inside their homes. This great display of anti-viral fervor turned out to be, as we will see, in large part a charade, but it seems to have inspired the more totalitarian-minded bureaucrats in Washington, D.C.

It is true that if you isolate everyone in individual cells of fear, keeping them from contact with anybody—colleagues, friends, family members—a virus will not spread. And when the last person to fall ill recovers or dies, the virus will die with him. This may well be the dream of the Dr. Faucis among us, but it is a nightmare for the rest of us. Like the Spanish Flu, the mutated and less lethal descendants of the coronavirus will be with us forever. And we now know that even the most vigorously enforced societal lockdowns—short of putting us all in hermetically sealed bubbles—is not effective in stopping the spread of a highly infectious airborne virus.

Medical (Mis)Information

Virology was in its infancy in 1918, and so there was no understanding of variants. All three waves were attributed to the same strain of flu. Doctors were not always sure of what their patients were perishing of, and so sometimes they recorded secondary causes or other sicknesses as the cause of death on their death certificates rather than influenza.

It became clear that some groups were at much higher risk than others of dying of the Spanish Flu—the very old, the very young, and people in their twenties and thirties—and that these risks were "increased by such socioeconomic factors as poor nutrition, overcrowding, living conditions (such as poor heating) conducive to secondary infection with bacterial pneumonia, pre-existing infection with other diseases, and low access to health care."[21] Medical science was making advances, even though it had virtually no treatment to offer for the influenza itself.

Another discovery of the time was asymptomatic transmission. As a 1919 U.K. medical report noted: "An initial practical difficulty in such prevention is that the patient for several days may not fully recognize his condition, and it seems likely that infection is chiefly spread during these earlier stages."[22]

But the major advance was the discovery that survivors of the Spanish Flu, like survivors of the bubonic plague, had robust natural immunity. Medical practitioners in France were the first to report that Spanish Flu victims did not become ill if exposed to the disease for a second time. As one rather lighthearted news item in a small-town California newspaper declared:

Can't Catch the Real Flu Twice

If you had the real Spanish Flu back in 1918 and 1919, and didn't die of it, you won't have it again. You can start in the winter with a perfectly light heart and no worry whatsoever in the event of fresh attack—now that the time-honored whiskey and quinine cure is no longer integrally available. This is the solemn and scientific assurance of Professor C. Dopter of the famous Val-de-Grace hospital at Paris. He has just published the full statistics and reports of the hospital on the Spanish Flu epidemic since its original arrival in 1918 and which demonstrate conclusively that one attack of the disease establishes immunity.[23]

While an understanding of acquired immunity from previous exposure to disease has been known from classical times, the Spanish Flu gave

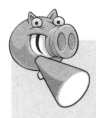

Then and Now: Quinine

Quinine, derived from the bark of the cinchona tree, has been used as a treatment for malaria since it was discovered in 1635. But the malaria wonder drug has also been widely prescribed for other ailments as well, including influenzas. And no wonder. Recent studies have shown that it has antiviral properties.[24] In fact, during the Spanish Flu, one of the remedies prescribed by doctors for those who became ill was a mixture of whiskey and quinine.

Quinine is not without occasional side effects, which have included loss of hearing, irregular heartbeat, and a lower blood platelet count. The search for a safer alternative treatment for malaria that could be manufactured in the lab led to the discovery of chloroquine (CQN) and hydroxychloroquine (HCQ), which are both synthetic modifications of quinine. Studies published years before the Covid-19 pandemic show that both CQN and HCQ preserve the anti-viral properties of their naturally occurring cousin and are effective against . . . coronaviruses.[25]

Quinine itself is currently being investigated as a nasal spray to stop Covid infections.[26] Since there are not massive profits to be made by Big Pharma, however, do not expect it to be approved any time soon.

modern scientists their first opportunity to observe in real time how "herd immunity" works. Herd immunity is the idea that when enough people have caught an infectious disease and thus acquired "natural immunity," that disease will slowly die out as it becomes increasingly more difficult for the pathogen to find new hosts who are susceptible to infection.

At the very same time as the world was struggling with the pandemic, bacteriologist W. W. C. Topley was creating epidemics in the lab among mice populations. As he reported in *The Lancet* in July 1919, he found that "unless there was a steady influx of susceptible mice, the rising prevalence of immune individuals would end an epidemic."[27]

So herd immunity was possible, but just how would it work in a human population? How high would the percentage of immune individuals have to be to stop the transmission of the Spanish Flu and end the pandemic? No one at the time knew. And how could they? Medical professionals in 1918 did not even understand what kind of pathogen they were dealing with, much less have any precise measure of its infectiousness and virulence. Waves of the pandemic seemingly came and went at will.

Only time would answer that question, and in time it did. The Spanish Flu pandemic came to an end when some 500 million people out of a total world population of 1,800 million had been infected. This means that we reached herd immunity vis-à-vis the deadliest virus the world has ever seen when only 28 percent of the population had come down with the disease. Fewer than one in three people had contracted the influenza virus when it—at least in its most virulent variant—died out forever.

Let me emphasize that it was not vaccines (which didn't exist for any respiratory virus at the time) or therapeutics that ended the Spanish Flu pandemic, but herd immunity.

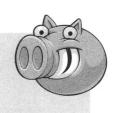

Then and Now: Herd Immunity

The initial estimates of what fraction of the U.S. population would need immunity to the China Virus for us to reach herd immunity and end the epidemic in the United States were between 60 and 70 percent, which is more than double the 28 percent that history tells us effected herd immunity to the Spanish Flu in 1918–20. Even more curious, as we shall see, Dr. Anthony Fauci continually raised the percentage that he claimed would be required to reach herd immunity, first from 70 percent to 75 percent, and then to 80 percent and 85 percent.[28]

Not Your Ordinary Flu Bug

Everybody—from personal experience—knows influenza (the "flu") as a common respiratory illness that causes a sore throat, headaches, fever, and muscle aches. The viruses that cause it are highly contagious and come in many different forms, one or two of which cause outbreaks nearly every winter.

But the influenza that laid the soldiers low in the summer of 1918 was an influenza that no one had seen before. While other flus target the ends

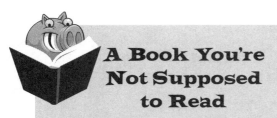

A Book You're Not Supposed to Read

If you want to get a sense of what a real American plague is like, read John M. Barry's *The Great Influenza: The Story of the Deadliest Pandemic in History*. Barry argues that the Spanish Flu pandemic of 1918–1920 killed as many as 100 million people worldwide, killing "more people in 24 weeks than AIDS has killed in 24 years, more in a year than the Black Death killed in a century." One caveat: Barry, writing in 2005, believed the Spanish Flu began with the outbreak in an army camp in Kansas. As we have seen, more recent evidence suggests that, like so many pathogens, it came from the East . . . the Far East.

of the age spectrum, putting the very young and the very old at particular risk, the Spanish Flu killed large numbers of healthy young adults. It was a terrifying disease—some of the sufferers actually turned blue as the fluid built up in their lungs and gradually suffocated them. The doctors called this unusual condition heliotrope cyanosis, but it was more commonly known as the "purple death" because patients went from blue to a deep blue-violet as they expired.

And die they usually did, because the medical science of the time had no antibiotics or other therapeutic drugs to offer them. Doctors could only watch, mystified by the fact that so many young and seemingly healthy adults were dying. As we now know, it was the very robustness of their immune systems that was killing them.

The deadliness of the Spanish Flu is often attributed to what is called a "cytokine storm"— as the virus infects lung cells, the body releases what are called cytokines into the lung tissue. These chemical messengers signal the body that an invader is present, prompting leukocytes in large numbers to head into the lungs to attack and absorb the virus. Unfortunately, the immune systems of the young sometimes produce so many leukocytes that the normal inflammatory response rages out of control, destroying not only the virus but a massive number of lung cells as well, clogging the air sacs and airways of the lungs with mucus and blood. The victim has trouble getting enough oxygen and, in the end, turns purple and suffocates to death.[29]

The immune systems of the young and healthy members of the U.S. military—and other young people in the United States—mounted such a strong defense against the Spanish Flu that it ended up killing them. The relatively weak immune systems of the old and the very young, on the other hand, rarely generate cytokine storms. Their bodies do not overreact to the invader, and the damage to their lungs from the overprotective leukocytes is minimal.

Medical science in 1918 simply had no idea what was causing the deadly influenza. Researchers knew from experiments that "invisible" infectious agents must exist but, until the invention of the election microscope in the 1930s, they weren't even able to see a virus, much less begin to identify which particular one was causing the carnage. Unlike a bacterium, a virus is not alive. It cannot grow, breathe, move, or reproduce. It is simply a minuscule capsule containing a genetic blueprint for its own manufacture. A virus repro-

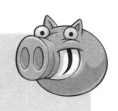

Then and Now: Age Matters

The age-specific mortality of the Spanish Flu and the China Virus—the percentage of people in each age group who died—are almost mirror images. The Spanish Flu in 1918 was especially dangerous to the young. This is why it devastated the ranks of otherwise healthy young men who were serving in the military.

The coronavirus that causes Covid-19 targets the opposite end of the age spectrum. The elderly are at far greater risk of dying of the China Virus than younger cohorts. In fact, the risk for infants and children is effectively zero, while for those in their twenties, thirties, and forties the risk posed by the China Virus is roughly comparable to that of the annual flu.

duces itself by hijacking the cellular machinery of a host cell it has invaded and using it to make hundreds of copies of itself. The host cell then dies, releasing a swarm of virus "offspring" to repeat the process.

It was not until 1995 that geneticists, piecing together small RNA fragments of the virus obtained from autopsies done in 1918, began to reconstruct the influenza's genome. The virus had only eight genes, but it was ten years before the last of them had been completely analyzed.[30] To the scientists' surprise, the Spanish Flu virus turned out to be not that much

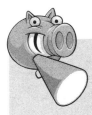

Then and Now: To Lock Down or Not to Lock Down, That Is the Question

The limited government response in 1918–1920 was not responsible for the spread of the pandemic across the United States or for the deaths of 675,000 Americans. Even if a total lockdown had been put in place by Washington, the highly infectious airborne virus would have made its way across America anyway. And locking people in their homes for extended periods of time would have increased, not decreased, the death toll from the Spanish Flu.

The case against lockdowns was best made by D. A. Henderson, an internationally recognized expert in virology who served as the dean of the Johns Hopkins Bloomberg School of Public Health. Henderson won the Presidential Medal of Freedom for leading the successful effort to eradicate smallpox from the planet. A 2006 paper he co-authored explained in detail why lockdowns are counterproductive. Indoor environments are a breeding ground for contagion, he argued, while the healthiest environment is outdoors in the open air, with no mask. But instead of "following the science," a lot of countries in 2020–2021 instead attempted lockdowns. All those lockdowns proved was that while you can attempt to confine people in their homes, people will find a way around these restrictions, and the virus will go where it wants. It was those who were already locked down—such as the elderly confined in senior care centers—who died in the largest numbers.

different from other varieties of influenza A they had come to recognize, which is the most common cause of flu in humans. We now know that the 1918 virus is the likely ancestor of all four of the human and swine lineages later identified, including the H1N1 Influenza A virus, the strain that caused the 2009 swine flu.

But even after we had completely sequenced the viral genome, the question remained: Why is this particular virus roughly one hundred times as deadly as other flus? Scientists knew that, because it was transmitted by air, sneezes and coughs could spread it quickly through a company of soldiers or a schoolroom of children. But this is true of most flus. What was different about the Spanish Flu is that it was a new arrival. This particular flu bug had just recently mutated in 1918—its immediate ancestor is thought to have been a bird flu—into a strain that could infect human lungs, which goes a long way towards explaining its infectiousness.

In other words, in 1918 a novel virus and man were encountering each other for the first time. Human immune systems were initially unprepared to deal with the new invader. No one had even partial immunity—what's called "crossover immunity"—from exposure to previous closely related strains of the virus, because there weren't any such strains. To mount an effective response to this new viral threat, people's immune systems would need time—but time is precisely what they did not have. The virus killed them too quickly.

This was a mistake on the virus's part. It is a poor virus that kills its host too quickly, limiting its opportunity to spread to other people via sneezes and coughs. Most viruses become less deadly over time for precisely this reason. But the newly mutated Spanish Flu virus was clumsily efficient: it was attacking a new host that it had not yet fully adapted to, and it killed too many soon after infecting them. Only its high infectiousness allowed it to continue spreading despite how imprudently it was slaughtering its hosts.

The average influenza pandemic registers a case fatality rate of less than 0.1 percent, which means that of a thousand people who have confirmed cases of the flu, more than 999 survive it, usually with nothing more than a cold and sniffles. But if you contracted the Spanish Flu, you were playing Russian roulette with viral bullets: you had a 1 in 10 chance of dying from it. The math is not complicated. The pandemic is estimated to have infected 500 million people around the globe, of whom perhaps 50 million succumbed to the disease.[31] The Spanish Flu's case fatality rate was roughly 10 percent, which is *100 times* as high as the ordinary flu.

The Spanish Flu was so deadly that births—around 13 million a year worldwide at the time—were eclipsed by deaths for two years, which means that the population of the world actually shrank over this period. Life expectancies were also dramatically shortened. Because many of those who lost their lives were healthy young adults between the ages of fifteen and thirty, the pandemic lowered the average life expectancy in the United States by more than twelve years.

If we accept the estimate of 50 million deaths overall published by Johnson and Mueller, the Spanish Flu killed 2.8 percent of the world's population of 1,800 million. And if it was in fact higher—perhaps as many as 100 million, a possibility the same authors contemplate—then the global death rate would have been 5.6 percent.[32] Demographers have lately come in with lower estimates, which generally run from 20 to 40 million, but I am inclined to think that these are underestimates. The data on which to base a detailed demographic analysis simply does not exist.[33]

The fact is, the numbers even in Western countries are suspect. There were no diagnostic tests for the virus itself, so the cause of death had to be ascertained from the symptoms alone, which would tend to produce an undercount, especially at the outset of a previously unknown illness. This is why, even in developed countries with fairly well-developed public health systems that collected vital statistics, widely varying numbers are offered of the number of people who succumbed to the Spanish Flu.

Take the United States, for example. While the commonly accepted number of deaths from the Spanish Flu is 675,000, both higher and lower estimates have been offered. At 675,000 deaths, the United States—which had what passed for a modern medical system at the time—would have suffered an overall mortality rate of 0.6 percent. But the mortality rate in poor countries, with poor nutrition, poor hygiene, and no public health system, would have been much higher, with up to 20 percent of those who became infected dying.

For African, Asian, and Latin American countries, the estimated numbers of cases and deaths are nothing more than guesswork, and often not very well-informed guesswork at that. I don't want to pit anthropology's poor spears against demography's statistical juggernaut, but for all their theoretical elegance modern demographers completely miss the reality of life and death in peasant villages of the time. No one really knows how many deaths from the influenza occurred in Indian, Chinese, or African villages from 1918 to 1920, although the mortality rate in such places was certainly much higher than in, say, the coastal cities of China and India where there was a Western presence. The latter had higher living standards and at least limited access to the Western medical services of the time. So, did 50 million, and perhaps up to 100 million, die from the Spanish Flu, as Johnson and Mueller proposed? I rate this as "True."[34]

A Trail of Infected Armies— and Chinese Laborers

From the Spanish Flu's inception, experts have struggled to pinpoint its point of origin. For a time, the prevailing theory was that it came from Kansas, with John Barry and others pointing to the fact that the first known American case was recorded at Camp Funston, a U.S. Army base in Kansas, on March 11, 1918.[36]

Then came an epidemiological study of mortality rates in New York City that showed an early wave of the influenza pandemic had hit the city from February to

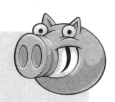

Then and Now: Mortality Rates

At the time of the 1918 outbreak of the Spanish Flu, there were no laboratory tests available to assist doctors in making their diagnoses. Neither were U.S. doctors required to report the disease to the public health authorities. The cause of death had to be determined symptomatically, and the diagnostic criteria for influenza, as opposed to bacterial pneumonia, were poorly defined. This led doctors to record secondary infections rather than the influenza as the cause of death, so that both case rates and death rates from influenza in the United States were almost certainly undercounted at the time.

In counting cases and fatalities from the China Virus in 2020–2021, we faced exactly the opposite problem. All patients who tested positive for Covid-19 and then died—whatever the actual cause of death—were counted as Covid fatalities.[35] Obviously, this practice grossly overcounted the number of deaths from Covid.

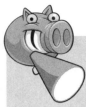

Then and Now: War and Pestilence

As we saw in the Antonine Plague of the second century, disease has always followed in the wake of armies. As Guy Carleton Jones, who would go on to be the Canadian surgeon general, wrote presciently in August 1914, "The trail of infected armies leaves a sad tale of sickness amongst women and children and non-combatants. Laws and regulations may govern the conduct of war, but disease and infections recognize no such law and refuse to single out the combatants only."[37] But China's release of an unrestricted bioweapon on the world's population reminds us that an infectious disease may be also used in a preemptive strike on one's enemies. In that case, as well, such a disease does not "single out combatants only," but kills indiscriminately without regard to age or sex.

China's actions also demonstrate once again that the Western effort to use international covenants to "govern the conduct of war" is a relic of a bygone age. It has been replaced by China's concept of unrestricted warfare, which dates back to Sun Tzu's *The Art of War*. The China Virus pandemic is proof of that.

April 1918. This meant that the virus could not have come from Kansas, the authors concluded, pointing to Europe instead. They hypothesized that wartime troop movements back and forth across the North Atlantic had brought it to New York City.[38] Other researchers concurred, noting that once the United States had entered the war on April 6, 1917, British and French advisors were sent over to advise and train the American Expeditionary Force in the winter of 1917–1918. They suggested these detachments probably carried the virus to New York City—and Kansas. They didn't attempt to unravel the mystery surrounding its point of origin, however.[39]

If the Spanish Flu did not originate in the United States, did it mutate into being in Europe? After all, there had been localized outbreaks of what was then called a "purulent bronchitis" in French army hospitals near Etaples in France in 1916–1917.[40] The young soldiers who died there suffered the same "purple death" from suffocation (heliotrope cyanosis) that would befall later victims of the Spanish Flu. Some have suggested that this may have been a milder variant of the virus that would explode into the influenza pandemic in early 1918.

In 2014 Canadian historian Mark Osborne Humphries weighed in on the origins question with a detailed study that traced the exact route the Spanish Flu had followed from East to West—all the way back to China. The story begins in North China in 1917 where, Humphries recounts, "a strange, contagious, and deadly disease of unknown origin began to spread" in rural villages. If not for the war, this killer influenza variant might have stayed there. Epidemics follow people, and the people of rural China in those days rarely went farther than the nearest market town. But that was about to change.

Half a world away, Europe was at war. The carnage had been tremendous, and the French and British armies that had taken the field at the outset of the war were quickly decimated. Historian Paul Fussell has written that by the middle of November 1914—only five months into the war—the huge casualties "had all but wiped out the original British army."[41]

By 1916, the western front had long since settled into grueling trench warfare. Troops on both sides stayed hunkered down in trenches for months on end, except for occasional bloody forays against the enemy in which they were often thrown back into the same muddy holes they had just crawled out of. Yet ammunition, food, and other supplies still had to be delivered to the front—and the elaborate system of trenches had to be constantly maintained, fortified, and extended.

It was the French who came up with the idea of recruiting additional manpower from China. In May 1916 the Chinese authorities agreed to supply fifty thousand laborers, and within two months the first shipload was on its way from Tianjin to the French port of Marseille. The British soon followed suit, setting up a recruiting base for their own "Chinese Labour Corps" (CLC) at the British colony of Weihaiwei in Shandong province in October 1916.[42]

Regular contingents of Chinese laborers were sent over the next two years, until there were roughly 140,000 men aiding the allied cause.

They were all illiterate peasants, whom Western officials of the time referred to as "coolies." The Chinese understood the term as a transliteration of two Chinese characters, 苦力, pronounced "ku li," which stand for "bitter labor." It was an apt description of their lives on the western front. Digging the multiple lines of trenches, with their earthworks and their underground command posts—all without modern earthmoving equipment—was "bitter labor" indeed. These laborers were recruited from villages in North China, the same places that suffered annual bouts of what was locally called the "winter sickness," and which in late 1917 were in the grip of a particularly vicious one.

It is not surprising that some of the new recruits to the Chinese Labour Corps turned out to be carrying the influenza virus. They were sent on to Canada and Europe anyway, and the cases continued to mount. By March 1, 1918, the British were forced to stop local recruitment because of what they called "the plague." British officials in Weihaiwei reported that they had "2,480 coolies not yet free from infection and probably ready to embark in about six weeks' time."[43] The official added that another ship had just set sail.

The British had routed their initial shiploads of laborers from Weihaiwei to Europe via Africa around Cape Horn, or through the Mediterranean by way of the Suez Canal. But as vessels became scarcer, the British decided that it would be much faster to transship them to France via Canada. Some of the Chinese laborers arrived in Canada sick and had to be quarantined on an island off of Vancouver.

Great Britain finally decided to cancel the program because of the danger of importing the Chinese influenza.[44] The French military also abruptly terminated its recruitment program in China in early 1918, probably for the same reason.[45] But it was too late.

As infected members of the Chinese Labour Corps traveled from China to France, they left behind outbreaks of the Spanish Flu wherever they went. When the laborers arrived in France they were sent to the "coolie camp" outside Etaples, close to the base that had seen the outbreak of purulent bronchitis. They had arrived there from southern England, which also saw its own outbreak of the Spanish Flu. And, of course, they spread the deadly disease wherever they worked along the Allied lines.

As Humphries writes, "The Mobilization of the CLC may have allowed a new disease to spread in fits and starts from China, across North America, to Europe, where it . . . exploded along the sinews of war. In this way influenza followed the same path carved by previous epidemics. The result was the most deadly disease event in history."[46]

Humphries's work has not been without its critics. One, arguing against a Chinese origin, pointed out that Canada did not experience an early outbreak of the Spanish Flu, despite tens of thousands of Chinese laborers who were shipped across Canada beginning in early 2017.

But, as Humphries notes, the program was a closely guarded secret: to avoid alarming the Canadian public, sealed trains guarded by railway police were initially used to move the imported workers across Canada. The Chinese were not allowed to have any contact with ordinary Canadians. Even so, the Canadian authorities grew so concerned about the possibility of a contagion arising from the arriving Chinese that after a few months they began diverting the arrivals south. Contingents arriving in Vancouver were sent down to Seattle so they could be shipped East on American, rather than Canadian, trains.

In Britain, contingents of the Chinese Labour Corps traversed the south of England on their way to the channel crossing and the front lines, and southern England did have an early outbreak. But the same is not true of the French shiploads of Chinese workers. The French disembarked their CLC workers in the Mediterranean port of Marseille and then transported

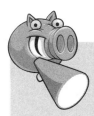

Then and Now: It Couldn't Have Come from China

After Humphries published his findings, the *Journal of the Chinese Medical Association* was quick to print a refutation. Its 2016 study, which was based on Allied war records, found that mortality rates from the 2018 influenza pandemic were far higher among the Western soldiers than among the imported Chinese laborers. This suggests to me that the Chinese laborers had already had the Spanish Flu (or an earlier variant) back in China, and had acquired natural or crossover immunity as a result. But the author of the Chinese journal article doesn't see it that way—concluding instead that the virus did not come from the East, but must have been circulating in Europe before the pandemic.[47]

Similarly, when the evidence began to mount that the China Virus had actually been constructed in, and released by, the Wuhan Institute of Virology, the CCP propaganda apparatus immediately launched a counternarrative. It began spreading the rumor that, while the coronavirus *was* a bioweapon, it was not China's. Rather it had been secretly bioengineered at the U.S. Army's biolabs at Fort Detrick, Maryland, and released on an unsuspecting China at the Military World Games in Wuhan in October 2019.

No matter how overwhelming the evidence, do not expect Chinese Communist Party leaders to embark upon an apology tour any time soon.

them north by train. But no detectable spread of the influenza along their route has been found, leading some to conclude that the Chinese could not have brought the disease to Europe.[48]

There is a simple explanation for the difference, however. While the British did their recruiting in North China, which was suffering from the plague, the French did most—though not all—of theirs in the Cantonese-speaking provinces of the far south, which was not.

And what about the early outbreaks of a "purulent bronchitis" in Etaples, France, that seemingly predate the 1918 pandemic? It turns out that the main "coolie camp" was near Etaples. This is where all the CLC laborers arriving in France, from the first contingents in late 1916 to the last, were first sent. It's reasonable to think they brought one or more varieties of the "winter sickness" with them.[49]

If many of the Chinese laborers had already had the Spanish Flu—or an earlier variant of it—back in China, they would have had acquired natural immunity, or some protection from crossover immunity, as a result. This would explain why studies of Allied war records have found that mortality rates from the 2018 influenza pandemic were far higher among the Western soldiers than among the imported Chinese laborers.[50] That would also explain why China was one of the few countries to come through the 1918 pandemic relatively unscathed.

Although reliable data is sparse—warlords ruled China in those chaotic days—studies suggest that the flu season there that year was relatively mild. Demographer Christopher Langford has written that "influenza was widespread in China in 1918–1919, but that, although severe in some parts, it was mild in many places compared with elsewhere in the world. . . . The most plausible explanation is that the 1918–1919 influenza virus, or a closely related precursor, originated in China, so that many Chinese had prior exposure and hence some immunity. . . . Chinese workers en route to France would have carried this virus with them, leading to the pandemic."[51]

If a European war hadn't brought millions of strangers from all corners of the globe together on the battlefields of France, the Spanish Flu would never have happened.

Flu in the Time of Air Travel: The Asian Flu (1957–1958) and Hong Kong Flu (1968–1969)

The invention of the electron microscope in the 1930s brought viruses into human view for the first time. But it wasn't until the 1950s that we discovered how they were structured, and thirty years after that that we were able to begin mapping their genes. It was then that we began to discover—to our surprise—that the Spanish Flu has never really gone away.

The first genetic analysis of the Spanish Flu was done in the late 1990s, using viral RNA from the body of an Inuit woman that had lain frozen in the Alaskan permafrost for eighty years, as well as from tissue samples from American soldiers autopsied at the time of the original pandemic.[1] That analysis revealed that an avian flu had crossed over to humans sometime before 1918, creating a novel virus a hundred times more lethal than the seasonal flu.

The deadliest variant had vanished shortly after 1920, of course. It had committed the unpardonable evolutionary sin of killing off too many of its hosts, inadvertently killing itself off in the process. The rest of the human herd that had been infected but survived had developed permanent, lifelong immunity. You might say that the original Spanish Flu was a victim of its own success.

But before it committed the viral equivalent of *hara-kiri* it had spun off—viruses have high mutation rates—a number of less lethal forms. Still infectious but much less deadly, these were variants that humanity could live with, which meant that the variants would live on inside the human population as well. They survive today among the very young

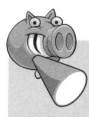

Then and Now: Naming and Shaming

From the first outbreaks in the cities of Singapore and Hong Kong, the new influenza was named the Asian Flu after the vast region from which it had come. Some years later, however, the "sensitivity" police at the Centers for Disease Control and Prevention decided that calling it the Asian Flu was racist. They now wish you to call it the "1957–1958 Pandemic."[2]

Believing that names that point to countries or regions of origin are *not* racist, and also that they are especially appropriate where the country of origin bears some responsibility, I continue to use the term Asian Flu. The Chinese Communist Party played no role in its creation—in this case the offending virus truly did have a natural origin—but the CCP certainly did play a role in its spread. The CCP deliberately chose not to warn the world about the new and deadly influenza that had arisen in Guizhou province in early 1957. China stayed silent even as the Asian Flu spread throughout the country in the months following. By deliberately withholding this information from the World Health Organization and other public health authorities, the Chinese Communists set the stage for the virus to go global.

And not for the last time.

and the very old—in other words, among those who have no preexisting natural immunity and those whose immune systems are growing weaker with age.

This is why the scientist who first sequenced the genome of the virus, Jeffery Taubenberger, calls the Spanish Flu "the Mother of all Pandemics."[3] Every single pandemic humanity has suffered until Covid-19 has been a direct descendant of the Spanish Flu, and nearly every seasonal flu as well. As Taubenberger says, "[A]lmost all cases of influenza A worldwide . . . have been caused by descendants of the 1918 virus, including 'drifted' [mutated] H1N1 viruses and reassorted H2N2 [Asian Flu] and H3N2 [Hong Kong Flu] viruses."[4]

Even today, the annual flu season is almost entirely populated by the sons and daughters of the Spanish Flu (actually viruses are gender-neutral, but you understand what I mean). The only major exceptions are avian viruses such as H5N1 and H7N7—and, of course, the China Virus.

The seasonal flu comes and goes, but once every decade or so something emerges out of nature's vast laboratory that is especially dangerous. Somewhere—usually a place where large numbers of people live cheek by jowl with pigs and fowl—an existing mild influenza A virus will recombine with a bird virus or a pig virus. And, just like that, a novel virus will be born that is not only highly infectious, but is also far deadlier than the ordinary flu. Another potential pandemic has arrived.

This is exactly what happened in 1957 with the Asian Flu, and then again in 1968 with the Hong Kong Flu, the next two pandemics to hit humanity.

The Asian Flu (1957–1958)

By 1957 the Spanish Flu of almost four decades past was fading from memory. Influenza remained a yearly occurrence, but no new virulent influenza type had emerged for decades. Instead of looking down into microscopes, the world was looking up into space. Russia had shocked the world in August by launching the first intercontinental ballistic missile, following up in October by launching Sputnik, the world's first artificial satellite. The space race was officially underway.

For most of the year, all had been quiet on the American epidemiological front. The Center for Disease Control's only available tool for monitoring infectious diseases was a weekly report, sent in those days by telegraph, from the public health departments of 108 large cities. The data that was reported to its National Office of Vital Statistics (NOVS) included codes for deaths caused by "pneumonia" or "influenza." In the early months of 1957, the numbers being reported indicated a normal flu season.[5]

Then, in June, the numbers coming through on the telegrams from the West Coast suddenly began to climb. Another pandemic had arrived from China.[6]

At least 45 million people in the United States were infected by the Asian Flu, and by the time the second wave subsided in March 1958, 116,000 Americans had died. The second worst pandemic that the United States had ever experienced had struck, and its death toll easily eclipsed the other tragedies of the time. It was more than three times the number of soldiers killed in the Korean War, and double the number that would be lost in Vietnam in the years to come.

The population of the United States has almost doubled since 1958. Were a pandemic of equal deadliness to have swept across America in late 2021, it would have cost 221,000 American lives.

In that same time the global population has grown from 3 billion to 7.8 billion people. The global death toll from the Asian Flu was estimated at 1.1 million. An equivalent pandemic today would kill 3 million people around the world.

The Singapore Flu?

In April of 1957, the WHO received reports from Singapore that a new influenza virus was on the loose. News of a major outbreak of that same flu in Hong Kong soon followed. "An influenza epidemic has affected thousands of Hong Kong residents," the *New York Times* reported on April 17.[7] Within days, estimates of the number afflicted grew to a quarter million. From those two cities, Hong Kong and Singapore, the Asian Flu—as it was already being called—spread rapidly across the Asian continent. Taiwan was reporting a hundred thousand cases by mid-May, and India over a million cases by June.[8]

The global network of laboratories linked to the World Influenza Research Centre in London had been tracking the Asian Flu as it spread from Hong Kong, and the centre itself became a clearing house for research on the new virus.[9] This was the first time that the rates of infection of a modern influenza virus could be carefully monitored. Like all flu viruses, the Asian Flu spread through the air, often impelled on its journey by a cough or a sneeze.

It also spread with incredible rapidity, since it did not have to find its way to a port and board a ship to get from place to place, as previous bacteria and viruses had to do. By 1958 air travel was common enough that the virus was able to travel in a matter of hours from country to country and continent to continent. This meant that shipboard quarantines, which had been around since Venice imposed them in the Middle Ages, were no longer effective.

Indeed, since the flu's incubation period was one to four days, travelers might not know they were already infected when they boarded a flight, only to arrive at their destination some hours later with a runny nose and a sore throat, having infected their fellow passengers on the flight on the way. It was soon evident that the rapidity of the influenza's spread far outpaced those of earlier pandemics, since it was not only highly infectious in close quarters, but was also being carried long distances by air by its unsuspecting host—us.

The Asian Flu reached Japan and the Middle East by May. It made landfall in the United States and United Kingdom in June. By the end of that month more than twenty countries were reporting cases.[10] South American and African countries were infected by July and August. Within five months of the Hong Kong outbreak, the virus had succeeded in circumnavigating the globe.

By September, there were widespread epidemics raging in the United States, the United Kingdom, and Europe. The second biggest influenza pandemic of the twentieth century, fueled by an entirely new strain for which no one had any natural immunity, was well underway. The pandemic that would come to be known as the Asian Flu would peak in two waves, with the first arriving in October and November of 1957 and the second following in early 1958.

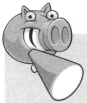

Then and Now: Worries about Germ Warfare

The sheer speed of the Asian Flu's advance, combined with the fact that the first Americans to suffer its effects were serving in the U.S. military in the Far East, gave rise to questions about whether it was a biowarfare attack by Communist China. An August 26, 1957, article in the *Evening Star* (Washington, D.C.) read:

"Planting" of Flu Germs by Reds Held Impossible

Dr. Leroy E. Burney, United States Surgeon General, said today the presence of Asiatic flu in this country is not the start of germ warfare by the Communists.

"Is there any possibility that the Communists have planted these germs?" Burney was asked in a copyrighted interview in the magazine U.S. News & World Report.

"No," he replied. "I don't believe that is a possibility. We have epidemics occasionally and have had them in the past."[11]

The CCP's biowarfare capabilities in 1957 were quite primitive. By the twenty-first century that was no longer the case.

Ask the same question today about the Covid-19 pandemic—"Is there any possibility that the Communists have planted these germs?"—and, as we shall see, the answer is quite different.

From the beginning, there was no question that it had entered America from Asia. Well before the first cases were reported in the continental United States in early June, outbreaks of the disease had already occurred in April and May on America's overseas military bases in Japan and South Korea, as well as on ships assigned to the U.S. Seventh Fleet, whose home-port was Tokyo Bay. The evidence available at the time suggested that Hong Kong had been the epicenter of the disease. But the suggestion by some in the West that it had originated there irritated the Hong Kong Chinese business community—they knew quite well that it had come over the border from mainland China.

It wasn't until the following year that information about the true location of the first outbreak leaked out of China. It was revealed that the first cases of the highly infectious flu had been recorded by Chinese health authorities around the third week of February deep in the South Chinese hinterland, in rural Guizhou province.

An international "Symposium on the Asian Influenza Epidemic" held in 1958 confirmed: "[The Asian Flu] originated in Guizhou province between the provincial capital of Guiyang and the city of Qujing, which is just across the provincial border in Yunnan Province. In early March the outbreak had spread to Yunnan Province and by the middle of March it had spread all over China."[12]

When Dr. Leroy E. Burney, the surgeon general of the United States, was asked in August of 1957 whether the entry of the Asian Flu into the United States could have been prevented, he said no. "There are about 1,800 people who disembark on the West Coast from the Pacific areas every day from planes, ships and otherwise. You can carry the virus and there's no way of detecting who has it and who doesn't have it."[13]

Speaking in August, Dr. Burney could not have known that six months before, the Chinese Communist Party had had an opportunity to warn the world about the novel influenza. Had the CCP been forthcoming about the epidemic when it was still confined to Guizhou, or even to China, a timely travel ban would have slowed down the spread of the Asia Flu, although it wouldn't have stopped it entirely.

In a pattern that would become familiar, however, in early 1957 the Communist authorities said nothing about the spread of the new influenza. China apologists claim that the CCP did not inform the WHO in timely fashion because it was not yet a member of that organization, but this is clearly just a dodge.

Even after China joined the WHO in 1981, it would prove to be equally tight-lipped about potential pandemics. When Covid-19 broke out in Wuhan in the fall of 2019, as we shall see, Beijing kept the epidemic quiet for as long as possible. It's almost as if the Communists *wanted* to infect the world.

Etiology

The first cases of the Asia Flu in the United States cropped up in military barracks on the East and West Coasts, and on U.S. Navy vessels, which reported anywhere from one-fifth to one-half of their crews down with the flu. The Asian Flu then spread to the population at large, causing localized outbreaks in institutional settings such as schools, conference centers, migrant worker barracks, and old-age homes, but not generally triggering community-wide outbreaks. Similar to the outbreaks in military barracks and on naval ships, the transmission rates in such closed settings ran as high as 40 percent to 50 percent.

Overall, according to a 2009 article in *Biosecurity and Bioterrorism* whose lead author was Dr. Donald Henderson, the man responsible for the eradication of smallpox, the flu spread swiftly across the United States: "[The] CDC estimated that approximately 45 million people—equivalent to about 25% of the population—had become infected with the new virus in October and November 1957."[14]

Then, after a month-long hiatus, an unexpected second wave hit the United States. For three months, from January to March of 1958, the Asian Flu returned, bringing with it more deaths from pneumonia, mostly among older Americans. By this time a sizable percentage of the American population had come to enjoy natural immunity, however, and the second wave was much smaller than the first. As Henderson notes, "There were no communitywide epidemics being reported, the National Health Survey revealed a normal winter occurrence of febrile respiratory illness, schools were not closing, and industrial absenteeism was not elevated."[15]

Most of the cases in both waves were mild, but the Asian Flu attacked its victims with great speed and put school-aged children—along with the younger children and the very old—at no little risk.[16] "Patients were often able to pinpoint the start of Asian flu to the very minute with wobbly legs and a chill followed by prostration, sore throats, running nose, and coughs; together with achy limbs (adults), head (children), and a high fever following," reported a British doctor at the time. "Young children, particularly boys, suffered nose bleeds."[17]

Doctors' offices and hospital emergency rooms saw overflow crowds during the first wave, although the vast majority of the patients were not severely ill and did not require hospitalization. These were sent home with instructions to go to bed, take aspirin if they spiked a fever, and drink plenty of fluids.[18]

In about 3 percent of cases, however, there were complications. About half of these were pneumonia and bronchitis brought on by the flu, while the rest were related to preexisting conditions, usually cerebrovascular and cardiovascular disease. Patients with underlying cardiovascular diseases tended to have severe complications, although the most frequent cause of death remained pneumonia.[19] Because antibiotics were now available to eliminate secondary bacterial infections, doctors discovered for the first time that viral pneumonias, even in the absence of bacterial co-invaders, could kill on their own.[20]

The case fatality rate in developed countries was 0.3 percent, meaning that the Asian Flu was three times as deadly as the annual flu. Globally, the case fatality rate was about twice that, running about 0.6 percent. Autopsies done on school-aged children who died rapidly of the Asian Flu showed the same kinds of "purple death" pathologies as the Spanish Flu victims of a half century before,[21] although it would be several more decades before the genetic linkage between the Mother of all Pandemics and the Asian Flu would be discovered.

A Pandemic without Panic

Perhaps because the sitting president Dwight D. Eisenhower was a former general, he understood that panicking the public, especially about a matter over which the federal government had little immediate control, was a bad idea. Soldier or civilian, anyone who is overwhelmed by fear is prone to hysterical, irrational behavior, which can kill him or her just as surely as a bullet—or a virus.

So it was that President Eisenhower had little to say about the Asian Flu. While he himself received a flu shot on August 26 to set an example for the nation, he did not attempt to impose a vaccination mandate—or lockdowns, quarantines, or masks—on the American public. In fact, no government anywhere ordered such measures put in place.

In large part because of the absence of lockdowns, quarantines, and store closures, there was very little effect on the U.S economy. Henderson concluded, "Despite the large numbers of cases, the 1957 outbreak did not appear to have a significant impact on the U.S. economy. . . . A Congressional Budget Office estimate found that a pandemic the scale of which occurred in 1957 would reduce real GDP by approximately 1% 'but probably would not cause a recession and might not be distinguishable from the normal variation in economic activity.'"[22]

Eisenhower's refusal to shutter businesses or prevent people from leaving their homes has lately come in for criticism from those who believe a more activist approach was needed. Critics even suggest that Eisenhower was more interested in "protecting markets than in protecting public health . . . [and] refused to initiate a nationwide vaccination program."[23] But these accusations are unfair. It is true that the Eisenhower administration wanted to avoid the pandemic panic and economic downturn that lockdowns and the like would have surely provoked. But this sensible approach was taken in the knowledge that a failure on either front would impose its own set of costs—paid in part in the coin of human lives—as anyone who has lived through the China Virus pandemic knows.

What about vaccines? In August 1957 Eisenhower asked Congress for funding to fight the outbreak and set a goal of 60 million vaccine doses.[24] But by the time the vaccine became widely available, the pandemic was already losing steam.

America's public health professionals concurred with the administration's approach. On August 27, 1957, a special meeting of the Association of State and Territorial Health Officials (ASTHO) was convened in Washington, D.C., to discuss the looming pandemic and decide on a course of action.[25] Although they didn't know how soon the pandemic would peak—some thought that it might happen as early as September, as it had in 1918, while others suggested that the worst period would coincide with the usual December–February influenza season[26]—they all agreed upon a markedly low-key response.

The vast majority of those who fell ill should be cared for at home, ASTHO stressed, with "hospital admissions . . . limited as far as possible to those cases of influenza with complications, or to those with other diseases which might be aggravated by influenza." Acknowledging that there was no reasonable way to limit the spread of the highly infectious virus, these sober-minded health professionals also recommended against lockdowns: "There is no practical advantage in the closing of schools or the curtailment of public gatherings as it relates to the spread of this disease. However, in some instances there may be administrative reasons for closing schools due to illness of teachers, bus drivers, large absentee rates, and so forth."[27]

What was the real-world effect of such politics? Did factory floors and church services become breeding grounds for the pandemic? Were hospitals overwhelmed with the sick and dying? In her overview of the Asian Flu, Kaitlynn Allen says no: "During the peak of the disease, absenteeism from

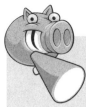

Panic Then and Now

The media in Britain were generally careful to avoid spreading panic, but some of the tabloids could not resist using hysterical headlines to sell newspapers. The medical community was outraged at these exaggerations. Several doctors wrote to the British Medical Association demanding that it release a statement correcting the record. One physician complained,

> Sir, my partners and I feel very strongly that it is time the British Medical Association took urgent steps to counteract the ridiculous and hysterical exaggerated publicity given in the daily press and magazines to the present epidemic of Asian Flu. Although so far there have been no cases of Asian Flu recognized as such in this [our] neighborhood, patients have already started sending for us urgently on most inadequate grounds. One woman in the best of health had obeyed instructions given her in a woman's magazine and had sent urgently because she felt hot. I gather that even television has been used to encourage patients to send for their doctor at once

if they think they are starting flu. It is difficult to imagine any more efficient way of encouraging unnecessary calls.[28]

And another wrote,

> Sir, I wish to protest against the highly sensational reports of the national press about the present influenza epidemic. Patients get worried unnecessarily and so do their doctors. A statement by the B.M.A. declaring that the influenza epidemic, whether Asian or 48-hour Flu, is highly contagious but quite harmless, without evidence of serious complications, might help. Perhaps the press could instead devote their pages to the publication of names and addresses of victims of carcinoma of lung, with the average number of cigarettes smoked.[29]

One looks in vain for statements from the American Medical Association in 2020–2021 urging the media not to exaggerate the severity of the China Virus. Indeed, the chief role of leading medical professionals, at least those in the employ of the federal government, seemed to be to spread confusion, fear, and panic, not allay it.

work only reached around 3 to 8 percent, and, though there were economic impacts, there was no severe recession, and economic recovery in the wake of the pandemic was rapid. Hospital admissions shot up, but extra capacity was achieved by cancelling elective surgeries and repurposing beds."[30]

It wasn't as if the United States was an outlier in these matters. Government officials in most other countries, supported by their own health officials, adopted a similar approach. Take the example of the United Kingdom, where the Asian Flu pandemic peaked at the same time as it did in the United States.

"General practitioners were 'amazed at the extraordinary infectivity of the disease' and the suddenness with which it attacked younger age groups," writes Mark Honigsbaum. "Yet, while some members of the College of General Practitioners called for the UK Government to issue a warning about the dangers presented by the virus and coordinate a national response, the ministry of health demurred. Instead, the virus was permitted to run its course."[31]

Even as Asian Flu deaths in the United Kingdom were peaking at around six hundred a week, no one in the media was calling for social distancing or lockdowns. "Instead, the news cycle was dominated by the Soviet Union's launch of Sputnik and the aftermath of the fire at the Windscale nuclear reactor in the UK."[32]

Although governments around the world tried to mitigate the economic effects of the pandemic, it did lead to a global economic slowdown. By the end of 1957, the stock market had fallen and consumer sentiment and spending were on the decline. The following year would see the United States enter a very brief recession. Nevertheless, the crisis caused by the Asia Flu was relatively mild, and despite the disease most Americans carried on with their normal activities throughout.

A Vaccine Not in Time Saves None

Those who want to relitigate President Eisenhower's actions claim that tens of thousands of lives could have been saved by a nationwide, government-supported vaccination campaign. Among these is historian Max Skidmore, who in his 2016 book was highly critical of President Eisenhower's response, calling it "an example of inaction in the face of a public health emergency." Skidmore claimed that the president's initial reluctance to get behind a vaccine campaign was catastrophic: "[A]s a result, the death rate was perhaps about doubled what it might have been otherwise."[33]

But is it true that a vaccination campaign could have cut the death toll in half and saved fifty-eight thousand lives?

On the other side of this argument is Dr. Maurice Hilleman, who has long claimed that the vaccine—*his* vaccine—did stop the pandemic. Hilleman was the man who first identified the new virus and played a key role in pushing for a vaccine to counter it.

Hilleman was chief of respiratory diseases at the Walter Reed Army Institute of Research when he got his first inkling that a new virus was on the loose. The article that tipped him off was in the April 17, 1957, edition of the *New York Times*, entitled "Hong Kong Battling Influenza Epidemic."[34]

"In 1957, we all missed it," Hilleman would later admit. "The military missed it, and the World Health Organization missed it. But I saw an article, mind you, in *The New York Times* that said all these children were being taken to the dispensaries in Hong Kong. 20,000 people lined up, and I looked at that, they said, babies had glassy-eyed stares [and I thought], my God this is the pandemic, it's here."

A few weeks later Hilleman was on his way to Japan. There he collected virus specimens from U.S. servicemen who had come down with what he called the Asian Flu and brought them back to his lab to analyze. After he confirmed that most people lacked antibody protection for this new virus, he was certain that a new pandemic was on the way.[35] "I was able to announce to the world," he recalled. "I had guts at that time. I said that there would be a pandemic which would start when school began in the Fall and it didn't let me down, the pandemic of '57 of Asian Influenza began on time."

If the production of a vaccine was delayed by inaction on the part of the Eisenhower administration, it doesn't come through in Hilleman's account. He maintains that because he was alerted by the *New York Times* and was able to detect the epidemic "very early," he was able to directly "go to the

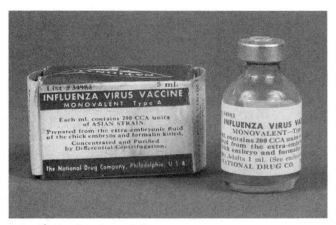

Asian Flu vaccine. *Leroy E. Burney*

manufacturers and get them going on an immediate basis without having to go through the bureaucratic red tape." He sent samples of the novel virus to the manufacturers and urged them to develop a vaccine in four months, so that it would be ready in time for the fall outbreak that he was sure was coming.

Once a vaccine was approved in August 1957, Eisenhower asked Congress for $500,000 in funding and for authorization to shift an additional $2 million, if needed, to fight the outbreak. His goal of 60 million doses of vaccines was enough to vaccinate a third of the U.S. population. He even took the vaccine himself, to set an example for others.

Hilleman continued to "help the manufacturers along" as they sought to develop and gain approval for an effective vaccine, and then to ramp up the production of the tens of millions of doses that would be required. In the end, the problem was not the lack of an early government-supported vaccination program, or lack of support from Eisenhower himself. Rather, it was simply the time it took to develop and produce the vaccine in sufficient quantity.

Some 40 million doses of the vaccine had been administered by the end of the year, an accomplishment that Hilleman claims was responsible for

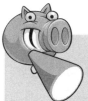

Then and Now: If You Can't Stop It, Treat It

The best summary of the measured response to the Asian Flu pandemic comes from the pen of the doctor who eradicated smallpox, Dr. Donald Henderson:

> The 1957–58 pandemic was such a rapidly spreading disease that it became quickly apparent to U.S. health officials that efforts to stop or slow its spread were futile. Thus, no efforts were made to quarantine individuals or groups, and a deliberate decision was made not to cancel or postpone large meetings such as conferences, church gatherings, or athletic events for the purpose of reducing transmission. No attempt was made to limit travel or to otherwise screen travelers. Emphasis was placed on providing medical care to those who were afflicted.... Respiratory illness brought large numbers of patients to clinics, doctor's offices, and emergency rooms, but a relatively small percentage of those infected required hospitalization.

> School absenteeism due to influenza was high, but schools were not closed.... The course of the outbreak in schools was relatively brief, and many could readily return to activities within 3 to 5 days. A significant number of healthcare workers were said to have been afflicted with influenza, but hospitals were able to adjust appropriately to cope with the patient loads.... There was no interruption of essential services or production. The overall impact on GDP was negligible....[36]

Dr. Henderson was writing in 2009. But a decade later, when another highly infectious influenza arrived from China, every last one of these lessons from a past American pandemic would be set aside. Instead, we slavishly modeled our public health response on the measures adopted by the same totalitarian dictatorship that, as it turns out, had created both the China Virus and the global pandemic.

Was that response justified? The answer hinges on whether the China Virus was the second coming of the Spanish Flu, or merely a reprise of the Asian Flu.

ending the Asian Flu pandemic. In his words, "[The vaccine] was used, that was the only time we've ever averted a pandemic with a vaccine."[37]

Others disagree with this assessment. While immunology had advanced to the point where vaccines could be produced, they inevitably lagged behind the spread of the disease. In the case of the Asian Flu, "the first vaccines were not distributed until August in the US and October in the UK, and then on an extremely limited basis."[38] Even by the end of November, enough vaccines had been produced to inoculate only 17 percent of the population.

Despite the low percentage of Americans vaccinated, the first wave of the pandemic was rapidly ebbing by the end of November. Nor did the numbers of the vaxxed climb much after that point, since as the pandemic receded interest in the vaccine sharply declined as well. The second wave of Asian Flu, arriving two months later, was much smaller and did little to change the public perception that the pandemic was over.

Reviewing the evidence, Dr. Donald Henderson, the man who eradicated the scourge of smallpox, discounted the impact of the vaccine. "Given the limited amount of vaccine available and the fact that it was not more than 60% effective, it is apparent that vaccine had no appreciable effect on the trend of the pandemic," Henderson wrote.[39] Others concur that the vaccine simply arrived "too little and too late to thwart the epidemic."[40]

So if the vaccine didn't stop the pandemic, what did? We are left with only one explanation: herd immunity. By the end of the first wave a full quarter of Americans had already been infected by and recovered from the Asian Flu. One in four Americans now enjoyed some degree of natural immunity.[41]

Although it was herd immunity that largely stopped the pandemic, one cannot completely discount the vaccine. To the 25 percent of the population that had developed natural immunity, one can add—if the vaccine was 60 percent effective—perhaps another 10 percent or so who had vaccine-induced immunity.[42]

These numbers suggest that America may have reached herd immunity vis-à-vis the Asian Flu when only about a third of the population was actually protected against it.

President Eisenhower encouraged vaccinations while refusing to impose harsh restrictions. His leadership during the Asian Flu provides an excellent example of how to balance a global viral respiratory pandemic with other concerns—including other public health issues—and the value of going on with everyday life, which, sadly, has been largely ignored or even denigrated by later politicians and public health officials.

The Anthony Faucis of our day are so obsessed with targeting and destroying viruses that they are willing to subjugate their fellow Americans in order to do so. They are seemingly oblivious to the collateral damage to the health and well-being of the public caused by their single-minded focus on vaccines *über alles*. And, sadly, in this case the vaccines, using an experimental mRNA technology, did not work well at all.

CHAPTER 7

"Fiasco": The Great Swine Flu Hoax of 1976 (1976–1977)

The year was 1976. America was celebrating the bicentennial anniversary of the Declaration of Independence. Gerald Ford, the thirty-eighth president of the United States, was in the political battle of his life with a Southern Democrat by the name of Jimmy Carter. Two tiny tech companies that would be household names one day—Microsoft and Apple—had just been incorporated.

The country's major pharmaceutical companies, on the other hand, were already billion-dollar businesses. And they were about to grow even larger by manufacturing a vaccine for a swine flu pandemic that never happened.

The late sixties and early seventies had already been a banner decade for the manufacturers of vaccines. A vaccine for mumps had been approved in 1967, a new attenuated vaccine for measles in 1968, and one for rubella (also known as German measles—in those days when it never occurred to anyone that it was xenophobic, let alone "racist," to call a disease after its reputed place of origin) in 1969. The MMR combination vaccine—for measles, mumps, and rubella—followed in 1971. The DPT vaccine—against diphtheria, pertussis (whooping cough), and tetanus—was being administered worldwide by the World Health Organization, greatly reducing the incidence of those deadly diseases among children.[1]

But the crowning achievement of the vaxxers was the complete elimination of smallpox. The last wild case of the deadly *variola major* virus, which killed 30 percent of those it infected, occurred in Bangladesh in late 1975.[2] The scourge of centuries was gone, and medical researchers, increasingly confident in their prowess, looked around for other infectious diseases to eliminate by universal vaccination.

They didn't have long to wait.

The Only Thing We Have to Fear Is Fear Itself

In mid-January 1976, a number of soldiers in training at Fort Dix, New Jersey, came down with a respiratory illness that was initially diagnosed as influenza. A few weeks later one of them, a private by the name of David Lewis, died.

The New Jersey Department of Health collected samples from the Fort Dix soldiers and found something unusual. While most of the samples proved to be the common influenza A Victoria strain, four could not be identified. These were sent on to the Centers for Disease Control, which identified them as a swine influenza A subtype H1N1 that was a close relative of the Spanish Flu.[3] None of the infected soldiers had been around pigs, so human-to-human transmission was assumed. Another bastard child of the "mother of all pandemics" was apparently stalking humanity.

These findings caused panic among the CDC's senior leadership, who feared a reprise of the Spanish Flu spreading across the globe, causing tens of millions of casualties. Worryingly, tests revealed that no one born after 1925—that is, after the Spanish Flu had receded—had any antibodies to the new strain.

On February 13, 1976, David Sencer, the head of the CDC, notified all fifty states of the outbreak of a new swine flu. An emergency meeting was convened at the CDC the following day at which the participants concurred that a vaccine was needed. They also agreed that, to avoid alarming the public, no mention should be made of the suspected origins of the new influenza.[4]

That unofficial gag order lasted only five days. The CDC called a press conference on February 19 to discuss the swine flu outbreak at Fort Dix. Bruce Dull, the CDC's assistant director for programs, admitted that the swine flu in question was closely related to the Spanish Flu. That news made the front page of the *New York Times*, which breathlessly reported "the possibility . . . that the virus that caused the greatest world epidemic of influenza in modern history—the pandemic of 1918–19—may have returned."[5]

> ## A Book You're Not Supposed to Read
>
> *The Swine Flu Affair: Decision-Making on a Slippery Disease* by R. E. Neustadt and H. V. Fineberg (Washington, D.C.: National Academies Press, 1978).

Dull added fuel to the fire by telling the assembled reporters that "it might take about six months to develop and produce large amounts of a new vaccine effective against the virus."[6] That sparked fears that if a major swine flu outbreak did occur somewhere in the United States, the vaccine might never catch up with the spread of the virus.

Samples of what was being called the Fort Dix virus were delivered to America's four vaccine manufacturers the following day, while the CDC sent state epidemiologists on a nationwide hunt for other cases of the swine flu. The search produced nothing but a few cases involving human–pig contact; no cases of the dreaded human-to-human transmission that could ignite an epidemic were reported.

But through round after round of CDC meetings in early March, the outlook of the assembled epidemiologists and virologists grew increasingly gloomy. They were convinced that a dangerous swine flu was on the loose that could plunge the United States into a pandemic. It was not enough merely to support the research and production of a vaccine, or even to stockpile it in the eventuality that a major outbreak occurred. What was needed, the experts concluded, was a preemptive strike against the virus:

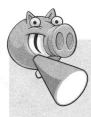

Then and Now: Scientific Hubris

Many of the medical researchers involved in the 1976 vaccination scheme, from CDC director David Sencer on down, were anything but neutral arbiters. They were eager to showcase their institutions and expertise. Dr. Harvey Fineberg, the former president of the Institute of Medicine and co-author of the 1978 *Swine Flu Affair*, revisited the events of 1976 in a 2008 article in the *Journal of Infectious Diseases*. Fineberg concluded that many of the senior scientists involved had their own agendas. Some researchers saw the chance to improve the credentials of their institutions or field on the national stage, he wrote, while others held a "conviction that prevention of disease by vaccination was an achievable perfection of the human condition."[7]

It is hard not to see our own public health authorities, such as Dr. Anthony Fauci, as the heirs of the other experts responsible for the deadly errors of the swine flu vaccine campaign. The gain-of-function research that Fauci has funded and defended is clearly a latter-day expression of this same scientific hubris, the idea that man can create dangerous viruses in the lab and then engineer their defeat before Nature can create a pandemic.

the vaccine should be administered to as many people as possible as soon as it could be readied.

So in 1976 the U.S. government set out to immunize every man, woman, and child in the country against what they were told was a dangerous descendant of the Spanish Flu.

In *The Swine Flu Affair: Decision-Making on a Slippery Disease*, R. E. Neustadt and H. V. Fineberg detail how more than 45 million Americans received a vaccine for an influenza pandemic that never happened. The vaccination campaign was accompanied by endless controversy, misleading ads, legal complications, bureaucratic wrangling, and unforeseen vaccine side effects, the end result of which was a blow to the credibility of public health authorities that would resonate for a generation. A more accurate title for their book would have been *The Swine Flu Affair: A Pandemic of Panic.*

The authors call the virus "slippery," but this appellation should really apply to the public health bureaucrats, politicians, media organizations, and manufacturers who pushed the vaccine. In one way or another—reputationally or financially—they all sought to profit by creating the perception that a pandemic was brewing.

Sound familiar? It should.

CDC director Sencer put the experts' recommendations into a March 13 action memo to the White House calling for an emergency campaign to vaccinate all Americans. Sencer's memo claimed that the public would not be safe from the swine flu scourge until at least 80 percent of the population had received the jab. Among its recommendations were that Congress appropriate $134 million so that the federal government could buy the vaccine, the states could distribute it, and public health agencies and private physicians could administer it.

On March 24 President Gerald Ford met with a blue-ribbon panel of vaccine experts, including Dr. Jonas Salk and Dr. Albert Sabin of polio vaccine fame and Dr. Maurice Hilleman, who helped develop the Asian Flu vaccine (although too late to stop that pandemic). Those present unanimously endorsed the CDC director's call for a mass vaccination campaign. Here was a chance for the virologists to show their quality.

> ★ ★ ★
> ## Dr. Fauci Makes a Losing Bet—with Other People's Lives
>
> "In an unlikely but conceivable turn of events, what if that scientist becomes infected with the virus, which leads to an outbreak and ultimately triggers a pandemic? Many ask reasonable questions: given the possibility of such a scenario—however remote—should the initial experiments have been performed and/or published in the first place, and what were the processes involved in this decision? Scientists working in this field might say—as indeed I have said—that the benefits of such experiments and the resulting knowledge outweigh the risks. *It is more likely that a pandemic would occur in nature, and the need to stay ahead of such a threat is a primary reason for performing an experiment that might appear to be risky*" [emphasis added].[8]
> —Anthony Fauci, October 9, 2012

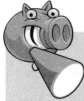

Then and Now: Pandemic Panic

Even before the beginning of the vaccination campaign, critics were raising questions. The *New York Times* noted, "This unprecedented effort is based on evidence whose significance is hotly disputed. Critics consider the campaign a panicky overreaction to a minimal threat. They see little likelihood of a swine flu pandemic this year and don't believe the disease would be especially lethal even if it did reappear. They also suggest that the vaccine may be a worse threat than the disease—that it won't offer much protection against swine flu and will inevitably cause adverse reactions in some recipients. There have even been allegations that the campaign was contrived as a political ploy to bolster President Ford's chances for re-nomination and re-election, or was engineered by vaccine manufacturers who saw a chance to make enormous profits. (Such allegations seem wide of the mark. The prime movers in the campaign have always been Federal health officials and their advisers in the universities and medical institutions.)"

When the China Virus arrived on our shores in 2020 the *Times* and other media would have a much different take. To be sure, Covid's arrival was preceded by a sustained propaganda campaign out of China that featured horror stories about its infectiousness and lethality, and the early death rates in states like New York and New Jersey, especially in assisted living facilities, were shocking. (It would take time for it to emerge that those deaths had resulted from misguided policies that seemed almost designed to drive up the death rate among the helpless elderly confined there.)

But, looking back, it remains surprising that so few in the media expressed concerns along the lines that the "vaccine may be a worse threat than the disease—that it won't offer much protection . . . and will inevitably cause adverse reactions in some recipients." Such concerns should be—and had been—a given whenever new vaccines are introduced. Why were the usual critics of capitalism and Big Pharma, including the *Times*, silent in the face of the enormous profits being made by vaccine manufacturers? Just as in the case of the 1976 swine flu, their profits are once again guaranteed by a combination of government purchase contracts and legal protection against lawsuits from those harmed by their vaccines.

Following the meeting, and flanked by his vaccine experts, the president immediately went before the television cameras to warn that a new and deadly swine flu pandemic might be coming to America. To head off this possible calamity, he went on, it was necessary "to inoculate every man, woman and child in the United States."

And just like that, the debate over whether to vaccinate everyone in America against the newly detected virus was over. It was no longer a matter of if, but only when, a vaccine would be ready, and all 221 million Americans would have to line up to get the jab. As the *New York Times* reported, "This was to be the largest immunization drive ever launched in this country, dwarfing even the polio immunization campaigns of the 1950's and 1960's."[9]

It is important to note that, while all this was taking place, not a single additional case of the Fort Dix swine flu had been discovered. Nor did anyone bother to take note of the fact that the only supposed victim of the swine flu, Private David Lewis, had risen from his sickbed to take part in a forced nighttime march. After marching for five miles on a bitterly cold midwinter's night, he had collapsed and died. Rather than dying *of* the swine flu, it is more likely that Private Lewis died *with* the swine flu.

But if the much-feared Fort Dix swine flu—to the extent that it even existed—may not have been particularly dangerous, the same cannot be said of the vaccine.

Vaccines Have Consequences

Congress quickly appropriated $135 million for a sweeping vaccination scheme, and President Ford signed into law the federal government's "National Swine Flu Immunization Program." The FDA did its part, rushing through approval for a new swine flu vaccine by June 21. The manufacturers cut corners as well, choosing to use an "attenuated live virus" for the vaccine instead of an inactivated or "killed" form—increasing the risk of adverse side effects among susceptible groups of people receiving the vaccination.[10]

Worried about liability, however, manufacturers hesitated to ramp up production.[11] They were willing to manufacture the tens of millions of doses that would be required, they told Washington, but only if two conditions were met: they wanted a guaranteed profit margin and, equally important, they wanted Congress to pass legislation indemnifying them against any lawsuits that might arise from side effects of the vaccine.

In the heated atmosphere of the time, arguments flew back and forth about the safety of the vaccine and whether a mass vaccination campaign was even necessary. In July an FDA researcher was fired for questioning the safety of influenza vaccines and subsequently went public with his doubts. The proposed legislation stalled in Congress, and the manufacturers threatened to stop manufacturing the vaccine.

At the same time, however, reports of alleged swine flu outbreaks in other countries were continually surfacing. Although testing would later reveal that every case was a false alarm, these reports added to the public perception that a pandemic was brewing. The fear was brought even closer to home in early August, when Philadelphia experienced an outbreak of a pneumonia-like illness that the newspapers suggested was caused by the swine flu, but was later found to be Legionnaires' disease.

On August 6, 1976, President Ford held a press conference, saying that he was "dumbfounded" by the unwillingness of Congress to act on indemnification legislation so that the vaccination campaign could get rolling. Congress responded to the president's public arm-twisting just four days later, sending legislation to his desk stating that all claims arising from the vaccination campaign were to be filed with the federal government.

Still, public enthusiasm for the immunization program continued to wane as no epidemic appeared on the horizon. A Gallup poll conducted in late August showed that although 93 percent of Americans were aware of the looming program, only slightly more than half—52 percent—actually intended to get the jab. To boost public participation, a massive public relations campaign was kicked off, with pictures of smiling celebrities and politicians getting the shot, including actress Mary Tyler Moore. But when she was later interviewed by Mike Wallace of *60 Minutes*, she insisted that she had never actually been vaccinated.

The first swine flu shots were given at the Indiana State Fair on October 1, 1976, and adverse reactions to the vaccine began to be reported almost immediately. The most serious came from a Pittsburgh clinic where three elderly people died shortly after receiving the vaccine.

The news was enough to convince not only Pittsburgh health officials but officials in nine other states to shut down the immunization program until the cause of the deaths could be determined. CDC director Sencer claimed at a press conference that the deaths were a coincidence, and autopsies showed that two of the three had suffered heart attacks. Within days, all of the states that had suspended their vaccination campaigns had resumed them. But public enthusiasm for the program had waned noticeably.[12]

In an effort to reassure the public of the vaccine's safety, President Ford and his family personally went before the television cameras to receive shots on October 14. But by that time even some leading experts were beginning to have doubts about the wisdom of the campaign they had initially supported.

Among these was oral polio vaccine inventor Albert Sabin, who in early November published a critical *New York Times* editorial entitled "Washington and the Flu." The initial decision to create the vaccine had been correct, he said, but given that in the months since

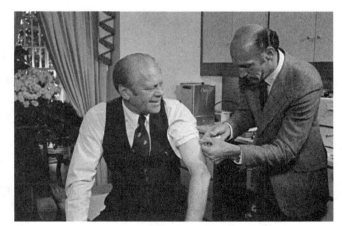

President Ford is inoculated against the 1976 swine flu by White House physician Dr. William Lukash. *Ricardo Thomas*

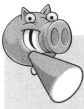

Then and Now: Pushing the Vaccines

Dr. Albert Sabin, inventor of the oral polio vaccine, was highly critical of the "scare tactics" that were being used by Washington in the fall of 1976 to frighten people into submitting to a vaccination for the swine flu. But it was not Washington's politicians but its medical researchers that had originally panicked at the possibility of a deadly influenza pandemic. Sabin himself had stood next to President Ford at the original press conference, in effect lending his scientific credibility to the mass vaccination campaign that the president announced. The same scenario would play out in early 2020 when a new generation of medical researchers and virologists would panic over the outbreak of Covid-19 in Wuhan, China. They would again convince a sitting president that a deadly pandemic was on the march and, once again, a new set of vaccines relying on a novel technology would be fast-tracked through the approval process with predictable results.

One wonders what Sabin would think of the Covid vaccination campaign in 2020 and 2021, which relied not just on "scare tactics" to get people to line up for the jab, but on open government coercion.

there had been no actual outbreak, Washington should stop using "scare tactics" to force people to line up for their vaccinations. Instead the vaccine should be stockpiled and a mass vaccination campaign undertaken only if the feared pandemic actually materialized.[13] Sabin's warning came too late. By the time his article was published the campaign was underway in all fifty states, and it would take more than a warning—even from America's most famous living virologist—to derail it.

Then, on November 12, Minnesota reported that a vaccine recipient had developed Guillain-Barré syndrome, a potentially fatal disease in which the body's own immune system attacks the peripheral nervous system. This autoimmune disease can result in acute muscle weakness that lasts months or even years and, in severe cases, paralysis, respiratory arrest, and death.[14]

Cases of Guillain-Barré continued to multiply over the next few weeks, with the CDC reporting on December 14, 1976, that it had been notified of fifty-four cases in ten different states.[15] Two days later, CDC director Sencer announced that he was suspending the vaccination program for one month. It would never be resumed.

Cases of Guillain-Barré continued to pile up, and public criticism mounted. CDC director Sencer was the senior official most closely identified with the campaign, and it came as no surprise when the incoming president, Jimmy Carter, asked for his resignation soon after taking office in January 1977.

In all, some 45 million people, roughly 20 percent of the U.S. population at the time, had received the vaccine by the time the campaign was called off. Of these, 362 people came down with Guillain-Barré within a few weeks of receiving the jab, which meant that the incidence of the disease was roughly four times higher in vaccinated people than in those not receiving the swine flu vaccine.[16]

Over the same period of time, how many cases of the Fort Dix swine flu were discovered? Aside from the four cases that sparked the panic in the first place, exactly zero. Never have so many been vaccinated for an influenza that caused so few infections and (maybe) one death. The swine flu vaccination campaign was one of the largest public health initiatives ever undertaken by the U.S. government—and a total "fiasco."[17]

Lesson Learned—and Forgotten?

Any drug or biopharmaceutical introduced into the body is going to produce side effects. Now if you're suffering from an illness, especially one with serious symptoms, side effects don't matter so much. You're willing to take acetaminophen for your headache even though you know that

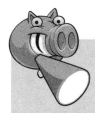

Then and Now:
Exaggerating the Danger

Mike Wallace of *60 Minutes* interviewed Sencer, who attempted to justify the mass immunization campaign against a nonexistent swine flu during his tenure as the head of the CDC by saying that "several" unconfirmed cases of swine flu had been reported around the world at the time. But when Wallace asked him if any actual outbreaks of the disease had occurred, the former director of the CDC simply answered, "No."

Nevertheless, based on this meager evidence and a false equivalence with the Spanish Flu, Sencer and his colleagues modeled a swine flu apocalypse of global proportions and used it to justify a crash vaccination campaign.

Ashley Sadler has pointed out, "It's a chain of events at least mildly reminiscent of last March's [2020] Imperial College London COVID-19 model, in which epidemiologist Neil Ferguson projected a cataclysmic number of deaths from the virus, leading to public hysteria and the lockdown of both the United States and the U.K. under draconian and unprecedented shutdowns. The model turned out to be based on faulty data and Ferguson himself was discredited after violating his own social distancing recommendations to engage in an extramarital affair."[18]

continually taking the drug over time may cause liver damage. The immediate benefit outweighs the possible costs.

But the calculation is very different with vaccination. With a vaccine you are giving a healthy person something that produces no immediate benefit. The hope is that, should that person one day be exposed to the disease being targeted by the vaccine, the vaccine will reduce his risk of catching it, or reduce the severity of the symptoms if he does contract the disease. If the person never encounters the disease, the lifetime benefit of the vaccine is effectively zero.

Since the benefit that people derive from a vaccine is much smaller—or more speculative—than the benefit they derive from a drug for an existing condition, the risk of side effects from a vaccine has to be much, much smaller.

The 1976 swine flu vaccine failed this test. The risk from vaccination was real, while the benefits were totally illusory. No one in America actually encountered the Fort Dix swine flu after the initial handful of cases, so the 45 million people who were immunized received zero benefit from the vaccine, and some were actually harmed.

For Big Pharma, however, it was a win-win. They profited from selling shots under guaranteed government contracts while at the same time enjoying complete immunity from liability for adverse medical consequences. It was a lesson they would never forget.

PART FOUR

THE CHINA CORONAVIRUS

CHAPTER 8

A Pandemic Unlike Any Other: The China Virus (2019–2022)

In the closing months of 2019, there were signs that all was not well in Wuhan, China. In October, there was a sudden increase in traffic at hospitals throughout the city of 14 million. As the U.S. deputy consular chief in Wuhan, Russell Westergard, would later report, "By mid-October [we] . . . knew that the city had been struck by what was thought to be an unusually vicious flu season."[1]

The epidemic continued to worsen in November, by which time U.S. intelligence officials were warning that a contagion was sweeping through China's Wuhan region. A report by the military's National Center for Medical Intelligence (NCMI) that month reportedly concluded that "it could be a cataclysmic event."[2]

By December city officials were closing public schools in an effort to control the spread of the disease, Westergard would later note. Regular reports on the worsening situation in the city were being sent by the consulate to the U.S. Embassy in Beijing, although they wouldn't reach the president until a month later.

Throughout these first few months of the spreading epidemic, Chinese Communist officials maintained a Sphinx-like silence. It wasn't until December 31 that the Wuhan Municipal Health Commission released a warning on its website that a previously unknown pneumonia was spreading in the city. At the same time, it attempted to downplay the severity of the outbreak, falsely claiming that there had been only twenty-seven cases, no fatalities, and no human-to-human transmission.[3]

Taiwan, always alert to threats coming from Communist China, immediately began screening all incoming passengers from Wuhan for fever or other symptoms of the flu.[4] With the Chinese authorities mum about the nature of the new pneumonia, Taiwan erred on the side of caution, screening passengers for no fewer than thirty-six known viruses. When tests for all thirty-six came back negative, the island nation concluded that a dangerous new disease was on the loose. It warned the World Health Organization within hours, pointing out that, despite China's denials, the virus was in fact spreading by person-to-person transmission, and spreading rapidly.[5]

Appeasing China

The warning went unheeded by the WHO, which—not for the last time—decided that playing nice with Beijing was more important than public health. The UN agency, which knew that Beijing would be upset if it took the slightest notice of its "renegade province" (as Communist Chinese refers to the nation of Taiwan), decided to ignore this urgent warning. In a clear dereliction of its duty, the WHO did not share the evidence of person-to-person transmission with other countries.[6]

On January 3, 2020, Communist Chinese officials formally notified the World Health Organization about a "cluster of cases of 'viral pneumonia of unknown cause' identified in Wuhan," and the next day the WHO tweeted out a statement, lifted virtually word for word from China's, that "China has reported to WHO a cluster of pneumonia cases—with no deaths—in Wuhan, Hubei Province." The critical fact of person-to-person transmission was not mentioned.

Long after it was evident that the novel coronavirus was a highly infectious airborne virus, the WHO was still parroting the Chinese authorities' claim that "there is no clear evidence of human-to-human transmission." Even when, on January 30, the U.S. Centers for Disease Control reported the first clear case of person-to-person transmission in the United States, the WHO immediately responded that "outside of #China" such transmission was "limited." By then, it was obvious that it was anything but.[7]

The Original Lockdown

Just the week before, the Chinese authorities had announced the biggest lockdown in the history of the world.

On January 23, 2020, after months of minimizing the outbreak, Beijing placed the entire population of Wuhan, some 14 million people, under indefinite lockdown. The city and the surrounding countryside would be quarantined from the rest of the country, the authorities said, until the epidemic could be brought under control.

In order to combat the worsening coronavirus epidemic, Communist Party leader Xi Jinping declared a "People's War" against the virus. The Communist leader mobilized the entire machinery of the state—the military, the government, and the party—and put the entire country on a war footing.

The province of Hubei, the epicenter of the epidemic, was cordoned off from the rest of China, while an invading army of "veteran Party members," medical personnel, and military units were sent to the province to take control. Their orders were to arrest all persons found to be carrying the disease and put them into containment centers.[8] They were authorized by Xi himself to use force against anyone who resisted; he personally threatened anyone who disobeyed government orders with severe punishment.[9]

Videos out of China showed the police dragging people with symptoms of the Wuhan Flu from their apartments and welding shut the doors of other apartments whose residents were suspected of having been exposed to the virus.[10] Pictures circulated of hospital wards overflowing with the sick and hallways crowded with the bodies of the dead. Vans loaded with body bags were filmed heading toward crematoria, where the local Communist authorities were offering "free cremation for the corpses of coronavirus victims who died on January 26 or later." The ovens, we learned from on-the-ground reports, were going 24/7 in a frantic effort to incinerate the growing piles of corpses.[11]

These measures were justified by CCP officials in the name of public health. "In the event of a public-safety threat, it is OK to sacrifice some privacy for the benefit of society," one was quoted as saying.[12]

The pictures and videos convinced some Western officials that a new Spanish Flu was on the loose, and they began to advocate for some of the same extreme measures to be adopted in their own country, with the same justification: to protect public health.

Up to that point in time few in America had been paying attention to the Wuhan Flu. The crisis at the southern border that President Trump had inherited from the Obama-Biden administration was easing. Mile after mile of border wall was going up, blocking off criminals, drug cartels, and human traffickers from easy access to the heartland. The flow of unskilled illegal alien labor was also subsiding, greatly benefiting blacks and Hispanics whose wages had been depressed by a flood of illegals willing to work for less. Unemployment rates, especially for minorities, had fallen to historic lows, reflecting the booming economy and the more secure border. The production of oil and natural gas had increased to the point where America was energy independent for the first time in decades. Gas prices at the pump had fallen to a mere $2 a gallon—which had the practical effect of giving most Americans a raise. The economy was surging under Trump's tax cuts, exports were strong, and the dollar was the envy of the world.

Adding to these happy circumstances was a further distraction: 2020 was a presidential election year. Most Americans pay little enough attention to events overseas in ordinary times; in election years they pay even less.

But the Wuhan lockdown got everyone's attention. As travel restrictions expanded to include the entire province of Hubei, some 67 million Chinese were soon languishing under some form of quarantine.[13] Many in the West were shocked by the draconian lockdowns, not realizing that they themselves would soon enough lose their freedoms to copycat measures.

The Trump Travel Ban

Taiwan, again, was the first country to respond to the plague raging in China, banning all flights from Wuhan on January 26. The Trump administration followed on January 31 with its own travel restrictions, announcing that it would deny entry to all foreign nationals traveling from China to the United States and require returning U.S. citizens to quarantine for two weeks.[14] No one had accused Taiwan of "hysteria, xenophobia, and fear-mongering" for banning flights, but when President Trump took the lesser step of banning foreign nationals, he was accused of all that and more.

History shows that Trump's decision to impose travel restrictions was the correct one. It undoubtedly kept several thousand, and maybe many more, carriers of a fast-moving respiratory virus out of the country. If anything, it was imposed too late. But with China first denying and then dissembling about the epidemic—and aided in its cover-up by the WHO—how was anyone to know the truth about what was happening behind the bamboo curtain?

The Trump travel ban elicited harsh criticism, including from three significant people: an immunologist by the name of Anthony Fauci, a presidential candidate named Joe Biden, and a spokesperson for the Chinese Communist Party.[15]

Trump advisor Peter Navarro has described a January 30 meeting in the White House Situation Room at which Dr. Fauci threw a temper tantrum when he learned of the imminent travel ban. "Two minutes in I'm in a shouting match with this SOB," recounts Navarro. "And all he can keep saying is 'Travel bans don't work.'"

Navarro recalls responding, "Dude, you mean to tell me that if China is sending us 20,000 Chinese nationals a day coming in to LAX and O'Hare and Kennedy and Pittsburgh, and some of them are lit up like a Christmas tree with the virus, that we would be better off simply saying, come on in?" But Fauci kept fighting him.[16]

Joe Biden, Trump's opponent in the 2020 presidential election, immediately went on the attack, tweeting out: "We are in the midst of a crisis with the coronavirus. We need to lead the way with science—not Donald Trump's record of hysteria, xenophobia, and fearmongering. He is the worst possible person to lead our country through a global health emergency."[17]

Chinese Communist officials were scarcely less intemperate. Foreign ministry spokesperson Hua Chunying blasted President Trump's travel ban, saying that "the U.S. comments and actions are neither based on facts, nor helpful at this particular time."[18] The WHO had advised against travel bans, she huffed, suggesting that Washington had "unceasingly manufactured and spread panic" about the Wuhan Virus from the beginning.[19]

What to make of these critics?

Anthony Fauci's bizarre insistence that "travel bans don't work" flies in the face of human experience. But it was only the first of many public health issues that the guy in the white lab coat would get catastrophically wrong. From masks and natural immunity to school closures and protecting the elderly, following Fauci's advice invariably made things worse, not better. As Navarro thought to himself at the time, "[Fauci] was going to hurt not only the President, but the country. . . . He could have saved millions of lives."[20]

Joe Biden, canny old pol that he was, was simply playing the pandemic for his own political purposes. Had Trump not put travel restrictions in place on January 31, and instead continued to allow people from plague-ridden

China to freely enter the country, Biden would not have hesitated to accuse him of putting American lives at risk, probably within the week.

Spokesperson Hua Chunying had the more difficult assignment. At a time when China was in the grip of a massive epidemic—why else would you quarantine 67 million people?—she had to argue that President Trump's travel ban was part of a devious plan to "spread panic" about the novel coronavirus. The Chinese regime media went into overdrive, criticizing "hostile foreign forces"—by which it principally means the United States—for creating panic in China by "overreacting."[21]

But neither Hua Chunying nor Joe Biden batted an eye as they slammed Trump for "hysteria," "fear-mongering" and "spread[ing] panic."

Throughout the early stages of the pandemic—indeed, all the way up until the election—Fauci, Biden, and the Chinese Communist Party were *de facto* allies in the effort to take down Trump.

China Virus, China PSYOP

The only way that the epidemic could possibly have been contained to China is if the Chinese authorities had acted promptly the previous fall, when the first cases of the Wuhan Flu appeared. But they chose not to. By the time they belatedly placed a cordon sanitaire around Hubei province on January 23, hundreds of thousands of infected citizens had already left Wuhan for other parts of China and destinations overseas. This was how Covid spread so rapidly to the rest of the world. The Chinese Communist Party itself is the biggest superspreader on the planet.

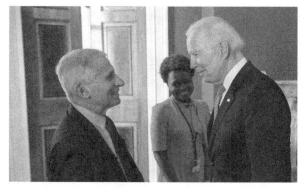

Dr. Anthony Fauci with President Joe Biden, May 17, 2021.
The White House

In the weeks leading up to January 23, 2020, hundreds of flights left from Wuhan for cities around the world. There were nineteen flights from Wuhan to either New York or San Francisco alone, for example.[22] Each carried hundreds of passengers, at least some of whom—given the rapidly rising infection rates in Wuhan—had been exposed to the virus. Some of them were feverish already. Many of the cities that were on the receiving end of these virus-laden flights from the epicenter of the epidemic, such as New York City, went on to become hot spots of their own.

It is hard for Westerners to imagine that any government would deliberately sow the seeds of a global pandemic this way, but what other explanation is there? For several months after the initial cases in Wuhan, the Chinese authorities did everything in their power to create the impression that the novel coronavirus was neither highly infectious nor particularly deadly. Everything was under control, they continually assured the world.

Actually, as someone who has studied Chinese politics for almost a half century now, I can affirm that Communist Chinese Party officials lie even when they don't need to lie, and count themselves clever for doing so. As members of an atheistic party organized along conspiratorial lines, it's in their political DNA to manipulate and deceive "the masses"—and "hostile foreign forces" such as the United States. But CCP officials, and President Xi himself, at the very least knew that their lies would result in the rapid spread of Covid-19 around the world, and they were willing to live with that result.[23]

Dr. Tedros Adhanom Ghebreyesus, director of the World Health Organization, played along. Even as he declared on January 30, 2020, that the novel coronavirus outbreak was a global public health emergency, he continued to praise China: "The speed with which China detected the outbreak, isolated the virus, sequenced the genome and shared it with WHO and the world are very impressive."[24]

He somehow failed to mention that Beijing was continuing to allow its citizens to carry a dangerous pathogen to the four corners of the world, in effect enlisting them to serve as human disease vectors.

As the virus was being seeded around the world in late 2019 and early 2020, it was accompanied by a psychological warfare campaign intended to spread fear about the coming plague on Main Street, U.S.A. A torrent of propaganda videos and pictures flooded out of China purporting to show people dropping dead in the streets from Covid, lying dead in the streets from Covid, or shot dead for trying to flee from the Covid quarantine in Wuhan.

These videos quickly went viral (irony intended). Americans, hungry for information during the early stages of the outbreak in the United States, watched them in grim fascination and then sent them on to friends. Western news media rebroadcast them as well, ensuring that the CCP's PSYOP campaign reached—and traumatized—an even larger audience with its intended message: a deadly contagion is coming, and many of you are going to die.[25]

At the same time, Chinese agents were barraging Americans with text messages warning them that the government would soon impose a nationwide lockdown with little notice to prepare.[26]

All of this helped create the state of fear on Main Street, U.S.A., that leveled resistance to Anthony Fauci's lockdowns. It gave ambitious politicians such as governors Andrew Cuomo of New York, Gavin Newsom of California, and Phil Murphy of New Jersey carte blanche to carry their belief in Big Government to its logical conclusion: total control over every man, woman, and child who lived in their domains. Finally, it

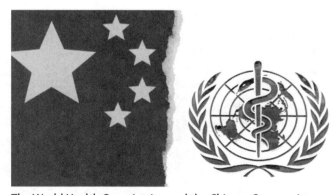

The World Health Organization and the Chinese Communist Party were on the same page when it came to Covid. *Courtesy of Katarina Carranco and Rnh-co2 molecular respiration*

helped produce the outcome most hoped for by Beijing: it vaulted Joe Biden into the White House.

It was, all things considered, one of the most successful PSYOP campaigns in history.

Once the leaders of the CCP realized that they had an uncontrolled epidemic on their hands, they appear to have made a conscious decision to spread panic and disease to the rest of the world, especially to China's chief geostrategic rival, the United States of America. Both the disease and the panic were, as we will see, manufactured—the former in a lab and the latter in the propaganda department of the Chinese Communist Party.

That explains why party hacks celebrated as if China had won a great victory when the number of deaths in New York City supposedly eclipsed the number of deaths in Wuhan.[27] As the editor of the CCP's *Global Times* put it, the "Chinese government has adopted scientific and effective control measures. Loose political system of the U.S. allows more than 3,000 people [to] die of pandemic every day."[28]

The panic spread by China's propaganda campaign was perhaps even more damaging than the China Virus itself. The hysteria was picked up and amplified by the media in the United States. And throughout 2020 the Democrats often seemed to take their talking points directly from the pages of the CCP's propaganda outlet, the *Global Times.* Many in the government followed suit, particularly Anthony Fauci and his colleagues at the CDC and FDA. The vaccine manufacturers, as in the 1976 swine flu hoax, hungrily anticipated billions in profits. For some of these players it was never

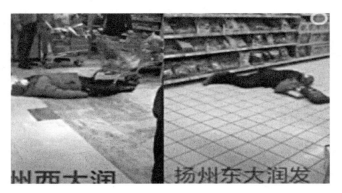

Screenshot from YouTube video "Coronavirus Has People Keeling Over in Streets." Courtesy of TomoNews US[29]

about public health at all, but rather about political power and pandemic profits.

As a result, Americans would spend much of the next two years in pandemic hell.

"The World Is Not Prepared"

On September 18, 2019, the Global Preparedness Monitoring Board, a group of fifteen scientists associated with the World Health Organization and including Anthony Fauci, Jeremy Farrar, and George Gao, the head of China's CDC, had issued a warning about a possible future global pandemic. The report, titled *A World at Risk: Annual Report on Global Preparedness for Health Emergencies*, was based on a September 10 study by Johns Hopkins.

The board said, "A rapidly spreading pandemic due to a lethal respiratory pathogen *(whether naturally emergent or accidentally or deliberately released)* poses additional preparedness requirements" [emphasis in the original] and warned, "The world is not prepared for a fast-moving, virulent respiratory pathogen pandemic."

The timing of the report was remarkably . . . prescient. Only a couple of weeks after it was published, just such "a lethal respiratory pathogen" that would lead to "a rapidly spreading pandemic" would appear in Wuhan. Despite the claims of Fauci and others that it was naturally emergent or accidentally released, as we will see in the next chapter, the evidence indicates that it belongs to the *third* category of pathogenic threats mentioned by the GPM Board: "deliberately released."[30]

In late January—after the great Chinese New Year diaspora sent infected travelers from Wuhan flying to cities around the world—cases of the novel coronavirus begin popping up outside of China. Reports came in from Taiwan, Hong Kong, Japan, South Korea, Singapore, and Thailand in rapid succession, with all the cases traceable back to travelers from Wuhan. The

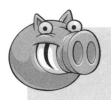

Then and Now: Naming Rights

Stop calling it the Wuhan Flu or the China Virus, insisted the WHO. The proper name for the disease that came from China, the UN agency informed us, is Covid-19. Why? Because we say so.

Never mind that, until now, we have always called pandemics by their place of origin. The West Nile virus, for example, came from the Nile Valley. And Lyme disease from Lyme, Connecticut. Even the infamous Dr. Anthony Fauci initially referred to mutated versions of the novel coronavirus as "the U.K. variant" and "the South African variant." And he didn't stop for fear of offending the sensibilities of the British or the South Africans, but because he must have realized that he was creating a precedent for calling the original strain after its mother country: China. Oops.

There is a sinister aspect to the WHO's insistence that the coronavirus not be connected to China by name. This clumsy effort to obscure the origins of the pandemic is just a small part of the WHO's larger effort to cover up China's culpability in general.

first case of the new virus that was diagnosed in the United States, on January 20, was also connected to the plague-ridden city: a thirty-five-year-old American from Washington State fell ill after returning from a visit to Wuhan.[31]

Even as the first deaths outside China began to occur, the total numbers of infected stayed small throughout most of February—perhaps depressed by the lack of an accurate test for Covid-19. The first fatality in the United States came on February 29, 2020, and the CDC said it was connected with a suspected cluster of cases in a long-term care facility in the state of Washington.[32]

If that didn't make it obvious to the CDC that the elderly, especially those confined in retirement homes, were at particular risk from the China Virus, then what happened next certainly should have. On March 1, an epidemic exploded in Italy, which because of a decades-long birth dearth has one of the most geriatric populations in Europe. By March 3 there were seventy-seven deaths and thousands of confirmed cases, mostly in northern Italy. On March 8 the Italian government put the entire Lombardy region, some 16 million people, into quarantine. But still the numbers continued to climb. The government-run health care system, which has a difficult enough time simply coping with the annual flu season, was overwhelmed, as thousands of elderly Italians fell ill every day. The daily death toll rose into the hundreds.

As it happens, Italy is an important European terminus of China's New Silk Road, also called the Belt and Road Initiative, which is the CCP's effort to recenter the world's commerce away from Europe and North America to China. This means that Italy, besides being the leading tourist destination for Chinese traveling to Europe, is also home to Europe's largest population of illegal Chinese immigrants.[33] It is no wonder that Italy was particularly hard-hit by Covid-19. By November 3, 2021, out of a population of some 60,367,000, the country had reported 132,161 deaths from the China Virus.[34]

Another terminus of the New Silk Road was Iran, China's closest partner in the Middle East. The country's close commercial ties to China made it another early epicenter of the China Virus. It's hard to know exactly how many Iranians paid with their lives for the privilege of being a way station on the Belt and Road, but at one point in late March the mullahs were digging mass graves the length of football fields. By November 3, 2021, the regime had reported 126,616 deaths to the WHO, but Iranian dissidents say that the actual number of deaths is almost four times that number.[35] Given that Iran's population is estimated at 85,422,000, that estimate of 469,700 deaths as of November 3, 2021, would mean that it had one of the highest death rates in the world.

Beijing touted its New Silk Road as a highway to riches. But as the China Virus followed the road to country after country around the world, it looked more like a one-way ticket to an early grave.

Who can forget the pictures of smiling young Chinese men and women standing on street corners in Milan, Florence, and other Italian cities holding signs saying, "Give me a hug, I'm not a virus"? Or the kindhearted elderly Italians lining up to do exactly that? One after another they would come up and embrace the sign-holders in sympathy for the epidemic that was ravaging their mother country.[36]

To the casual Western viewer, it was a heartwarming picture of international solidarity in the face of an invisible enemy of humanity.

To me, as a China Hand of long standing, it was clearly political theater. I immediately thought the stunt was probably staged by local Chinese consulates through local CCP-controlled organizations to elicit sympathy for China.

Which it was. It turned out that the videos were put out by the Unione Giovani Italo Cinesi (Union of Young Italian Chinese), a group funded by the Chinese government.

One tip-off for me was that this was *very un-Chinese-like* behavior. The Chinese simply do not go around hugging people, especially not in public, and most especially not strangers of the opposite sex. *It just is not done.* Traditionally, the Chinese don't even shake hands when meeting strangers. They practice what might be called an early form of social distancing, bowing towards each other from a safe distance. Hands never touch, arms never embrace, and kisses are never exchanged in public.[37]

Viewing videos of these strangely intimate encounters, however, another thought occurred to me. What if these well-dressed, attractive young Chinese men and women who were baiting Italians into giving them affectionate hugs and squeezes were actually superspreaders, who requited the love they were receiving with a breathy load of a highly infectious—and, for the elderly, very dangerous—pathogen?

What organization would possibly be evil enough to use its own people as human disease vectors in this way, you may be asking yourself. The Chinese Communist Party, I answer. The same international terrorist organization that deliberately released a deadly virus on the world in the first place—using human disease vectors.

America's Doctor

Back in America, the highly communicable airborne virus continued to spread like wildfire—as it was designed to do. And a diminutive doctor by the name of Anthony Fauci, the longtime head of the National Institute of

Allergies and Infectious Diseases (NIAID), was the expert that the deep state recommended the White House rely on in this time of crisis. Joining the Coronavirus Task Force, Dr. Fauci instantly became a media favorite at President Trump's China Virus press conferences, for the most part because he made for very good headlines: he did not hesitate to tell anyone who would listen that we might be facing a viral Armageddon.

Early on he warned us in his raspy voice that we were facing a disease so infectious that a single droplet in the air could infect and kill us.[38] Stopping the spread of this disease would not be easy, he said, but nothing else mattered because this was the kind of pandemic that comes along once a century or so. CNN broadcast an interview with Fauci in which he suggested that if we didn't follow his instructions to the letter, millions of Americans could die from this previously unknown virus for which there was no cure.[40] CNN summarized the interview thus: "Dr. Anthony Fauci tells Brianna Keilar that in a worst-case scenario millions of people in the US could die from the coronavirus." Lest anyone miss the point, the chyron running below Fauci's talking head read, "Coronavirus Spreads Fear and Transforms Life across America."

Actually, it would have been more accurate had it read, "Fauci Spreads Fear and Transforms Life across America," because that's exactly what he was doing, and would continue to do for the next two years.

During past plagues, we had no effective therapeutic drugs to treat those who became infected, and they often died. By the time of the Covid pandemic, we had several effective therapeutic drugs available, but—thanks

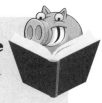

A Book You're Not Supposed to Read

Peter Navarro's *In Trump Time* is a gripping, behind-the-scenes look at a White House grappling with a sudden pandemic. Navarro, a longtime confidant of President Trump, was director of the Office of Trade and Manufacturing Policy in the Trump White House. He went toe-to-toe with Fauci on countless occasions in an effort to inject some economic sanity and public-health common sense into the diminutive doctor's wrecking operation.[39]

largely to the malign influence of Big Pharma, wild-eyed at the thought of tens of billions in profits, and Anthony Fauci, eager to test mRNA vaccines on tens of millions of unsuspecting subjects—doctors were ordered not to prescribe them.[41]

The only solution, Fauci told us on March 15, 2020, was for the entire country to go into lockdown,[42] which meant leaving (losing) your job, closing your business, picking up your kids from school for the last time, and then going home and locking yourself in. At the outset he warned us that we might have to "hunker down" in this way for "several months." But by early April he was saying that the lockdown would have to continue until there were no "new cases" of coronavirus.[43] That is to say, indefinitely.

For many Americans, it was nothing short of an open-ended sentence of house arrest. Yet Fauci was absolutely insistent, in interview after interview, that we had to make this collective sacrifice. Over and over again he demanded that the lockdown continue, warning that "suffering and death" awaited America if it opened too soon.[44]

Fauci was all over the media all the time with this grim message.

The entire country panicked, especially the Democratic governors in blue states. Following Fauci's advice, they abused their authority to impose unheard of restrictions on Americans' liberty. They put job-killing lockdowns in place, along with a whole host of other new rules. People were allowed out of their homes only to buy "essentials" such as food, hand sanitizer, and toilet paper, and only at their local big-box store—the only place they could shop anyway, since the mom-and-pop stores were padlocked. You could not visit your elderly mother in the seniors' home, see your sick friend in the hospital, or even spend time with God in his churches, which were also closed.

Few dared question Fauci's dictates. He was assumed to be the voice of scientific rationality. Surely, most people apparently thought, he must have reams of scientific evidence to back up the claims he was making—about the lethality of the coronavirus, about the ease of its spread, about masks, social distancing, and testing—to justify such draconian restrictions on their lives. Those who questioned him were questioning science itself, Fauci declared loftily.[45]

Most of us felt that we had no choice but to go along. America's leading infectious disease expert had assured us that it was either his way or the graveyard. To avoid breathing our last in a hospital room locked away from our families, dying a slow painful death from the twenty-first-century equivalent of the bubonic plague, we all dutifully kept our homes shuttered against the killer virus lurking outside. As weeks went by with no end in sight, Fauci continued to demand that the shutdown be extended.[46] In May, when President Trump began praising states that were reopening after the prolonged lockdown, Fauci doubled down, warning of the danger that awaited Americans if they ventured outside too soon.[47]

Liberty Lost

Those who violated the quarantine had the full weight of the law dropped upon them. An elderly barber in Michigan was cited by police, required to defend himself in court for the crime of cutting hair, and had his license yanked when he persisted in trying to earn a living.[48] A salon operator in Texas was humiliated by a judge for having dared to defy a local lockdown order.[49] A Maine restaurant owner had his business license revoked by his governor for daring to serve food—outdoors.[50]

The governors of red states such as Georgia who wanted to allow their people to go back to work were accused in a hate-filled screed in the left-leaning magazine *The Atlantic* of conducting an "experiment in human sacrifice."[51] If the governors of such states let their people out of lockdown, the magazine warned, they would jeopardize the public health of the entire nation. Fauci himself endorsed this view, saying on April 3 that the entire country "really should be" under a stay-at-home order and that he didn't "understand" why it wasn't.[52]

But the real vitriol was reserved for those who dared to come out and protest the Fauci-inspired lockdowns in places such as New York, California, Virginia, and Michigan. These crowds of normal Americans who simply wanted to get on with their lives were attacked as "racists," "fascists," and "extremists." Their overwhelmingly peaceful protests had nothing whatsoever to do with racism or fascism, of course, and everything to do with the way they were being deprived of their liberty. This distinction was ignored by the Left and its media attack dogs, who instantly resorted to name-calling.

The real extremists were politicians such as Michigan governor Gretchen Whitmer, who, as The Political Insider reported, "want[ed] to extend" the lockdown "to punish protestors" who were discontented by her bizarre orders.[53] How dare the deplorables disobey her dictates?

These tremendous infringements on our liberty were possible only because our white-coated scientific savior, Dr. Anthony Fauci, had solemnly informed us that they were absolutely necessary. He could save us from this pestilence, he intimated, but only if we heard and obeyed his Delphic voice.

Some Protests Are More Equal than Others

Then, on May 25, 2020, an African American man named George Floyd died in Minneapolis, Minnesota, while being arrested by the police. Urged on by the leftist media and Democratic politicians, and fueled by anarchists, Antifa, and Black Lives Matter activists, people who had been confined to their homes for weeks surged out into the streets. City after city saw huge crowds of protesters flowing down city streets practically touching one another. Not only that, they were chanting at the top of their lungs, potentially releasing clouds of China Virus into the surrounding air that others would breathe in. It was Fauci's worst nightmare. Everything that he had achieved with his dire warnings was being swept away in an instant in an orgy of anger.

In the starkest display of hypocrisy I have seen—and we live in an age of hypocrisy—the same politicians who had been ordering everyone to stay home now took to the streets in solidarity with the demonstrators. Even Governor Whitmer blew off her own stay-at-home order to march with the protesters.[54] One week she's throwing the book at a self-employed barber for not social distancing,[55] and the next she's mixing and mingling with thousands of people.[56] And she was not the only one.

I expected Fauci to instantly take to the airwaves to sternly denounce this reckless behavior and to call upon the nation's governors to reimpose the lockdowns. The demonstrators would be ordered back into their homes and told to once again shelter in place lest they unleash a "second wave" of the China Virus upon the land. The governors would be told to ensure that those few who are allowed to go out must continue to wear masks, practice social distancing, and, above all, not congregate in large groups. Or so I thought.

But the man who had been constantly hectoring us suddenly went silent. Instead of haranguing this wave of demonstrators—the way he had harangued those protesting against the loss of their liberties to the lockdowns—about the danger that their activities posed to themselves and others, he simply fell off the radar. For two long weeks, as tens of thousands of demonstrators continued to march through the streets of dozens of American cities, he remained hidden from public view.

There can only be one explanation for the difference. Obviously, in Fauci's eyes, some protesters were more equal than others. When small business owners and liberty-loving deplorables in red and blue states alike broke quarantine, he hyperventilated over their lack of social responsibility and predicted epidemiological disaster.[57] But when the elite media and

Democratic politicians not only sanctioned protests but actually participated in them, he looked the other way.

Fauci claimed to be an objective, unbiased scientist. Eventually, he would go so far as to identify himself with science itself, declaring in June 2021, "Attacks on me, quite frankly, are attacks on science."[58] But his silent approval of the Black Lives Matter demonstrations the year before had made it obvious that he was playing politics with people's health.[59] Senator Tom Cotton called Fauci "a Democratic activist in a white lab coat," which seems a fairly apt description of the diminutive lab rat.[60] And Dr. Fauci was only one of the numerous left-wing ideologues who made it clear that they were cloaking their political opinions in the mantle of science by condoning the BLM protests. Those were the phrases Betsy McCaughey used to call out hypocritical "experts" who "proposed a draconian lockdown without assessing its side effects on the rest of us. They demanded rigorous adherence to it, until suddenly they decided marching against racism was more important than preventing virus deaths. Americans won't forget."[61]

Fauci seems to have made a habit of bending science to his own political ends. This may have been why, at the very beginning of the pandemic, he promoted a model from the Imperial College London that predicted millions of deaths in the United States. It later turned out that the model, authored by the now disgraced Professor Neil Ferguson, was "highly flawed"[62]—which is a polite way of saying that it was algorithmic garbage, a fact that America's most famous virologist apparently only discovered at the same time the rest of us did. In other words, the man we had trusted to make critical decisions about the entire country didn't even bother to do his homework.

Much of the actual science seems to have eluded our white-coated savior as well. He often expressed conflicting opinions about the China Virus itself. He didn't know how lethal it was. He didn't know how contagious it was. He didn't know whether it could be spread asymptomatically, whether wearing masks could help contain it, or whether it was possible to be reinfected. He was all over the map on whether there would be a second wave. He didn't know—or he couldn't stick to his story.[63]

Fauci did not let his ignorance (or deliberate obfuscation) of essential facts stop him from recommending in mid-March—again on the basis of the Imperial College's sham model—that the economy of the entire country be shut down indefinitely, 40 million people be put out of work, tens of millions of children be denied an education, and millions of "non-essential" small businesses be shuttered, many never to reopen.

One by one, all of his predictions came to naught. Millions of Americans did not, in fact, die of the virus. Actually, as the numbers came in, the mortality rate of the China Virus kept dropping until it bottomed out at a fraction of 1 percent, more in line with the Asian Flu of 1958 than the Spanish Flu of 1918. Yet throughout the two years of the pandemic, Dr. Fauci remained indifferent to the tremendous human cost of his policies. He didn't seem to notice that the China Virus wasn't the only thing killing Americans, and that maybe destroying the economy and closing schools wasn't the best approach. He put tens of millions of Americans through hell on the basis of a flawed model and a complete misunderstanding of the nature of the thing he is supposed to be an expert on: viruses.

Error Prone

Under Dr. Anthony Fauci's influence, the U.S. Coronavirus Task Force committed every epidemiological error in the book. Among his mistakes were:

MISTAKES ON CONTACT TRACING: At the outset of the U.S. outbreak, Fauci insisted on contact tracing. An enormous amount of valuable time and resources were wasted trying to track down every last person who *might* have come into contact with every person who *might* have had Covid.

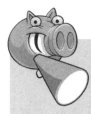

Then and Now: Dr. Fauci

As Dr. Anthony Fauci snaked his way through the pandemic, his twists and turns on masks, vaccines, natural immunity, therapeutics, and more made him the subject of mockery in many quarters. But the flipping and flopping of the longtime NIAID director was really no laughing matter. These are all issues that have deeply divided the country. Even worse, they cost hundreds of thousands of lives.

Fauci vs. Fauci on Masks: According to emails obtained by BuzzFeed, Fauci did not believe that the ordinary paper masks that most people wear offered any protection to healthy people from catching Covid.[64] As he candidly told Sylvia Burwell, the former secretary of the U.S. Department of Health and Human Services, in a February 2020 email: "Masks are really for infected people to prevent them from spreading infection to people who are not infected rather than protecting uninfected people from acquiring infection. The typical mask you buy in the drug store is not really effective in keeping out virus, which is small enough to pass through the material."[65]

He said that same thing in a March 8, 2020, interview on *60 Minutes*, assuring people, "There's no reason to be walking around with a mask. When you're in the middle of an outbreak, wearing a mask might make people feel a little bit better and it might even block a droplet, but it's not providing the perfect protection that people think that it is.

And, often, there are unintended consequences—people keep fiddling with the mask and they keep touching their face."[66]

But a month later he was singing a different tune, insisting that masks should be worn "in public settings when around people outside their household, especially when social distancing measures are difficult to maintain." When he was called on the contradiction a full year later—for a long time no one dared question the pronouncements of Saint Fauci—he claimed he had been simply trying to prevent people from buying up masks and depriving medical professionals of the much-needed supplies.[67] His diminishing number of defenders called this a "noble lie." But whatever his motivation, he had actually been telling the truth at the outset. It was only after he realized that masks could be *weaponized for political gain* that he began to dissemble.

Once Fauci had decided that he would force everyone to wear face coverings, he went all in. Soon he was recommending wearing not just one, but two masks. Here is Fauci in January 2021: "So if you have a physical covering with one layer, you put another layer on, it just makes common sense that it likely would be more effective."[68] (*Why not three or four masks?* wags asked. *Or ten? Or a hazmat suit for everyone?*)

The following month Fauci warned that Americans might still need to wear face masks through the end of 2022 to protect against emerging Covid variants.[69] (Or whatever other superbug might emerge from one of the gain-of-function labs he funded in China, I am tempted to add.[70])

But by then the widely detested masks were being used not to keep the virus from spreading—a task which they performed poorly, if at all, studies showed[71]—but to get the vaccine into the arms of the hesitant. "Get the jab, ditch the mask," was the new refrain. As the Centers for Disease Control promised on May 13, 2021, "People vaccinated against Covid-19 can go without masks indoors and outdoors."[72]

The CDC was even clearer on the connection between masks and vaccines in its July 27, 2021, updated guidance:

> If you are fully vaccinated, you can resume activities that you did prior to the pandemic.
>
> Fully vaccinated people can resume activities *without wearing a mask* or physically distancing, except where required by federal, state, local, tribal, or territorial laws, rules, and regulations, including local business and workplace guidance.
>
> If you haven't been vaccinated yet, find a vaccine. [Emphasis added.]

The message was clear: Americans would be gagged until they submitted to the jab.

Fauci vs. Fauci on Natural Immunity: When oncologist Dr. Zeke Emanuel, who had been a health advisor in the Obama administration, privately asked Fauci via email if people who had recovered from Covid-19 were immune to getting the virus again, Fauci replied in the affirmative: "No evidence in this regard, but you would assume that there would be substantial immunity post infection."[73]

That would be a safe assumption, since every major pandemic in human history, from smallpox and the bubonic plague to the Spanish Flu and the Asian Flu, has been ended by natural immunity. As a virologist, Fauci knew quite well that the survivors of these plagues had lived fearlessly ever after, since they now possessed lifetime immunity.

But in public Fauci flipped the script and spread fear and uncertainty. He told Americans who had had Covid that they still needed to get the vaccine.[74] People who had had Covid should get at least one dose of the vaccine,[75] he said on numerous occasions, suggesting that the vaccine might give them more protection from "highly contagious variants."[76]

We now know that people who have recovered from Covid-19 have robust natural immunity to the virus, which means that they generally don't need to be vaccinated for it.[77] The CDC admitted that it had no records of a recovered person infecting another person.[78]

According to CDC guidelines, "Contact tracing will be conducted for close contacts (any individual within 6 feet of an infected person for a total of 15 minutes or more) of laboratory-confirmed or probable COVID-19 patients."[79] Fauci actually arranged Zoom calls with groups of hundreds of "contact tracers" to give them pep talks.[80]

For sexually transmitted diseases such as HIV/AIDs, syphilis, and gonorrhea, tracing and treating contacts is very effective in disease prevention. For a highly infectious airborne viral infection, however, it was a criminal misuse of public health resources that did nothing to stop the spread of the disease.[81] That's why we've never tried to prevent the spread of commonly circulating influenzas using contact tracing, even though they kill an average of twenty thousand Americans each year, and sometimes, as in the Hong Kong Flu of 1968, up to one hundred thousand or more.

MISTAKES ON PROTECTING THE ELDERLY: As the China Virus produced a cascade of corpses in geriatric Italy, but merely gave the young the sniffles, it was already clear by early March 2020 which demographic was at high risk. The vulnerability of the elderly was shockingly confirmed in the following weeks by the speed at which the virus decimated the population of long-term-care centers in New York City and New Jersey—its spread accelerated by Governor Andrew Cuomo's insane policy of confining the sick with the healthy.[82]

At the same time, the evidence showed that the mortality risk was dramatically lower in younger age cohorts, and that for the very young the risk approximated zero. For children, as the Great Barrington Declaration pointed out, "Covid-19 is less dangerous than many other harms, including influenza."[83]

From the beginning, public health professionals such as Scott Atlas, who joined the Coronavirus Task Force in August 2020, tried to get Fauci to focus on protecting the vulnerable. The idea of "focused protection" was to let young, low-risk populations carry on with their lives and naturally become infected with a virus that—to them—posed little or no threat, while protecting those at high risk.

Fauci rejected this sensible idea out of hand, arguing that it would be impossible to protect the elderly, the obese, and others with health problems who live outside of nursing homes.[84] As an immunologist who had spent his professional life working on viruses and vaccines in a lab, he had no idea how to implement "focused protection" and was unwilling even to listen to those who did. When Scott Atlas and other public health scientists tried to lay out how such a program could be successfully carried out—and, in fact, was being carried out in places like Taiwan and Sweden—Fauci publicly attacked their ideas as "nonsense and very dangerous."[85]

How many lives could have been saved if vaccination efforts had been quickly targeted at those over sixty who had not yet contracted and recovered from Covid, instead of being delayed and dissipated in a scattershot effort to vaccinate every man, woman, and child in America?[86]

MISTAKES ON MASKING: As we have seen, Fauci was against masks before he was for them. His flip-flop on mask mandates flies in the face of the science. Two randomized studies on the efficacy of masks have been carried out, and neither suggests that masks work. A study carried out in Denmark concluded that masking offered no statistically significant protection against Covid.[87] A later study in Bangladesh suggested that masks reduced transmission between 0 and 18 percent. If masks are of little benefit to adults who are at some risk from Covid, as these studies show, they are of even less benefit to children, who are at almost no risk from the disease.

MISTAKES ON CLOSING THE SCHOOLS: From the first, Fauci was calling for nationwide school closures.[88] On March 12, 2020, for example, he said, "One thing I do advise . . . [is] mitigation. And what was done when you close the schools is mitigation."[89] And he did not hesitate to criticize those who questioned his prescriptions, as when he slammed Florida's governor Ron DeSantis on April 13 for merely remarking that he wanted to get schools back open as soon as possible. Fauci responded by saying that opening the schools would get children infected with the coronavirus. "If you have a situation where you don't have real good control over an outbreak and you allow children together, they will likely get infected," Fauci insisted.[90]

Few dared to question the all-knowing Dr. Fauci in those days, but the proper response to his fearmongering about infections among children would have been: So what if children get infected? Their risk of dying from the China Virus is effectively zero, far lower than their risk of dying from the seasonal flu, which itself is minuscule. And in fact schools, which are hotbeds of transmission for the annual influenza, turned out not to be hotbeds of transmission for Covid.[91]

We know this because not every country shut down its schools in a panic when the China Virus hit. Sweden, for instance, kept its schools and daycares open throughout 2020. Neither did it mandate any testing, masks, or social distancing for its nearly 2 million students and preschoolers ages one to nineteen. Neighboring Finland did follow the "Fauci protocol," closing its schools and testing widely—*and it made absolutely no difference.* Sweden's Public Health Agency later compared the two approaches and concluded, "Severe Covid-19 disease as measured in ICU admittance is very rare in both countries in this age group and no deaths were reported. Outbreak investigations in Finland has [*sic*] not shown children to be contributing much in terms of transmission and in Sweden a report comparing risk of Covid-19 in different professions showed no increased risk for teachers."[92]

In a final slap in the face to Fauci, the Swedish agency reported: "Closing of schools had no measurable effect on the number of cases of Covid-19 among children."[93]

The Swedish study suggests that closing America's schools did not save lives of either students or teachers. But it did have a measurable effect on both the academic performance and the emotional health of children—both destructive. Many children went a year with virtually no schooling or social interaction at all, suffering severe learning losses that will stunt their lives and even shorten their lifespans.[94]

As professors Martin Kulldorff and Jay Bhattacharya wrote at the end of 2021, "Considering the devastating effects of school closures on children, Dr. Fauci's advocacy for school closures may be the single biggest mistake of his career."[95]

MISTAKES ON LOCKDOWNS: Anthony Fauci's "original pandemic sin," as it might be called, was convincing President Trump that he had no choice but to put the entire country under lockdown. Relying upon the faulty computer model produced by now-disgraced Neil Ferguson of the U.K.'s Imperial College, he told the president that without a society-wide lockdown to slow the spread of the coronavirus, 2.2 million Americans would die over the next three months, and 65 million people worldwide. As Ellen Sauerbrey pointed out at American Thinker, Ferguson had previously predicted "that up to 200 million people could be killed from bird flu," whereas "[t]he actual number was several hundred." And he had ventured "an estimate of 65,000 deaths from the Swine Flu in the U.K.," but U.K. deaths actually topped out at five hundred, meaning that he was off by a factor of more than a hundred.[96]

Then and Now: No Christians Need Apply

From the Antonine Plague onward, Christians have always been on the front lines, risking their own lives caring for the sick and the dying. When the third outbreak of the Black Death hit Siena in 1374, city officials fled, but the great St. Catherine of Siena stayed behind with her Christian companions to open hospices and care for the sick. The Crown encouraged the churches to stay open in Daniel Defoe's London during the plague year of 1665, and the pews were filled with people seeking solace there.

★ ★ ★

A China Virus Success Story

We would have been far better off if we had followed Taiwan's example.

Taiwan lies only about a hundred miles off the Chinese coast, and its economy is more closely intertwined with the Communist giant's than any other country's. From the island's airports you can fly directly to every major Chinese city, including, of course, Wuhan.

Yet despite huge cross-border traffic with neighboring China, the 24 million people of this island nation remained virtually free of the Wuhan Flu in 2020, suffering only seven deaths. A second wave in 2021 was quickly controlled, and Taiwan remained among the countries with the lowest number of confirmed cases and deaths per million from the China Virus.[97] Only China, which fabricates its numbers, and some countries in sub-Saharan Africa where the anti-malarial drug hydroxychloroquine (HCQ) is in everyday use as a malaria prophylactic, reported lower numbers.

In other words, Taiwan stopped the deadly invader from China in its tracks. How is that even possible? One reason is that the democratically elected government of Taiwan reacted to the epidemic in Wuhan promptly, imposing a travel ban on foreign nationals on January 19, 2020. Over the next few weeks, it put in place no fewer than 124 sensible mitigation measures without, however, ever imposing a nationwide lockdown.[98] Then, in early 2021, in a decision that flew in the face of the WHO's "strong advice" against using HCQ for the treatment or prevention of Covid-19,[99] Taiwan's Food and Drug Administration distributed massive amounts of the drug to more than 6,600 community pharmacies around the island for free.[100]

The picture with regard to vaccines is much more mixed. Vaccines were slow to be accepted by the people on Taiwan, many of whom felt that the risk of an adverse reaction outweighed the benefit of protection from a coronavirus that seemed to be under control and posed little threat to their health.[101] Their concerns were validated soon after the vaccination campaign got underway in earnest in April 2021, as reports of adverse reactions began to come in. By October, the number of people who had died after their Covid-19 vaccination—865— had exceeded the number of deaths from the virus itself, which stood at only 845.[102]

One final point: Democratic Taiwan, which is always alert to threats from Communist China, is the canary in the coal mine that can tip us off about future CCP viruses and pandemics. It is not just a scandal that opposition from China has kept Taiwan out of the WHO; it endangers global health—and that means everyone's.

During the China Virus, however, the secular authorities not only kept chaplains and ministers out of hospitals, but locked Christians out of their churches as well. Democratic governors used the cover of the pandemic to impose a sanitary dictatorship on their people—and to shut down all activities they disapproved of, which turned out to include going to church or synagogue.[103]

But the hysterical, fearmongering projection had its desired effect. Urged on by Fauci, on March 16, 2020, President Trump announced "15 days to slow the spread."[104] But the two weeks stretched into months. And the drastic restrictions placed on work, schools, and social gatherings worked their predictable results: a massive destruction of commerce, the loss of tens of millions of jobs, and a rise in non-Covid-related deaths. Moreover, as public health experts Kulldorff and Bhattacharya note, "After more than 700,000 reported COVID deaths in America, we now know that lockdowns failed to protect high-risk older people."[105]

America was not the only country that followed the China model of hard-core lockdowns to deal with the disease. The political and professional classes in many countries in Europe and Asia imported the same totalitarian "public health" regime from China, with the same dismal results—high mortality rates and economic devastation.

MISTAKES ON NATURAL IMMUNITY: Perhaps one day Fauci will tell us why, throughout the last half of 2020 and 2021, he ignored, dismissed, and even ridiculed the idea that those who had recovered from the China Virus had acquired natural immunity. This wasn't the way he was talking at the outset of the pandemic, and not just in private emails to political allies such as Zeke Emanual.

In a March 2020 interview with Trevor Noah of Comedy Central, for example, Fauci asserted that it was highly likely that those who had been infected with the coronavirus were now immune. "Tests haven't confirmed it yet," said Fauci, "but I feel really confident that if *this virus acts like every*

★ ★ ★

HIV/AIDS: Lessons Learned . . . and Lost

The most deadly viral pandemic of the past half century is HIV/AIDS, which killed an estimated 36 million people worldwide from 1981 to 2020—far more people than Covid ever will.[106] Unlike Covid, HIV/AIDS is a disease of the young that radically shortens human lifespans.

HIV/AIDs is a disease that is spread primarily by people who have no symptoms of the disease, that has infected up to 100 million people to date, that has a high mortality rate, and for which there was—and is—no known cure. It was clear at the outset that it was primarily spread by sexual intercourse, but at the time there was widespread public concern that it could be transmitted by more casual contact as well in public bathrooms or public transportation.

Yet despite the seriousness of the pandemic, the public health authorities did not engage in mass testing; testing even in high-risk groups such as homosexuals, prostitutes, and the highly promiscuous remained entirely voluntary. Those who tested positive were not placed under any sort of restrictions, much less quarantine. The public health authorities of the time, far from sowing panic as Fauci so often did in the 2020–2021 Covid crisis, sought to damp down public concern.

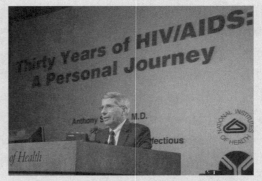

Dr. Fauci gives a talk: "Thirty Years of HIV/AIDs: A Personal Journey." *National Institute of Allergy and Infectious Diseases*

Billions of dollars were spent in a massive effort to develop an effective vaccine. But careful long-term trials showed that none was effective in creating an immunity to HIV/AIDS.[107] Over time, however, effective antiretroviral therapy (ART) was developed that, regularly taken, enables sufferers to live with the infection and enjoy a near-normal life expectancy.

Then the China Virus came along, and all of the lessons we had learned from our decades-long effort to defeat HIV/AIDS went down the memory hole, seemingly forgotten by those in charge of the nation's public health.

other virus that we know, once you get infected, get better, clear the virus, then you'll have immunity that will prevent you from reinfection" [emphasis added].[108]

You don't have to be an immunologist like Fauci to know this, of course. As we saw in chapter 1, medical practitioners have known about natural immunity since at least the time of the Antonine Plague that began in AD 165—in other words, for a very long time. Everyone who's had high school biology knows about natural immunity from disease.

Once Fauci went all in for mandatory vaccination of every man, woman, and child in the United States, however, natural immunity became an inconvenient truth. Paradoxically, this was at the very time that evidence was accumulating that acquired immunity provided long-lasting and robust protection from reinfection. A study out of Israel, for example, showed that the vaccinated were twenty-seven (!) times as likely to be reinfected with the China Virus as the unvaccinated who had recovered from a prior infection.[109] Fauci pushed forward with his mandates regardless, even though disaster awaited.

CHAPTER 9

A Pandemonium of Errors

Unlike the authorities in China, Australia, and New Zealand, who from the beginning of the pandemic were monomaniacally focused on eradicating the China Virus from within their borders, Anthony Fauci never explicitly endorsed "Covid Zero." But he came close.

His initial weapons of choice against the virus were masks, social distancing, and especially lockdowns. And it is true that if you kept everyone under house arrest for weeks on end, preventing them from coming into contact with others, the virus would be unable to find new hosts and would presumably die off.

Once Fauci believed that he had an effective vaccine on hand, he grew even more certain that he could defeat the virus. He began insisting, for example on May 20, 2021, that the vaccines could not just contain Covid, but could "essentially eliminate" it. In an interview with the *Washington Post*, he laid out how this could be accomplished: "With good vaccination programs, [nations could] essentially eliminate the presence of a particular pathogen. . . . That's called elimination, and the other is control [which means] you have a very, very low level in the community. . . . With Sars-CoV-2 and with Covid-19, I would hope it would be much closer to elimination than just control."[1]

And in Fauci's view, mandates were an integral part of a good vaccination program. As he told NBC News on September 10, 2021, "We hope when those mandates get implemented it would also trigger a number of people to voluntarily come forward to get vaccinated, because we can end this. We have the capability and the resources to end it. We just got to get people to step up and get vaccinated."[2]

This is very close to what we might call the Covid Zero Fantasy—the idea that you can "shut down the virus" by some clever combination of government restrictions and vaccine mandates.[3]

But Fauci's fantasy that Covid could be "essentially eliminated" caused enormous collateral damage, both to public health and to the economy. The prevention and treatment of other diseases was sidelined, while the cost in terms of non-health-care-related goods and services ran into the trillions of dollars. Moreover, for multiple reasons having to do with the China Virus itself, eliminating Covid was an impractical goal from the outset, which is why it was finally abandoned—as of November 28, 2021, even Dr. Fauci was saying that the virus was "not going to go away"[4]—although not before havoc was wreaked on people's lives and livelihoods for the better part of two years.

The "Covid Zero" Fantasy: The Impossible Dream

Consider that the seasonal flu is still with us, despite vaccination campaigns stretching back decades. The problem is not only that it is highly contagious, making it easy for it to escape quarantine, but also that it plays a kind of musical chairs with us: multiple strains descended from the Spanish Flu are circulating in humanity, and we never know what strains are going to predominate from year to year when the music stops each fall. The China Virus, with its proliferating variants, creates a similar problem, preventing a one-size-fits-all vaccine defense. The buzz about annual boosters[5] does not suggest that we are going to be "essentially eliminating" it any time soon—or ever.

Consider that the plague bacillus, *Yersinia pestis*—which caused the Plague of Justinian, the Black Death, the Yunnan Plague, and countless localized epidemics through the centuries—is also still with us. And, as we saw in chapter 4, because plague-carrying rodents were able to hitch a ride on human transport, *Y. pestis* now has natural reservoirs in animal populations in countries around the world. Cases of the plague now occur not just in China, its original home, but in places like Madagascar and other African countries, and even occasionally in the United States. Unless you were able to eliminate all these natural reservoirs, which would entail a vast slaughter of rodents and other animals of all kinds, you will never entirely eradicate the plague.

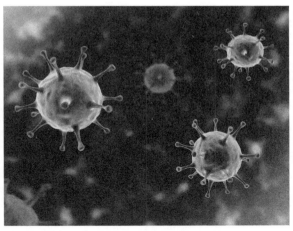

The Covid Zero fantasy. *Courtesy of Katarina Carrano, using an illustration of the Covid spike protein created by Alissa Eckert and Dan Higgins*

Finally, despite a century-long effort to develop a vaccine for the plague bacillus, these vaccines remain, much like the vaccines for Covid, limited in both effectiveness and duration. The bubonic plague was brought under control by therapeutic drugs, in this case antibiotics, and by public health measures such as putting bounties on rats, not by vaccines.

Smallpox posed none of these problems. It had no natural reservoir other than human beings. The vaccine worked so well that it provided almost complete immunity from the disease for up to a decade. Even mild breakthrough cases were rare post-vaccination, and severe cases requiring hospitalization were almost unknown. Because the vaccine was so effective, short-term quarantines, rather than long-term lockdowns, were sufficient to curb the spread of the disease. Even with all these advantages, the eradication campaign lasted decades and required a synchronized global effort. It was also very expensive, but even poor nations willingly collaborated because the disease, with a mortality rate of 30 percent, was so devastating.

The China Virus, on the other hand, poses all of these problems in spades. The China Virus has infected not just people since 2019, but also animal populations with which we have been in close contact—and the animals can now presumably return the favor. To get to Covid Zero we would need to eliminate not only rats—which pretty much everyone would be happy to do—but our beloved pets as well. Millions of dogs, cats, guinea pigs, and so forth would have to be euthanized, not to mention any other natural animal reservoirs we happened to discover along the way. Horses? Sheep? Cows?

Then there are the Covid vaccines which, unlike the smallpox vaccine, seem to be practically useless at preventing the spread of the disease.[6] Given the absence of a long-term highly efficacious vaccine, the China Virus could only be eliminated by simultaneously imposed global lockdown that might have to continue for years. The collateral damage from such an effort would be colossal, far outweighing any conceivable benefit from eliminating a virus that, with an infection fatality rate (IFR) of below 0.3 percent, is less than one-hundredth as lethal as smallpox.[7]

Those in charge of public health policy in the United States in the Covid era should also take note of the fact that Covid Zero policies have been tried in three countries—China, New Zealand, and Australia—and have failed in each case.

Communist China, with its brutal lockdown program in Wuhan, was the first out of the gate. On January 23, 2020, the entire population of the city was ordered at gunpoint to stay inside their homes for forty days. Many other cities were put under lockdown in the days following. Anyone with symptoms of Covid was rounded up and taken by force to hastily built "hospitals" that were in fact internment camps. Those who dared venture out in violation of quarantine, often in search of food, were welded back inside their apartments as punishment, often to starve. The effect on the physical and mental health of the population was devastating. To give just one example, by the end of the lockdown people were literally jumping off

★ ★ ★

Zero Covid in China—or Not

China, ground zero of the pandemic and the most populous country in the world, reported ridiculously low numbers throughout. As of November 9, 2021, for instance, its total reported cases of Covid—97,885—placed it down at country number 114 in the rankings of case rates, right between tiny Rwanda and Jamaica. But the real eye-opener was its claim, endlessly repeated by Western media, that over the entire course of the pandemic it had suffered only 7 cases and less than one death per 100,000 population.[8]

If these numbers were accurate, we would be forced to conclude that, whatever the human cost of the draconian lockdowns, China's pursuit of Covid Zero had been a spectacular success. These are, after all, by far the lowest case fatality rates and mortality rates reported by any major country. In fact, *they are the lowest case and mortality rates in the entire world* except for five tiny island nations in the South Pacific. If we were Jacinda Ardern or Tony Fauci, we might conclude that Beijing's top-down lockdowns were even worthy of emulation to some degree.

That would be a mistake. China's numbers were nothing more than a propaganda exercise intended to deceive the gullible.[9]

The reality on the ground in China could be seen in the smoke boiling out of the chimneys of Wuhan's crematoria, in the skyrocketing demand for funeral urns, and in the tears of the masses of people mourning their dead on the Qing Ming festival, the April day that the Chinese traditionally visit the graves of their ancestors.[10]

Yet some in the West suffer from bizarre blind spots where Communist systems are concerned.[11] The leftist editors of *The Guardian* in the United Kingdom, for instance, were happy to regurgitate Communist propaganda to score cheap political points against their domestic opponents. As late as October 2021 they claimed, "Since the first coronavirus cases were reported nearly two years ago, China has run a zero-tolerance Covid policy. Its success in preventing the virus from spreading across the vast country *serves as a stark contrast to the situations in many western countries*. Since last year, fewer than 100,000 cases have been officially recorded, among a population of about 1.4 billion" [emphasis added].[12]

Rated: Pants on Fire.

the balconies of high-rise apartment buildings to escape quarantine in the only way they could: by dying.

By March 13, 2020, Communist China was touting the success of its lockdown, claiming that only eleven new cases had been discovered in all of China, and that all but four of those had been brought in by travelers from the United States, Italy, and Saudi Arabia.[13] Then, just six days later, on March 19, it proudly announced to the world that its draconian lockdown had achieved its goal: not a single new domestic case of the virus had been found within its borders.[14] The Wuhan Flu had been completely eradicated. With the exception of a few infected foreigners who had brought the virus with them (and were being quarantined at their own expense), China had achieved Covid Zero. China's brutal, top-to-bottom quarantine had worked—or so Beijing claimed.

I could have told Jacinda Ardern, the prime minister of New Zealand, that the pathological liars who govern Communist China were not telling the truth. Among other pieces of evidence, the eighty-four ovens in Wuhan's seven crematoria were still incinerating corpses day and night at that point.[15] More broadly, statistics out of China were always based on political calculations rather than straightforward math. But the prime minister didn't ask me. She bought into China's lie that it had eradicated the virus—and decided that she would adopt the exact same policies in her island nation of 4.2 million people.[16] After all, the World Health Organization was repeatedly congratulating China on its successes.[17]

On March 19, 2020, the same day China bragged about reaching Covid Zero, New Zealand's Ardern began putting in place the most drastic lockdown that the Western world has ever seen. She began by closing New Zealand's borders to all but returning New Zealanders. By March 25 she had closed all the schools and imposed a national lockdown on all businesses except supermarkets, gas stations, and hospitals. Aside from essential workers, everyone was ordered to isolate themselves at home—and to keep careful watch on their neighbors, reporting any isolation breaches or illegal business openings to the New Zealand Police. To enforce the harsh lockdown, a controversial law authorizing warrantless house searches by the police was passed.[18]

Australia, once a proud member of the Free World, also imposed a dark dystopia on its population in the name of public health.[19] "Fortress Australia" slammed its borders shut on March 20, 2020, and required returning citizens to spend two weeks in supervised quarantine. Then the Australian states and territories followed suit, closing their borders to outsiders. On March 29, a restriction on all gatherings—indoor or outdoor—of more than two people was put in place.[20] Schools were closed, and most businesses were shuttered.

A large contact-tracing force was recruited to track down and quarantine anyone suspected of having been exposed to the virus. The police were on high alert for anyone who dared stay outside for more than the allotted one hour per day, or who ventured more than the legally permitted three miles from home. In Sydney, Australia's largest city, the military was brought in to help enforce the rules. Hectoring health officials cautioned people to avoid dangerous activities such as chatting with neighbors.[21]

Initially, the efforts to achieve Covid Zero seemed to be successful in both island nations. By shutting off arrivals, and by hunting down and killing the virus by—literally—imprisoning those who carried it, the authorities were able to achieve a decline in the number of cases. In May of 2020 Ardern announced that because New Zealand had reached Covid Zero she was partially lifting the lockdown. However, the police continued to carry out warrantless house-to-house searches to hunt down any secret carriers.

Case numbers in Australia declined as well, with only two reported for the State of Victoria on June 6, 2020, the lowest total since the beginning of the outbreak[22]—and, as it happened, the low-water mark of the entire pandemic.

Both countries began to relax their lockdowns and allow life to get back to near normal. The media and even some scientific journals celebrated their success. Prematurely, as it turned out.

For as soon as people were allowed to circulate, the virus did too, as it would again and again in both countries over the next two years. Australia and New Zealand have been in and out of lockdowns more than any other countries in the world outside of openly totalitarian states like China and North Korea. And over time, formerly quiescent populations have become increasingly restive.

New Zealand's Ardern locked down the entire country again on August 17, 2021, because a single China Virus case had been detected. It was the first and only locally transmitted Covid-19 case in the country since February, but that didn't matter. Everyone had to suffer harsh lockdowns and aggressive contact tracing.[23]

In the face of increasing public resistance and climbing infection rates, Ardern finally acknowledged that Covid could never be completely eradicated. She abandoned her Zero Covid policy on October 4, 2021, and lifted some restrictions—"You can now go to beaches and parks," she decreed—but warned the lockdowns would be completely lifted only when 90 percent of the population had been vaccinated.[24]

Across the Tasman Sea, protests had become a regular feature of life in Australian cities such as Sydney and Melbourne by mid-2021. These were brutally put down by the police, who in one unforgettable encounter shot fleeing protesters in the back with rubber bullets. In a further escalation, the military was brought in to patrol the streets and maintain order.[25]

Stories like these brought the insanity into focus:

- August 22, 2021: "Rescue dogs shot dead by New South Wales council due to Covid-19 restrictions." Volunteers from the nearest animal shelter had been forbidden to drive to pick them up.[26]
- September 18, 2021: "Police prevent mourners from watching funerals from their cars." The grieving family members

stayed in their cars some distance away with the windows rolled up, but they were still arrested for violating the rules on "gatherings."[27]

- October 18, 2021: "Police in Australia shake coffee cup to check Covid-19 rules being followed." A policemen grabbed the coffee cup of a maskless man sitting on a park bench to make sure he was actually drinking coffee—and not violating the mask mandate.[28]

Australia eventually had to throw in the towel, with Prime Minister Scott Morrison announcing that it was time to leave lockdowns and "come out of the cave." "With vaccinations accelerating," he said, "Australians will soon live with the virus." It was a tacit admission that Covid Zero had failed.[29]

If the two island nations, one small and one continent-sized, could not achieve Covid Zero, then it is obviously beyond the reach of other nations. Even if every country on earth locked down at the same time, and stayed locked down until such time as everyone sick with Covid had recovered, this would only eliminate the China Virus from humanity. A single encounter with an animal reservoir named Fido or Kitty, and the entire Covid Zero program would collapse.

Reflecting on the state of play in late 2021, Professor Jay Bhattacharya explained in the pages of the *Wall Street Journal*, "Much of the pathology underlying Covid policy arises from the fantasy that it is possible to eradicate the virus. Capitalizing on pandemic panic, governments and compliant media have used the lure of zero-Covid to induce obedience to harsh and arbitrary lockdown policies and associated violations of civil liberties."[30]

At the end of the day, vaccines will replace lockdowns, and vaccines will be replaced in turn by highly effective therapeutic drugs that will protect us against the ever weakening, but still highly infectious, variants of the original Covid strain. The ever mutating China Virus, like the Spanish Flu, will never really go away. It will be with us forever in one variant after another. But we will learn to live with it. We will have no choice.

SARS, or the Flu?

By the end of 2020, it was estimated that one in three Americans had already been infected with Covid.[31] Those who developed symptoms—and many did not—described a respiratory disease not all that different from the seasonal influenza or the Asian Flu:

- Fever or chills
- Cough
- Shortness of breath or difficulty breathing
- Fatigue
- Muscle or body aches
- Headache
- Sore throat
- Congestion or runny nose

There were a few twists. Many people lost their sense of taste or smell, while others reported nausea, vomiting, or diarrhea. A few developed novel circulatory problems. And some, as is always the case with the flu as well, developed a life-threatening pneumonia. But the vast majority survived.

This is not what the shocking early reports out of China at the end of January had suggested was going to happen. Wuhan's early numbers, which I would argue were calculated to spread terror in the West, suggested that the novel virus might kill up to 4 percent of those it infected.[32] Even if the infection fatality rate—the percentage of those who were sick and tested positive who died—was only 3 percent, it would be catastrophic. It would mean that if all of America fell ill, up to 10 million Americans might die from the disease. The global death toll might be well over 200 million. These were staggering, Spanish Flu–like numbers.

Within a month it was clear that, except for the elderly and people with severe comorbidities, this was a gross exaggeration. The projected infection fatality rate began to plummet, bottoming out at between 0.1 and 0.2 percent in most countries.[33]

As usual, Anthony Fauci was on both sides of this issue, repeatedly suggesting in public that Covid was far deadlier than the flu, while confiding in communications with his medical colleagues and political allies that it was probably more akin to a severe flu season.

Testifying at a high-profile congressional hearing on March 11, 2020, for example, Dr. Fauci famously compared the SARS-CoV-2 coronavirus to the earlier SARS virus, which he soberly announced "had a mortality rate of 9 to 10 percent." Then he declared to his shocked audience, "The stated mortality [case mortality rate] of this, if you look at all the data, including that which comes from China, is about 3 percent." Fauci was talking about the case fatality rate, or CFR, which is the ratio of deaths to symptomatic cases of the disease. He went on to give an infection fatality rate, or IFR (the proportion of deaths to the much larger number of total infections, with or without symptoms): "If you count all the cases of minimally symptomatic or asymptomatic infections that probably brings the [infection] mortality rate down to somewhere around 1 percent. Which means it is 10 times more lethal than the seasonal flu, I think that's something that people can get their arms around."[34]

Fauci's doomsaying had its intended effect: heads exploded across America. The nightly news led with the sobering news that America's chief infectious disease doctor had determined that Covid was "ten times more lethal than the seasonal flu." Headlines shouted that Fauci was predicting millions of deaths from Covid.[35]

Fauci became an overnight sensation in the mainstream media—prophets of doom are always popular with the media—where he continued to warn in interview after interview that a viral Armageddon was coming. Appearing on Comedy Central on March 27, 2020, for instance, he shared with host Trevor Noah the very unfunny news that Covid is "insidious and treacherous in that you can spread it easily . . . even though you are young, you are not absolutely invulnerable. . . ." He said it would be "devastating for the elderly" and "different from anything we've ever faced before." Again he warned that the new virus was something far worse than the seasonal flu: "The mortality of [Covid-19] is about 10 times [the seasonal flu]. It's at least ten times that."[36]

The message: be afraid, be very afraid.

Fauci was much more circumspect, however, in his communications with his medical colleagues. Writing in the *New England Journal of Medicine* that same month, he estimated that "the case fatality rate may be considerably less than 1%." And later: "This [evidence] suggests that the overall clinical consequences of COVID-19 may ultimately be more akin to those of a severe seasonal influenza (which has a case fatality rate of approximately 0.1%) or a pandemic influenza (similar to those in 1957 and 1968) rather than a disease similar to SARS or MERS, which have had case fatality rates of 9 to 10% and 36%, respectively."[37]

Nothing had changed between the times that Fauci uttered these wildly divergent mortality estimates—except his audience.

In fact, the China Virus was nothing like the second coming of SARS or the Spanish Flu. It was more like . . . a bad seasonal flu.

How Many People Really Died of Covid?

If you want to start an argument between two epidemiologists, just ask them how many people died of the Spanish Flu. One may say fewer than twenty-five million,[38] while the other may say "as many as a hundred million."[39] The truth is that no one, even the experts, really knows what the total global death toll was during the plague years of 1918 and 1919.

The same is true of every pandemic down to the present time. Did the Asian Flu kill 1 million people worldwide? Or did it kill 4 million? Did 116,000 people in the United States die of the Asian Flu, or only 66,000? Were there 100,000 Hong Kong Flu deaths in this country in 1968–1970, or only 33,800?[40]

Even today, these disputes over past pandemics rage on with no resolution in sight. Public health experts give different answers, in part because they answer a number of threshold questions differently: What starting and ending points should be used for the pandemic? Should the deaths of people who only had a short time to live anyway be attributed to the pandemic? In the case of multiple comorbidities, which should be counted as the underlying cause of death?

Yet during the China Virus pandemic, all uncertainty suddenly vanished. Almost every country—including the United States—claimed to be reporting the *exact number of deaths that had occurred in their country* from Covid, updated every single day. The WHO website purported to give you the *exact number of deaths that had occurred worldwide* from Covid, again updated every single day (5,070,244 as of November 8, 2021).[41]

Really?

Look at Italy, for example, the earliest country outside of China to experience a major outbreak of Covid. On November 3, 2021, Italy was reporting precisely 132,161 deaths from the China Virus, the highest total in the European Union.[42] But did they all die *of* Covid? Or did some die *with* Covid, but primarily from other causes?

The Instituto Superiore de Santita (ISS) of the Italian government (equivalent to the U.S. Centers for Disease Control) ignited a firestorm by releasing a study on October 19, 2021, showing that only a small fraction—2.9

percent—of those who had supposedly died of Covid had been healthy at the time they contracted the disease. The rest, the study said, had had one or more serious preexisting health conditions ("pathologies" in the Italian terminology, which are the same thing as "comorbidities"; researchers in the United States call them "comorbidities").[43]

Critics pounced, saying that the Italian government's own study proved that fewer than four thousand Italians had actually died *of* Covid. Many of the rest may have died *with* Covid, but the ultimate cause of their death lay elsewhere, they said. Just as in the United States, the sick in Italy had been hastily diagnosed with Covid using vague diagnostic criteria, and the death toll had been driven up by financial payments and other inducements to ensure that "Covid" was listed as the "ultimate cause of death" on as many death certificates as possible. As Professor Walter Ricciardi, scientific advisor to Italy's minister of health, once admitted, "The way in which we code deaths in our country is very generous in the sense that all the people who die in hospitals with the coronavirus are deemed to be dying of the coronavirus."[44]

So is it 132,000 or 4,000? Or does the truth lie somewhere in between?

The ISS study involved an in-depth analysis of the health records of several thousand Italians whose primary "cause of death" on their death certificates had been given as Covid-19. A total of 7,910 records, dated from February 2020 to September 2021, were reviewed in all.

Two-thirds of those who died had three or more comorbidities. While some of these were conditions such as hypertension, which, properly medicated, does not radically shorten lifespans, most of the others were combinations of life-shortening conditions such as dementia, diabetes, atrial fibrillation, coronary artery disease, and congestive heart failure. Many of those who contracted Covid already had one foot in the grave; the virus simply gave them a final nudge.

The ISS heatedly denied that the mortality rate from Covid was in any way inflated, claiming that it was common knowledge that having a preexisting health condition—or two, or three, or four—increased the risk of dying from the China Virus. At the same time, however, it admitted that its own review showed that "death certificates report Covid-19 as *the cause directly responsible for death* in 89% of deaths of SARS-Cov-2 positive persons" [emphasis in the original].[45]

This seems less like a defense than a confession, since what the ISS is saying is that in 11 percent of supposed Covid deaths, Covid was not listed as the primary cause of death on the death certificate by the attending physician. That's at least 14,500 questionable cases of some bureaucratic overseer overriding the judgment of the doctor on scene and recoding the deaths.

But while 132,000 deaths is probably far too high, 4,000 is undoubtedly far too low, since many of the comorbidities listed by the ISS are health issues that one can live with for many years, rather than die of over the short term. Again, the truth lies somewhere in the murky middle.

The official Covid death toll in the United States, which as of November 11, 2021, was said to be 755,201, suffers from all of the Italian data's shortcomings—and more.

Code It as Covid

Most of those who are said to have died from the China Virus had multiple comorbidities, or were approaching the end of their lives, or both. As the CDC notes, "There were co-morbidities or other conditions listed on the death certificate for as many as 95 percent of all Covid-19 deaths. The other 5 percent of death certificates in which Covid-19 was the only condition listed was likely related to a lack of detail listed about other conditions present at the time of death."[46] The average number of comorbidities listed was four.

The CDC has a simple solution for such complex cases: code everything as Covid on the death certificate. You can write whatever you want on the

★ ★ ★

Was Covid-19 a Population Control Program?

CNN perversely found a way to celebrate the Covid contagion, crowing: "There's an unlikely beneficiary of coronavirus: The planet."[47] The story rhapsodized about the suddenly blue skies over Beijing and the eerily empty highways. Unmentioned was the fact that no one was taking nature walks to enjoy it, since the Chinese were all confined to their apartments by the CCP's brutal lockdown. The story was completely tone-deaf to the human suffering and death caused not just by the virus, but by the closed factories, the shuttered businesses, and the social isolation. There have always been those who wanted to reduce human numbers, and many of them were not particular about how this was to be accomplished. British humanist Bertrand Russell bemoaned the fact that "war, so far, has had no very great effect on this increase [in the population of the world]. . . . [War] has been disappointing in this respect . . . but perhaps bacteriological war may prove more effective. If a Black Death could spread through the world once in every generation, survivors could procreate freely without making the world too full. . . . The state of affairs may be somewhat unpleasant, but what of it? Really high-minded people are indifferent to happiness, especially other people's."[48]

Those "high-minded people" would include Prince Philip, Queen Elizabeth's late husband. The queen's consort was a rabid population controller who once remarked, "In the event that I am reincarnated, I would like to return as a deadly virus, to contribute something to solving overpopulation."[49]

lines giving the contributing causes of death, it says. But by all means write Covid as the underlying cause of death, or UCOD for short.

Don't take my word for it. Here is the language from the CDC's own "Guidance on Reporting Deaths due to Coronavirus Disease 2019 (Covid-19)":

- If COVID-19 played a role in the death, this condition should be specified on the death certificate. In many cases, it is likely that it will be the UCOD. . . .

- The reported UCOD should be specific enough to be useful for public health and research purposes. For example, a "viral infection" can be a UCOD, but it is not specific. A more specific UCOD in this instance could be "COVID–19."
- Natural deaths are due solely or almost entirely to disease of the aging process. In the case of death due to a COVID-19 infection, the manner of death will almost always be natural. [That is to say, if Covid is suspected in a natural death, then list Covid as the UCOD.]
- Ideally, testing for COVID-19 should be conducted, but it is acceptable to report COVID-19 on a death certificate without this confirmation if the circumstances are compelling.
- In cases where a definite diagnosis of COVID-19 cannot be made, but it is suspected or likely (e.g., the circumstances are compelling within a reasonable degree of certainty), it is acceptable to report COVID-19 on a death certificate as "probable" or "presumed."[50]

Do you see a pattern here? The message of the CDC's "Guidance" is if you even suspect that the deceased had Covid, then report Covid as the underlying cause of death. And doctors, under pressure from hospital administrators, did exactly that. Natural deaths were no longer coded as such, and deaths from the flu cratered—likely just recoded to Covid so that the hospital qualified for the Covid bonus payment.[51] Deaths from the China Virus, on the other hand, skyrocketed. There were even traffic deaths reportedly coded as Covid.[52] As the CDC itself approvingly notes, "For the majority of deaths where COVID-19 is reported on the death certificate (approximately 95%), COVID-19 is selected as the underlying cause of death."[53]

Scott Jensen, who is both a doctor and a Minnesota state senator, criticized the new guidelines as a stark departure from past practice. Dr. Jensen said, "If it's COVID-19, we're told now it doesn't matter if it was actually the diagnosis that caused death. If someone had it, they died of it."[54]

How many of these deaths are not *from* Covid, but are merely *with* Covid—or, worse yet, are of people who merely tested positive for Covid at some point? We may never know.

It took nearly two years for the CDC to even acknowledge that this might be a problem. It was not until January of 2022 that CDC director Rochelle Walensky, in response to a direct question from Fox host Bret Baier, admitted, "In some hospitals we've talked to, up to 40 percent of the patients who are coming in not because they are sick with Covid, but because they are coming in with something else and have had to—Covid or the omicron variant detected." In other words, claiming that they are Covid patients is a misdiagnosis of their actual condition.

Are Covid deaths also exaggerated by 40 percent, as Dr. Jensen had claimed?[55] Walensky didn't say. When Baier asked her to break down the total number of deaths into those who actually died *from* Covid as opposed to those who died *with* Covid, she clumsily dodged the question.[56]

So the question remains: How many of the 911,145 Covid deaths that the CDC was reporting on February 15, 2022, were actually *from* Covid?[57] As opposed to people who were acutely or terminally ill with something else and just happened to test positive for Covid at some point during their hospital stay?

What we do know is that the current U.S. population, a little more than 330 million, is more than three times larger than the U.S. population in 1918, estimated at 105 million. The 675,000 deaths attributed to the Spanish Flu were 0.64 percent of the total population, that is to say, between 6 or 7 out of every 1,000 people died.[58]

By contrast, even using the CDC's numbers, the more than 900,000 deaths attributed to Covid are only 0.27 percent of the current population, or a little under 3 out of every 1,000 people. And if the misdiagnosis rate is 40 percent, as Walensky let slip, then the actual death toll may be far lower, perhaps around 500,000.

Had the China Virus caused deaths at the same rate as the Spanish Flu, we would have been digging graves for 2.2 million Americans. Thankfully, while Covid-19 was considerably more infectious, it was not nearly as lethal.

One final way to assess the gravity of a pandemic is to look at average life spans. The Spanish Flu, which swept away hundreds of thousands of healthy young adults, shortened the average American life span by a full twelve years. The China Virus, which largely targeted the elderly, only reduced the average life span by thirteen months in 2020.[59] In terms of life years lost, the Spanish Flu was many times as deadly as the China Virus.

This is not to make light of the deaths of those we have lost to the pandemic. Each one of its victims was someone's husband or wife, father or mother, grandfather or grandmother. Each one was a unique, irreplaceable human being of infinite worth.

The ones trivializing their deaths are those who used inflated numbers to gaslight the rest of us into a state of abject terror. The goal was to scare us into submission and, not incidentally, into getting a vaccine that the 200 million or so of us with natural immunity did not need.[60]

We are left with the obvious question: If a large number of those whose deaths were coded as Covid over the past two years did not die *from* Covid, but merely *with* Covid, then what actually killed them?

The CDC readily admits that, in addition to its advertised Covid death toll, there were over 200,000 "excess deaths" from a baker's dozen of other common ailments including heart disease, hypertension, and dementia. And it is willing to grant, as the chief of the mortality statistics branch of the CDC made clear in mid-February 2022, that "many of the people who died of Covid were elderly, sick or very frail" and "might not have survived across the two-year span of the pandemic."[61] But they were coded as Covid deaths anyway.

But even this is not the whole story. Beginning in 2021, the insurance companies began reporting a sudden, unexpected, and historically unprecedented spike in deaths and disabilities among otherwise healthy Americans in the prime of life. At a virtual news conference held on December 30, 2021, Scott Davison, the president of OneAmerica, announced that deaths were up 40 percent among people ages eighteen to sixty-four.[62]

As a life insurance company, Indiana-based OneAmerica is in the business of insuring people against death and disability, which means they have to accurately forecast the likelihood that those they insure will die or become disabled. Their forecasts, which rely on decades of actuarial data, are generally quite accurate. But in 2021, according to Davison, their forecasts turned out to be dramatically wrong. As the year went on, the working-age people his company insures suddenly started dying at a rate 40 percent higher than pre-pandemic levels. That means that for every ten people between the ages of eighteen and sixty-four who died in 2019 or 2020, fourteen died in 2021.

How statistically improbable is this? Davison explained, "Just to give you an idea of how bad [a 40 percent increase] is, a three-sigma or a 1-in-200-year catastrophe would be 10% increase over pre-pandemic. So 40% is just unheard of."

The effect on OneAmerica's bottom line must have been dramatic. In 2019, the company paid out $6 billion in claims. It paid out the same amount in 2020, despite the pandemic—presumably because most of those dying were quite elderly, or they were already at high risk because of pre-existing medical conditions.[63] Both age and health are already factored into the actuarial tables, so the company's payouts were not affected. But in 2021, to listen to CEO Davison, they will be paying out 40 percent more.

Apparently others in the insurance industry are seeing the same unusual rise in claims. According to Davison, "We are seeing, right now, the highest death rates we have seen in the history of this business—not just at OneAmerica. The data is consistent across every player in that business."

A quick check of a few of OneAmerica's competitors confirms Davison's claims. Prudential paid out 87 percent more in death benefits in the third quarter of 2021 than it did in the third quarter of 2020. Pacific Life and Annuity claims are up by over 80 percent. New York Life doesn't break down its data by quarter, but by September 30, 2021, it had paid out 27 percent more in death benefits than in 2020. Most of the excess deaths occurred in the last two quarters of the year.[64]

And the bad news does not end there. Davison said that his company was also seeing an "uptick" in both short-term and long-term disability claims, explaining that initially it was mostly short-term disability claims, but most recently the increase was in long-term disability claims. "For OneAmerica, we expect the costs of this are going to be well over $100 million, and this is our smallest business. So it's having a huge impact on that," he said.

At the same news conference where Davison spoke, Brian Tabor, the president of the Indiana Hospital Association, said that hospitals across the state were being inundated with patients "with many different conditions," concluding that "unfortunately, the average Hoosier's health has declined during the pandemic." In a follow-up call, Tabor said he did not have a breakdown showing the conditions or ailments for which so many people in the state were being hospitalized. But he did confirm that the extraordinarily high death rate reported by Davison matched what hospitals in the state were seeing.[65]

Davison blamed the rise in deaths on Covid, although he admitted that most of the insurance claims being filed do not indicate Covid as the cause of death. He blames poor reporting: "What the data is showing to us is that the deaths that are being reported as COVID deaths greatly understate the actual death losses among working-age people from the pandemic. It may not all be COVID on their death certificate, but deaths are up just huge, huge numbers."

The suggestion that Covid deaths are "underreported," however, which we also hear from government health bureaucrats, is simply not credible. As we have seen, the CDC and HHS have made enormous efforts, up to and including cash inducements, to ensure that Covid is listed as the underlying cause of death on as many death certificates as possible.

If we are seeing more excess deaths among the young and healthy than at any time since the Spanish Flu of 1918–1919, there must be a dangerous new pathogen on the loose. This novel pathogen not only leads to death from a wide variety of causes but also gives rise to an equally wide variety of short- and long-term disabilities. And it must have struck, curiously enough, not long after the new mRNA vaccination campaigns began in earnest in the beginning of 2021. And this leads us to another curious coincidence: if you review the tens of thousands of reports that have been filed with the FDA's Vaccine Adverse Event Reporting System (VAERS) about Covid vaccines, you will find listed an equally wide variety of side effects leading to death and disability that medical professionals and others believe were caused by the injections.[66]

So are the Covid vaccines themselves responsible for this alarming spike in deaths? Professor Spiro Pantazatos of Columbia University decided to find out.[67] In the first study of its kind, he and his coauthor Hervé Seligmann used vaccination data from all fifty states and twenty-two European countries to see if the wave of vaccinations that rippled across both continents in 2021 had been followed by a wave of deaths. After analyzing the data from the first nine months of the year, they concluded that the overall mortality rate jumped following injection and remained high for five weeks thereafter. Or, in their own words, "vaccination predicted all-cause mortality 0–5 weeks post–injection in almost all age groups."

Just how many people in the United States do Pantazatos and Seligmann calculate passed away unexpectedly as a result of the jab? For the months from February to August 2021 alone, they estimate that between 146,000 and 187,000 Americans lost their lives to the vaccines. The death toll for the entire 12 months of 2021 would, of course, be much higher.[68]

From these numbers they calculated a Vaccine Fatality Rate, or VFR, of 0.04 percent, which means that out of every 10,000 Americans who received the vaccine, 4 have succumbed to it. Needless to say, this finding put them at loggerheads with the CDC, which continued to claim that the vaccines were "safe and effective," and put the odds of dying from the vaccine much lower, at only 2 in 100,000, or 0.002 percent. The CDC based its numbers on its VAERS reporting system, which on February 11, 2022, was showing 12,899 deaths from the vaccines.

The fact that almost 13,000 vaccine-related deaths have been reported to VAERS is itself very worrisome, but it is undoubtedly only a small part of the picture. Because reporting a vaccine injury or death to VAERS is entirely voluntary, the service suffers from a well-known underreporting bias. Pantazatos and Seligmann have suggested that you have to multiply the vaccine-associated deaths reported in VAERS by "at least a factor of 20" to get the true number of fatalities.

What this meant for the Covid mass vaccination campaigns that were still underway at the time of their study was obvious: for most age groups, the risk of dying from the vaccine is greater than the risk of dying from the coronavirus. Or, as the authors put it, "the risks of Covid vaccination outweigh the benefits in children, young and middle age adults, and in older age groups with low occupational risk, previous coronavirus exposure [i.e., natural immunity], and access to alternative prophylaxis and early treatment options."[69]

The CDC has run advertisements touting a recent paper by Stanley Xu and coauthors that it says "found no increased risk of death among Covid-19 vaccine recipients," which would seem to ignore its own VAERS data. Pantazatos and Seligmann suggest, with typical academic understatement, that

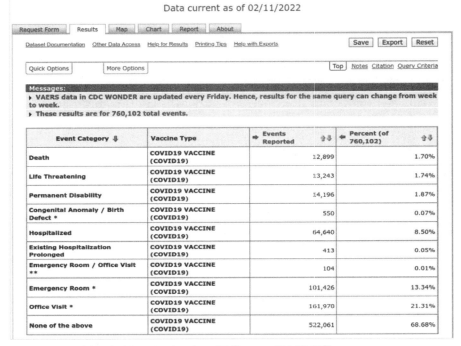

The Vaccine Adverse Event Reporting System (VAERS) Results

Data current as of 02/11/2022

Messages:
▸ VAERS data in CDC WONDER are updated every Friday. Hence, results for the same query can change from week to week.
▸ These results are for 760,102 total events.

Event Category	Vaccine Type	Events Reported	Percent (of 760,102)
Death	COVID19 VACCINE (COVID19)	12,899	1.70%
Life Threatening	COVID19 VACCINE (COVID19)	13,243	1.74%
Permanent Disability	COVID19 VACCINE (COVID19)	14,196	1.87%
Congenital Anomaly / Birth Defect *	COVID19 VACCINE (COVID19)	550	0.07%
Hospitalized	COVID19 VACCINE (COVID19)	64,640	8.50%
Existing Hospitalization Prolonged	COVID19 VACCINE (COVID19)	413	0.05%
Emergency Room / Office Visit **	COVID19 VACCINE (COVID19)	104	0.01%
Emergency Room *	COVID19 VACCINE (COVID19)	101,426	13.34%
Office Visit *	COVID19 VACCINE (COVID19)	161,970	21.31%
None of the above	COVID19 VACCINE (COVID19)	522,061	68.68%

VAERS Reported Covid-19 Vaccine Deaths – US (Source: CDC/VAERS)

COVID Vaccine Adverse Event Reports as of February 11, 2022. *Centers for Disease Control and Prevention*

the authors of the CDC-touted study may have committed "a technical or human error involving group labeling or coding. Note that the data used for their study is not publicly accessible (in contrast to our study), and *two authors report receiving funding from Pfizer*" [emphasis added].[70] I would add that two of the coauthors are also employees of the CDC.

Statistical analyses have their place, but by spring 2022 the risks associated with the mRNA vaccines were brought home to many Americans by personal experience. I myself can count five people—including one who died suddenly the day after the jab—who were injured by the vaccine throughout the course of 2021 among my own family and friends. And when

I speak of injuries I don't mean commonplace complaints like sore arms and mild fevers. One family member developed myocarditis, while three friends suffered partial paralysis, seizures, and blood clots, respectively.[71] Anthony Fauci would likely scoff that these five cases were merely "anecdotal," and they were, but multiplied by the hundreds of thousands they turned popular sentiment not only against the mandates, but against the vaccines themselves.

Those most aware of the adverse effects of the vaccines were medical professionals, although they faced disciplinary action—up to and including losing their jobs and their licenses to practice—if they spoke out. Dr. Scott Jensen, for instance, an outspoken critic of the vaccine mandates, has been investigated no fewer than five times by the Minnesota Board of Medical Practice.[73] Another doctor had his medical license suspended for suggesting that masking is more about theater than health.[74]

★ ★ ★

Pantazatos and Seligmann vs. Big Pharma

"Given that vaccines do not appear to reduce community spread and that the risks outweigh the benefits for most age groups, vaccine mandates in workplaces, colleges, schools and elsewhere are ill-advised. We do not see much benefit in vaccine mandates other than increasing serviceable obtainable market share for the vaccine companies."[72]

The vaccine mandates did little to improve public health, but greatly boosted the fiscal "health" of the companies that manufactured them.

But as we entered the third year of the pandemic, more and more questions began to be raised about the vaccines. When New York's health care workers were ordered to get a third shot by mid-February 2022, half of all nursing home workers said they would quit rather than comply. They were not interested in playing booster roulette. Governor Kathy Hochul was forced to scrap the mandate just days before it was to come into force.[75]

As we saw in chapter 7, this was not the first time that a dangerous vaccine had been hastily rolled out in a mass inoculation campaign. The great swine flu hoax of 1976 followed exactly the same trajectory. Politicians and

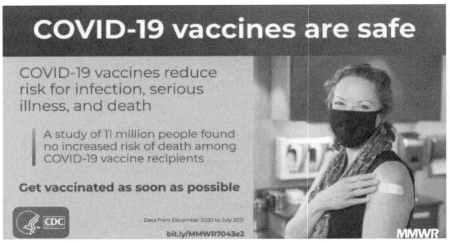

CDC advertisements touting a paper by Stanley Xu and coauthors published in late 2021,[76] claiming that the study "found no increased risk of death among Covid-19 vaccine recipients," a claim which would seem to contradict the CDC's own VAERS data.

the public were first stampeded into believing that a reprise of the Spanish Flu was on its way. Vaccine companies then quickly produced tens of millions of doses of a vaccine on government contracts on the promise that they would be granted immunity from liability.

The promised plague failed to materialize, but 50 million Americans were vaccinated before the jabs were called off. By that time, thirty-two people had died, and thousands had been injured by the vaccine.

We have, by even the VAERS numbers, far, far exceeded that number.

A Vaccine Unlike Any Other

Most vaccines contain either "attenuated" live viruses or "inactivated" dead viruses, in whole or in part. The dead viruses are, well, dead, while the live viruses have been attenuated—weakened and so rendered harmless to humans. Both are still sufficiently similar to the wild variety that the human immune system builds a defense against it. Jonas Salk's polio vaccine was an inactivated variety of the polio virus, while Albert Sabin's polio vaccine, which came along later, is the attenuated variety.[77]

The vaccines used in the fight against the China Virus were a different animal altogether. Some experts, such Dr. Robert Malone, have said that they are not vaccines at all—at least in the traditional understanding of the term—but are rather experimental gene therapy. Dr. Malone would know, of course, since he invented the gene therapy in question in the late 1980s while at the Salk Institute.[78]

But there is an even easier-to-understand way to describe the mRNA vaccines that were sold by Pfizer and Moderna to the American public. What was injected into the shoulders of hundreds of millions of people worldwide is best understood as a man-made virus.

As a recent article on mRNA vaccines put it, "Vaccination with non-viral vector delivered nucleic acid-based vaccines mimics infection or immunization with live microorganisms." Exactly.[79]

In other words, in order to stop a pandemic caused by a virus, we fashioned a kind of crude counter-virus in the lab. What could possibly go wrong?

Most drugs that we take are simple chemical compounds that attach to receptors on the outside of our cells, either blocking or activating them. They are used for things like controlling pain, regulating blood pressure, and lowering cholesterol levels. But to treat cancers, autoimmune diseases, and genetic disorders, a far more sophisticated approach is used: complicated proteins and enzymes are grown in the lab and then injected into the patient to target cancer cells or regulate other physiological processes.

But, scientists asked themselves, what if the body's own cellular machinery could be hijacked and used to produce these same proteins? If that sounds familiar, it's because that's exactly what viruses do—they hijack the cell's machinery and use it to produce copies of themselves. The new mRNA

★ ★ ★

The mRNA Vaccines: Fact and Fiction

The CDC assures us that "mRNA never enters the nucleus of the cell where our DNA (genetic material) is located, so it cannot change or influence our genes."[81] This may be true, but there is at least one study that suggests that the same is not true for the protein—the famous spike protein—that the mRNA forces our cells to make. The study, published in the journal *Viruses*, found that the spike protein migrates inside the nuclei of cells where our genes—the crown jewels of human creation—are kept. There, reportedly, it interferes with the activity of two proteins charged with keeping our chromosomes in good repair.[82]

vaccines are essentially man-made viruses that invade your body's cells and force them to manufacture the spike protein of the China Virus.[80]

Perhaps not surprisingly, the human body is not happy about being invaded in this way, and it mobilizes all of its defenses to prevent it from happening. That's why, as Alex Berenson writes, "the mRNA must be both disguised AND hidden inside a tiny ball of fat . . . or our bodies will likely destroy it before it can even reach our cells."

But it's hard to fool our incredibly sophisticated immune systems with such clumsy efforts, which may explain why the mRNA vaccines fail to confer permanent immunity and start wearing off within a few months. Before it was used as a vaccine, the mRNA biotechnology had been used in earlier trials to address other illnesses, but "failed upon repeated dosing."[83]

By September of 2021, the CDC was admitting that the protection against Covid offered by the vaccines was in decline, especially for the elderly—precisely the group most at risk from the disease.[84] Apparently acting on the principle "when in doubt, keep jabbing," we began to hear about the need for a third, a fourth, and even annual booster shots. As usual, Fauci led the way, suggesting on September 4, 2021, that three doses of Covid-19 vaccine were likely needed for full protection. The following month the CDC went even further, suggesting that a fourth shot might be advisable for those who are immunocompromised.[85]

As the vaccines were rolled out, the CDC published the infection fatality rates for various age groups, from which the survival rates from the disease can be calculated:[86]

Under 18 = 99.998 percent survival

18–49 = 99.95 percent survival

50–64 = 99.4 percent survival

65+ = 91 percent survival

Given these survival rates, one can make a good argument for vaccinating the elderly, since they are at significant risk of death. The argument for vaccination rapidly weakens as you move into the younger age cohorts, however, especially given the risk of adverse reactions to the mRNA vaccines themselves. Such considerations didn't seem to matter to Dr. Fauci, however. His one-jab-fits-all approach was to insist on vaccinating everyone, from the superannuated down to students and children.[87]

By now most of us know—despite the efforts of the legacy media and the Biden administration to hide the fact—that the China virus poses virtually zero risk to kids.[88] The vast majority of children who contract it will come down with no more than the sniffles, if they show any symptoms at all.

Even better, once they are exposed to it, their immune systems will ever after be alert not only for the original invader, but for nearly all of the variants that it spins off over time. This robust immunity will probably last their entire lives. After all, the survivors of the much more deadly Spanish Flu of 1918–1919 came away with life-long immunity.

"Original Antigenic Sin"

But the wonderful process by which the human body produces natural immunity to a novel virus it has never encountered before will be short-circuited in children if they are given an mRNA jab. The vaccine will violate their immune system's innocence by forcing it to commit what has been called the "original antigenic sin."

It turns out that the human immune system is not capable of an infinite number of responses to an infinite number of viruses. Rather, the strongest response to influenza viruses, for example, is produced by the body's first exposure to this disease class, which usually occurs in childhood.

But it is not only that subsequent immune responses to the influenza are weaker, which they are. That would be concerning enough. The problem is that the first childhood infection primes the immune system to respond to subsequent infections with antibodies specific to the original strain.[89]

The authors of a 2005 *Nature Medicine* article defined the "original antigenic sin" as follows: "After exposure to a new but cross-reacting antigenic variant, such individuals may respond by producing antibodies that are primarily directed at antigens characterizing influenza viruses encountered during earlier epidemics."[90]

In other words, their bodies are producing antibodies to the wrong variant. Instead of responding to the variant that is currently circulating in the population and to which they have newly been exposed, their immune system is producing antibodies to the variant—now long gone—that they were first exposed to in childhood.

Think about that in the context of the China Virus. This is a novel coronavirus that *no one on the planet* has ever before encountered. And when they are vaccinated with the mRNA vaccine, they are not fully exposed to it either—only to its spike protein.

Once that spike protein in the virus mutates, as it already has in, for example, the Delta variant, the body has no epitopes—parts of the virus—that it immediately recognizes and can use to produce appropriate antibodies against. So what does it do? It produces antibodies for the original China Virus's spike protein, because that's what it has been programmed to do.

A similar misallocation, as we might call it, of the body's immune resources may mute the development of the kind of robust, long-lasting immunity that results from a natural infection. This may have been why a large study published in the *European Journal of Epidemiology* found that higher vaccination rates did not lead to fewer Covid cases. In fact, the authors concluded from their sixty-eight-nation survey, "the trend line suggests . . . that *countries with higher percentages of population fully vaccinated have higher Covid-19 cases per 1 million people*" [emphasis added].[91]

Since the vaccines may weaken the body's immune response to new variants, the mass vaccination campaigns still being carried out by some countries may lead to repeated waves of infection—each of which will be met by a frantic and ultimately futile attempt to give everyone booster shots, which at best will offer only temporary and limited protection until the next variant comes along. Mass vaccination was presented as a vital matter of public health, but it turns out that it didn't bring us any closer to herd immunity. To vax or not to vax should always have been left up to the individual, since it is a matter of personal, not public, health.

Many, perhaps most, of those resisting the jab have already recovered from bouts of the China Virus, enjoy robust immunity, and realize that the mRNA vaccine has nothing whatsoever to offer them but an endless series of increasingly risky booster shots.

The best real-life illustration of original antigenic sin comes from the effort to develop a vaccine for dengue fever, which people get from the bite of an infected mosquito. There are four main variants of the dengue virus, and the original vaccine only covered one of them. Subsequent boosters for the other variants proved ineffective because the boosters only triggered "the immunological footprint of the first vaccination."

Authors of a study on this phenomenon concluded:

> Original antigenic sin has the advantage that a response can be
> rapidly mobilized from memory. However, the downside is that in
> some cases, such as dengue, the response is dominated by inferior-
> quality antibody. . . .

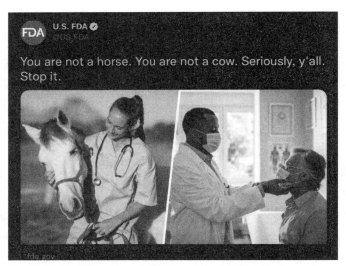

The FDA was not interested in repurposing existing therapeutic drugs for use during the Covid pandemic, but only in discouraging their use. Ivermectin was one of its targets.[93]

Once a response has been established, it is unlikely that repeat boosting will be able to change its scope, meaning that balanced responses against the four virus serotypes will need to be established with the first vaccine dose.[92]

The danger is not only that the mRNA vaccines may confer only narrow immunity to a specific variant, but that they may undermine our immune system's response to future variants, leading to longer and more severe infections.[94]

Something else that Fauci wasn't telling us (and there was always something else that Fauci wasn't telling us) is that an "emergency use authorization" for a vaccine cannot be granted if there is an effective therapeutic drug or drugs available.[95] So HCQ, and later ivermectin, had to be attacked and discredited—otherwise the emergency use authorizations for the Covid vaccines would be called into question.[96] And Big Pharma's hundred-billion-dollar gravy train would be derailed.

There has never been a vaccine that did not entail some risk. As we saw in chapter 7, we take vaccines despite the risk because of the "reward" we receive in terms of immunity from this or that infectious disease. But the China Virus is unlike anything we have ever encountered before. Because it is so highly infectious, and because simply being vaccinated does not protect you from being infected—as the CDC belatedly admitted[97]—it was

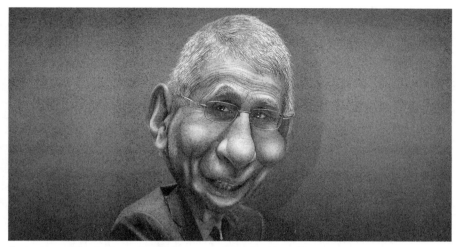

Caricature of Dr. Anthony Fauci. *Courtesy of DonkeyHotey*[98]

clear that, vaccinated or not, virtually everyone in the world was eventually going to contract the disease in one variant or another.

We found out even earlier—in the opening months of the pandemic, actually—that kids will survive the China Virus just fine, which means that they receive no "reward" for taking the vaccine. They are still exposed to the "risk," however—the real danger of myocarditis or other adverse medical consequences.[99]

Throughout 2021, health authorities were notoriously reluctant to talk about potential side effects from the experimental vaccines for fear that that would fuel "vaccine hesitancy"—instead endlessly repeating that the vaccines were "safe and effective." But reality soon intruded upon this narrative, as vaxxed professional athletes began collapsing on the field of play in front of tens of thousands of fans. An investigation by Israel's *Real-Time News* found a five-fold increase in sudden cardiac death among professional soccer players following the roll-out of the vaccines. In all, up to mid-November of 2021, they counted 183 professional athletes and coaches who had suddenly been stricken. Nearly all were male, and nearly all had

Vaccines vs. Treatments

Early on in the pandemic, evidence began accumulating about existing drugs that could potentially be used to treat China Virus infections. First came hydroxychloroquine, which had been approved for medical use in the United States in 1955. When the FDA issued emergency use authorizations for hydroxychloroquine and azithromycin to treat Covid-19 on March 21, President Trump was quick to celebrate the news in a tweet.[100] HCQ and Zithro taken together, Trump said, "have a real chance to be one of the biggest game changers in the history of medicine. The FDA has moved mountains—Thank You!" Trump even cited an article from the *International Journal of Antimicrobial Agents* showing the two worked better in tandem.[101]

Moving quickly, the FDA shipped 70,000 doses of hydroxychloroquine, 10,000 of Zithromax, and 750,000 doses of chloroquine to the states.[102]

But not everyone was celebrating. Least of all Anthony Fauci. In the absence of "definitive studies," Dr. Fauci suggested on April 3, we could not know whether hydroxychloroquine was "truly safe and effective" for this off-label use. And yet Fauci knew quite well that HCQ had antiviral properties. As Prabhash K. Dutta would note in early June, when an Indian study confirmed the effectiveness of HCQ as a Covid

treatment, "In the 1985–86 edition of 'Harrison's Principles of Internal Medicine' [a highly recommended book for students studying medicine in medical colleges], Dr. Fauci wrote that HCQ worked as an anti-viral agent despite being an anti-malarial drug. There was no COVID-19 back then. HCQ's anti-viral properties were known."[103] Despite this, Fauci called for "more studies." But if he, with his almost $6 billion annual research budget,[104] wasn't going to fund such studies, Big Pharma certainly wouldn't. HCQ was a cheap generic drug—there would be no big payday from its use. On June 15, 2020, the FDA revoked its emergency authorization.[105]

When ivermectin, another widely available drug, showed promise as a Covid-19 treatment, it met the same fate. In August of 2021 Dr. Fauci said, "Don't do it. . . . There's no clinical evidence that indicates that this works." He warned about "people who have gone to poison control centers because they've taken the drug at a ridiculous dose and wind up getting sick."[106] He was given an assist by an FDA tweet suggesting that ivermectin was only suitable for farm animals.[107] Just days earlier, the Centers for Disease Control had warned against taking "highly concentrated" ivermectin in the form of "'sheep drench,' injection formulations, and 'pour-on' products for cattle" to treat Covid-19.[108] Others disparaged it as horse-dewormer.[109]

Neither the CDC's health advisory nor Dr. Fauci mentioned that the inventors of ivermectin had been awarded the Nobel Prize on account of its safe and effective treatment of parasite-caused illnesses in humans[110]—or that ivermectin was proving to be a highly effective treatment for Covid-19 in India. On August 6, 2020, the Indian state of Uttar Pradesh had introduced ivermectin for the treatment of those infected with Covid-19, and also as a prophylactic for health workers and those in close contact with the infected. Its success there led the Indian government to add ivermectin to its national protocol for Covid treatment and management in early 2021. Within three months of Dr. Fauci's disparaging comments, ivermectin would have nearly eliminated Covid from the Indian state, which as of November 12, 2021, was reporting only 9 cases of Covid among its population of 241 million people.[111]

suffered heart-related problems, ranging from myocarditis and pericarditis to heart attacks and cardiac arrest. Of this number, 108 died.[112]

Nothing fueled concerns about the vaccines like seeing a superbly conditioned professional athlete at the peak of his career drop dead. Soon even the *New York Times* was reporting on the problem of vax-induced myocarditis, although the paper predictably called it "rare."[113] But when the CDC finally published its own study in January 2022—which for some reason took twice as long to find its way into print as the approval process for the mRNA vaccines themselves—it revealed a shocking increase in heart damage among young men.

The study, published in the *Journal of the American Medical Association*, revealed that Pfizer's Covid vaccine is associated with a 133-times increase in the risk of myocarditis for boys between the ages of twelve and fifteen. Older teenagers and young men were at higher risk as well, and most of the damage occurred following the second shot. The actual risk is undoubtedly many times higher, since the study relied solely upon VAERS data, which even the CDC admits may be an undercount. Yet all the CDC employees had to say about their startling findings was, "This risk should be considered in the context of the benefits of Covid-19 vaccination."[114]

Many parents followed the CDC's advice to the letter. And they decided that, since their children would receive little benefit from the mRNA vaccines, they would not subject them to the risk of myocarditis, or to any other of the numerous side effects that have been reported on VAERS.

But as we have seen, there is another problem with giving kids an mRNA jab that at best offers a few months of protection against a variant that is already dying out. Namely, it may cripple their body's immune response to future coronaviruses that their immune systems would otherwise handily vanquish.

So why in the world were our public health officials insisting that it was a good idea to vaccinate all children in the United States from five to eleven years of age? One argument was that even if children were at zero risk from Covid, vaccinating them would help to control the spread of the pandemic. The Swedish study discussed in chapter 8 soundly debunked that idea, however. It concluded that, with zero Covid deaths among children and teenagers, and no added Covid risk for their teachers, "keeping the schools open has a positive mitigating effect by helping the country reach herd immunity."[115]

In other words, there is a positive benefit to society as a whole from letting the highly adaptable immune systems of children take on and defeat the virus. The commenter who writes the Substack "A Plague Chronicle" under the pen name Eugyppius summed it up best: "The most dangerous thing to do, at this point, would be to vaccinate children. The virus is not a threat to them, and if they are infected by the new forms of SARS-2 that are sure to emerge every winter, we will begin to establish—through them and the as yet unvaccinated—the layered immunity that is the only way of coming to terms with SARS-2 in the longer term."[116]

This means that those who protected their children from the vax-mongers, and the states that have banned vaccination mandates, as Florida did, actually served the public interest by helping us to get ahead of the next Covid variant.

Fauci's quixotic attempt to eliminate Covid-19 was a fantasy from the first. The China Virus is not polio or smallpox to be eliminated or eradicated by universal vaccination. It is a highly infectious, highly mutable airborne virus that, like influenza and the common cold, will be with us forever. Basic evolutionary biology suggests that the over-ambitious vaccine campaign and mandates merely forced the virus to mutate in an effort to escape the limited immunity conferred by the vaccines. By mid-2021, the CDC was reporting that over 80 percent of the cases were now the Delta variant.[117] Then in November of 2021 a new variant, which would prove to be more contagious than the Delta but much less dangerous,[118] was officially named Omicron when the World Health Organization decided to skip Xi, the letter before Omicron in the Greek alphabet, on the excuse that Xi is a "common" name[119]—including, as it happens, the name of Xi Jinping, the president of China. And we wouldn't want to hurt the CCP dictator's feelings. What has he ever done to us?

From Two Weeks to Flatten the Curve to Two Years That Flattened America

If America had simply protected the vulnerable from the China Virus and relied upon the immune systems of the healthy to deal with the disease—as only the human immune system can—the economic impact of the virus would have been minimal. There would have been far fewer victims, and they would still have been overwhelmingly people in their seventies and eighties who were already retired and out of the workforce. On the other hand, the consequences of the misguided and interminable public health campaigns—the masking, the social distancing, the quarantines, the lockdowns, the vaccine mandates, and so forth—were devastating.

We went from two weeks to flatten the curve to two years that flattened America. The shutdown of society was a strategy that—in retrospect—obviously did far more harm than good. Not only did it prolong the most dangerous phase of the worst U.S. pandemic since the Spanish Flu, it put in train long-term consequences that will continue to cause harm for decades to come.

I will leave it to the experts—the honest ones cited in these pages—to explain the collateral public health damage from the lockdowns. Among these are Martin Kulldorff and Jay Bhattacharya, who write, "A fundamental public health principle is that health is multidimensional; the control of a single infectious disease is not synonymous with health. As an immunologist, Dr. Fauci failed to properly consider and weigh the disastrous effects lockdowns would have on cancer detection and treatment, cardiovascular disease outcomes, diabetes care, childhood vaccination rates, mental health and opioid overdoses, to name a few. Americans will live with—and die from—this collateral damage for many years to come."[120]

Concerns about the long-term medical consequences of the vaccines themselves are also growing. As Alex Berenson has pointed out, since April of 2021 vaccinated English adults under sixty have been dying at twice the rate of unvaccinated people the same age. At the same time, overall deaths in Britain are well above normal.[121] There may be some other explanation besides vaccine-caused mortality for this spike in mortality rates in the vaccinated. But as of this writing, the U.K. authorities have not offered one.

One possibility is that, apart from the vaccine itself, another cause of higher mortality rates among the vaccinated could be what might be called the "fear factor." Stoked by Fauci and other public health officials, exacerbated by incendiary reporting by an unhinged media, and reinforced by the overblown reactions of Democratic politicians in blue states, a climate of fear was created around Covid that completely overshadowed the actual danger that it posed to most people.

Nearly a year into the pandemic, well after everyone (even the public health authorities) following the actual course of the pandemic had concluded that the China Virus was not nearly as deadly as originally thought, a majority of voters polled still believed the exaggerated claims of Covid's lethality. A December 2020 Gallup–Franklin Templeton survey of thirty-five thousand Americans revealed that almost all Americans believed that having symptomatic Covid gave you a good chance of ending up in the hospital, with more than a third saying that the odds of hospitalization if you were infected were greater than 50 percent.[122] Just how wrong was this? In reality, over 99 percent of those infected with Covid-19 do not need to be hospitalized. On top of that, one-third of those who are admitted to the hospital have mild rather than severe cases.[123]

All of this panic porn—besides fueling the destructive lockdowns—exacted its own toll on Americans' mental *and* physical health. For inside the riddle of the China Virus, the mystery of the mRNA vaccines, and the enigma of the botched public health response was a very real pandemic of fear. Even at this late date, when it is clear we are dealing with nothing more than the equivalent of a severe flu, to which many of us now have natural immunity, some are still terrified by Covid. The real pandemic within the pandemic was a pandemic of fear.

It is well known that stress and anxiety can depress a person's immune system, making him more susceptible to an infection. But I believe that those same fears also drove many to the hospital as soon as the vaccine was available so they could be first in line to receive their promised salvation in a syringe. Others, with a better understanding of the modest danger that the China Virus posed to them, had to be herded to the hospitals—many months later—by the short-lived vaccination mandates.

So maybe the higher mortality that the United Kingdom is reporting for the vaccinated has to do with the irrational fears that put them at the head of the line for vaccination, rather than the vaccine itself. Fear itself is a killer with many faces.[124]

Speaking as an anthropologist, I suspect the biggest price in terms of life years lost will be paid by the young. Widespread masking deprived small children of the faces that they need to see to know that they are loved, and the opportunity to connect language to lips and sound—and all of that will extract a cost. Social distancing deprived people of all ages of affective touch, but it was especially harmful to children, since touching plays a key role in social bonds and attachment.[125] Lockdowns and school closures added to the harm suffered by children and teenagers, which was expressed in higher rates of depression, suicide, and drug use.

All of these consequences were predictable at the outset of the pandemic, yet for various reasons, many defended the masking, social distancing, quarantines, and lockdowns long after they were transparently indefensible.

Anno Domini 2020 was, of course, an election year. The Democrats, supported by their allies in the legacy media, seized the opportunity provided by the pandemic to relentlessly hammer President Donald Trump for every comment and every decision he made. The woke Left, driven by hatred for Trump no less than for freedom itself, gleefully joined in cheerleading the lockdowns. Those who criticized the endless lockdowns in states such as New York and New Jersey, as the president himself was soon doing, were reviled as heartless idiots who didn't care how many people died.[126]

It wasn't just that the lockdowns placed the burden of the elite's fears on the working class, which they did. They were also quite deliberately used to disadvantage ordinary people, the kind of deplorables who had overwhelmingly voted for Trump in 2016. The politicians made the political calculations and knew what they were doing. Big businesses made the financial calculations and knew what they were doing. It wasn't by accident that so many new billionaires were minted by the Covid pandemic and the middle class shrank. Under the cover of the pandemic, the biggest transfer of wealth in human history took place.[127]

The economic damage was tremendous, running into the trillions of dollars. And those hurt most by the targeted lockdowns were those who could least afford it—small and medium-sized businesses and the workers they employ. Those who benefited—the big-box stores and online retailers—did even bet-

A Book You're Not Supposed to Read

"Something in our nature cries out to be loved by another. Isolation is devastating to the human psyche. That is why solitary confinement is considered the cruelest of punishments."

Gary Chapman, *The 5 Love Languages*[128]

ter once their smaller competitors were crushed by the heavy hand of government. And it was no accident.

Democrats and their deep state allies made sure that not everyone suffered equally. Not a single government employee at any level of government lost his job, even though many stopped working. Blue-state governors seized the pretext of the pandemic to go after the economic base of their political opponents—the small business owners who mostly vote for their opposition—and close them down.[129]

Meanwhile, Big Tech, at least the titans who rule it, would have been happy to see the lockdowns continue forever.

The lockdowns forced us to spend far more time in a virtual world. If we were paying attention, we were already aware going into the pandemic that the platforms that we had been told were for free speech were actually controlled from behind the scenes by hidden puppet masters. But Big Tech's increasingly heavy-handed efforts to silence dissenters—and its unprecedented profit, even as debt, misery, and non-Covid deaths piled up for the rest of us—brought the issue of its enormous power over our lives out from behind the curtain. The success of open Sweden versus the failure of

Blame Capitalism (Not the China Virus)

America's economy tanked when it followed China into lockdowns, but the Chinese Communist Party was quick to explain that it was *all our fault*. The China Virus that Beijing had unleashed upon the world had nothing to do with rising unemployment rates and shrinking economic growth. Rather, as the CCP-run *Global Times* reported, the economic collapse was caused by our "wild-growing capitalism" that had "bred chaos."[130]

locked-down England, the success of open Florida and the failure of locked-down New York were obvious—to anyone who knew the facts. But the censorious minions of the Big Tech giants wouldn't let us share them, or sometimes even see them. No one was allowed to question what the government was doing in the name of "public health." That was "misinformation."

But what the boards of Apple, Facebook, Google, Microsoft, and Twitter weren't telling their "woke" employees is that they had baser motivations. They were in the business of extracting as much money and (what is the same thing in the Information Age) information as possible from those who ventured onto their domains. The longer the lockdowns continued, the more visitors they had, and the more money and information they could extract.[131]

The Covid pandemic was real, but the pandemic of fear that followed it was stoked by a pack of jackals who used it for political and material gain. Or should I say our corporate ruling class?

So where did the societal lockdowns originate? Who put out the initial grossly inflated mortality rates that justified massive quarantines? Who posted the pictures of people dropping dead in the streets to terrify the public? All of this panic porn, it turns out, was issued from the same dark corner of pandemic hell as the coronavirus itself: the People's Republic of China.

A Book You're Not Supposed to Read

"Some of the world's largest and most profitable companies also had reason to hope that lockdown continued. Giant chains such as Walmart profited from government-mandated lockdowns of their competitors.

"But even those gains paled compared to the riches won by big technology and social media companies—Apple, Facebook, Google, Microsoft, and especially Amazon. Even before the pandemic, these companies had become the world's most important. They were the Information in the Information Age. They were all among the world's largest companies in terms of market value, and enormously profitable, with more than $150 billion in earnings in 2019.

"Now they had an almost unthinkable advantage—a world in which people had to rely on the internet to connect socially, for work, and to shop. . . .

"The gains made billionaires of many of the [tech executives at the very apex of the wealth pyramid]—and supercharged the already vast fortunes of titans such as Facebook's Mark Zuckerberg and Amazon's Jeff Bezos. Suddenly the tech elite had both extra ammunition and extra motivation to support the lockdowns. They could live in comfort in their second or third homes, with food and everything else they wanted delivered, watching their fortunes mount from day to day.

"They had no reason to want anything to change."

—**Alex Berenson,** *Pandemia: How Coronavirus Hysteria Took Over Our Government, Rights, and Lives*[132]

CHAPTER 10

Made in China: Thanks, Bat Lady (and Thank Your American Colleagues)

It is typically difficult, if not impossible, to pinpoint a pathogen's point of origin. In previous pandemics, going all the way back to the Antonine Plague in second-century Rome, no little scientific sleuthing has been required to identify the country in which the disease first arose.

Not so in the case of the novel coronavirus. It is obvious to everyone that it came from Wuhan, China. Moreover, an increasing number of experts believe it was created in a lab, the Wuhan Institute of Virology, as the product of genetic engineering. The CCP's bat story doesn't fly.

The pandemic the world is now facing is thus a man-made disaster, and the men who oversaw the bioweapons research that gave rise to it are the leaders of the Chinese Communist Party, starting with CCP secretary general Xi Jinping himself. To ensure they get full credit for the virus, we should probably call their creation the "Chinese Communist Party Coronavirus." (The World Health Organization, for its part, prefers to obscure the origins of the virus by calling it SARS-CoV-2.) In the interest of brevity, however, I simply refer to it as the "China Virus." That's what it is.

Made in China

Both the China Virus and the pandemic that followed its release were "Made in China."

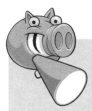

Then and Now: Chicom Cover-up

In the SARS epidemic of 2002–2004, patient zero was a snake seller in China's Guangdong province who came down with the disease on November 16, 2002. He died shortly thereafter, and hundreds of other cases were soon recorded by Chinese health officials. But the Communist regime lied about the disease for months, silenced whistleblowers, doctored data, duped global health authorities, and even accused "outside forces" of carrying out a "bioterrorist" attack. They did not inform the WHO about the outbreak until February 2003, three months later, and only after Canadian intelligence had detected a "flu outbreak" in progress in China.[1]

Like Covid-19, SARS—short for severe acute respiratory syndrome—is a viral respiratory illness caused by a coronavirus. But unlike its genetically engineered cousin, which can be spread through an entire room by a single person's cough, SARS was not an airborne disease.[2]

As a result of its relatively low transmissibility, by the time the SARS epidemic ended in June of 2003, there had been a total of only 8,469 cases reported, and there are no known cases after 2004. The SARS-CoV virus did stand out in one respect, however. It had the highest case fatality rate (CFR, which, as we have seen, is the proportion of deaths to symptomatic cases)—of any influenza since the Spanish Flu. Eleven percent of those who came down with SARS died.[3]

This case fatality rate no doubt impressed China's bioweapons experts.[4] If they could just make a deadly SARS-related coronavirus that was highly infectious as well . . .

In late 2017 a Chinese researcher named Dr. Shi Zhengli, with the help of British zoologist Peter Daszak of EcoHealth Alliance, a beneficiary of U.S. government funding and an ally of Dr. Anthony Fauci,[5] traced the original SARS virus back through an intermediary host to the original carrier: the cave-dwelling horseshoe bats of Yunnan province.[6] The rest is history.

Secret history. Because China didn't tell the world the truth about Covid-19 either.

As we saw in chapter 8, the Chinese Communist Party, true to form, hid the pandemic that was brewing in Wuhan in late 2019 for as long as possible. China flouted its international obligation to report the outbreak to the World Health Organization, which only found out about it on December 31, 2019, when its office in Beijing happened to "pick . . . up a media statement by the Wuhan Municipal Health Commission from their website" reporting a spate of cases of viral pneumonia in the Chinese city.[7]

Confronted with this information, Chinese officials claimed that there were only forty-four cases, and that many were linked to vendors at the Wuhan Seafood Market, which they blamed for the outbreak. They further insisted that they had not yet identified the pathogen responsible, that no health care workers had been infected, and that there had been no human-to-human transmission.[8]

Every single claim was a lie.

Time is of the essence in containing and combating an epidemic. And because of China's misdirection it took several precious weeks for the world to realize what Beijing had known all along, namely, that this was a highly transmissible airborne coronavirus of considerable pathogenicity. The CCP had withheld absolutely critical information. As past pandemics show, it is almost impossible to check the spread of an airborne virus.

Indeed, by the time WHO director-general Tedros Ghebreyesus visited Beijing on January 28, 2020, the China Virus had already gone global. Some 4,500 cases were being reported in 28 different countries.[9]

President Xi Jinping, however, in his meeting with the WHO head, did his best to pretend that the deadly coronavirus epidemic raging in China was completely under control. Xi insisted that he had "been in command of the situation from the beginning," and he promised to continue to "release information on the virus in a timely manner." "The epidemic is a demon," he grandly proclaimed, "and we cannot let this demon hide."[10]

The truth is that Xi Jinping and other Communist Party officials had been playing "hide the demon" for at least three months at that point. And they continued to insist—as they do down to the present day, against all evidence—that the novel coronavirus had come from wild game that was being slaughtered in an open-air market for sale to Chinese consumers who like their meat fresh.

The Investigation That Wasn't

For over a year after the outbreak, Beijing refused to allow the World Health Organization, or anyone else, to carry out an on-the-ground investigation of SARS-CoV-2's origins. Finally, in January 2021, the Chinese authorities consented to allow a carefully selected group of experts, including Peter Daszak of EcoHealth Alliance, to visit Wuhan. The visit did not begin well, as the members of the delegation were first unexpectedly quarantined in their hotel rooms for two long weeks. And the final ten days they had in China were spent for the most part in briefings by Chinese officials, who were intent on convincing them that the China Virus had come from nature. They would allow only one brief, perfunctory visit to Dr. Shi's lab at the Wuhan Institute of Virology. Their Chinese minders achieved what they wanted: the resulting 120-page report devoted only a couple of pages to the Wuhan lab and concluded that it was "extremely unlikely" the virus came from there.[11]

Jamie Metzl, who had served as a national security official in the Obama administration, remarked that he wouldn't call the WHO effort an "investigation" at all. "It was essentially a highly-chaperoned, highly-curated study tour," he said. "This group of experts only saw what the Chinese government wanted them to see. . . . It was agreed first that China would have veto power over who even got to be on the mission. . . . WHO agreed to that. . . . Imagine if we [had] asked the Soviet Union to do a co-investigation of Chernobyl [nuclear disaster]. It doesn't really make sense."[12]

Except as a cover-up.

Xi and the CCP not only misled the world, they also misled their own people. Information about the seriousness of the outbreak was withheld from the people of Wuhan, who went on contracting and spreading the virus among themselves for weeks. Then, just as the virus was reaching epidemic proportions in their city of 14 million or so, the Chinese New Year arrived.

Every year, the largest migration on the planet takes place in China. By long tradition, hundreds of millions of Chinese head back to their ancestral homes—or head off on vacations—for the lunar new year, which in 2020 began on January 25.

In the days leading up to the holiday, no fewer than *5 million* residents of Wuhan got in cars, buses, trains, and planes and went away for the holidays. Some were already ill when they left Wuhan; others came down with Covid on the road. This diaspora carried the coronavirus not only to every corner of China, but to all corners of the globe as well.

Even as the CCP banned flights from Wuhan to other cities within China, it continued to allow flights to other countries. By using their own people as innocent disease vectors, the Chinese leaders deliberately created a global pandemic in record time. The world has been battling this epidemiological nightmare ever since.

What Happened in the Wuhan Lab?

At first, Beijing blamed bats. China's original cover story was that the virus had leapt from bat to man at the Wuhan Seafood Market, an open-air abattoir where all kinds of exotic animals, not just fish, were slaughtered for food. Perhaps someone had gotten a bad bowl of bat soup at this "wet market."

I was among the first to question this highly implausible explanation. "Don't buy China's story," I wrote in the *New York Post* on February 22, 2020. I marshaled several pieces of evidence linking the virus to the lab:

- China had only one Level 4 lab that could "handle deadly coronaviruses," and that lab just happened to be located in Wuhan at the very "epicenter of the epidemic."

- Underlining China's shoddy lab-safety record, Xi Jinping himself had warned about "lab safety" as a national security priority in the early days of the crisis.
- Following Xi's guidance, "the Chinese Ministry of Science and Technology released a new directive titled: 'Instructions on strengthening biosecurity management in microbiology labs that handle advanced viruses like the novel coronavirus.'"
- As soon as the outbreak began, China's military was put in charge, and the People's Liberation Army's top biowarfare expert, Major General Chen Wei, was dispatched to Wuhan to deal with it.[13]

Even at the time, there was other evidence pointing to the lab—and to the involvement of the Chinese People's Liberation Army (PLA):

- On December 30, the director of the Wuhan Institute of Virology's high-containment lab went through and censored her lab's research records, in what looks like a clumsy effort to disassociate herself from the outbreak.
- On January 3, China's National Health Commission ordered all the early samples of the coronavirus that had been collected by private and university labs in China—vital for tracing the origin and early spread of the disease—to be destroyed, along with any records of the genetic sequence of the virus's RNA strand.
- China's civilian Center for Disease Control was completely shut out of the picture in favor of the PLA—suggesting a classified military program was involved.

- Military academies and installations in and around Wuhan were closed around January 1, 2020, well before the Chinese public was notified that there was a problem.
- China lied about human-to-human transmission, leaving the United States and other countries unprepared for the rapid spread of the virus, and thus virtually ensuring that more lives would be lost.[14]

It was still early days, and the evidence was circumstantial, but I was fairly certain even then that I could have convinced a jury of China's culpability. Even so, as I waited for more facts to surface, I was careful to call the "lab origin" just a possibility.[15]

Information was slow to come out because China had the Wuhan lab locked down tight. At the same time, the U.S. virology establishment, following the lead of its chief funder, Dr. Anthony Fauci, had closed ranks against the lab-leak theory. Both China and Fauci and his colleagues were strenuously denying that gain-of-function research—not to mention a PLA bioweapons program—had anything to do with the pandemic. It took over a year for the attempted cover-ups on both sides of the Pacific to unravel, but by the middle of 2021 the outline of the true origins of the China Virus was becoming clear.[16]

During that time China had burned through a half dozen increasingly implausible cover stories. After the collapse of the wet market fable, China tried to pin the blame on a wild succession of animals—bats and pangolins and raccoon dogs, oh my!—for harboring the virus.[17]

But it wasn't long before the story switched back to bats. The world was told that many years ago, in a cave in Yunnan province—far away from the Wuhan lab—miners had fallen ill from being peed on, pooped on, and bitten by those nasty, virus-harboring creatures. The Yunnan caves were the location where the "zoonosis"—a fancy word for the transmission of a disease from animal to human—occurred, the authorities confidently declared.[18]

Yet when scientists went to those caves and collected samples from the bats there—bats that Beijing claims were infected with the direct ancestor of the China Virus—the samples were confiscated by the police. The caves were placed off-limits to researchers and journalists by the authorities in November of 2020, and police and hired thugs were stationed along roads to block access to the caves.[19]

Soon the Associated Press was reporting that, "under direct orders from President Xi Jinping," the State Council—China's cabinet—must vet all research papers based on evidence from the caves.[20] Since Xi had made it impossible to gather such evidence, this was tantamount to saying that no one would be allowed to question the Communist authorities' claim that the novel coronavirus evolved in bats in a Yunnan cave.

No one except the authorities themselves, it seems. Communist officials have cast doubt on their own bat cave deception by simultaneously advancing another story about the virus's origins—namely, that it came from . . . America. As early as February 27, 2020, one of China's leading scientists, a party official by the name of Zhong Nanshan, held a press conference in the southern city of Guangzhou at which he suggested that the China Virus was a foreign import. "Though the COVID-19 was first discovered in China, it does not mean that it originated in China," Zhong insisted.[21]

This tale has grown more elaborate with the telling. In its latest rendition, CCP officials describe SARS-CoV-2 as an American bioweapon created in the U.S. Army's research labs in Fort Detrick, Maryland. As to how the "American Virus"—as they unabashedly called it—got to China, they have an answer for that too: it was secretly released on the unsuspecting Chinese population of Wuhan by the American soldier-athletes who participated in the October 2019 Military World Games in that city.[22] Chinese ambassadors and propaganda outlets around the world now parrot this absurd claim.

Then and Now: Baseless Accusations

The Chinese Communist claim that the novel coronavirus is an American bioweapon is not the first charge of germ warfare that the CCP has leveled against the United States. During the Korean War, the People's Liberation Army, echoed by the North Koreans and the Soviets, claimed that American troops were deploying biological weapons against its forces.

No such germ warfare attacks by U.S. forces on Chinese and North Korean forces ever occurred. On one level, the accusations were nothing more than straightforward anti-American propaganda, intended to discredit the United States in the eyes of the world. But the baseless claims also served as cover for the biological weapons programs of the PLA itself, which disguised its germ warfare units as "anti-plague units," under the pretense that they were stood up solely to defend against (imaginary) U.S. attacks.[23]

Beijing attempted a similar deception during the Covid pandemic.

China leveled false accusations that the United States had released a bioweapon on China—which would be an act of war—when in fact the reverse was true. The United States did not attack China. Rather, China attacked the world.

What this recycled Korean War propaganda tells you is that the Chinese Communist Party still considers itself to be at war with the United States. Fighting on the Korean peninsula ended on July 27, 1953, with an armistice—a temporary cessation of hostilities—but that ceasefire never gave way to a formal peace treaty. So our two countries are still technically at war, although for some decades the United States has preferred to pretend that we are not.

NOTE: If your enemy says you are at war, then you are probably at war, whether you want to be or not.

Who makes up such bat-sh*t crazy stories about secret bioweapons and superspreading soldiers? The same people, it seems, whose fever dream for decades has been to do exactly the same thing. There is copious evidence that Chinese labs were engaged in dangerous gain-of-function research, and that these techniques were being used in an active bioweapons program that included the Wuhan lab. It wasn't an innocent bat that produced the deadly virus, but highly classified gain-of-function research carried out under the direction of the Chinese People's Liberation Army.[24]

The Chinese Whistleblower

The big break in uncovering the origins of the China Virus came when a Chinese medical doctor and virologist by the name of Yan Li-Meng defected to the United States in April 2020. Dr. Yan, thirty-six, whom I interviewed shortly after her arrival, insisted that, based on her own research and experience, the coronavirus "did not come from a wet market in Wuhan. It did not come from nature at all. It was created in a lab."[25]

Dr. Yan was one of the first scientists to study the novel coronavirus. Before she defected, she worked at Asia's top virology lab—the P3 Lab at the University of Hong Kong. The lab was and is the global center for coronavirus research. Its famous "SARS hunters" cracked the code of the first SARS coronavirus outbreak in 2003. Now there was a second SARS virus on the loose.

In December of 2019 Dr. Yan's supervisor, Dr. Leo Poon, became alarmed at reports of a cluster of SARS-like cases centered in the city of Wuhan in central China and asked her to look into it. Yan sent out inquiries to her network of medical contacts in mainland China, and by December 31 she had confirmed that the infections were caused by a hitherto unknown virus and that it was spreading—quickly—by human-to-human transmission. "This key fact was suppressed by the Chinese Communist Party and, later, by the World Health Organization," she told me.

Yan took her concerns about the Wuhan epidemic to Poon, but he warned her that she must "keep silent." Do not criticize the CCP for its lies about the virus, and don't contradict the official line that the virus had come from wild animals at the Wuhan wet market. Poon told her repeatedly, "If you speak out, we will get into trouble and be disappeared."

Disappeared. As in secretly arrested, tortured, and killed.

For three months, Yan took her supervisor's advice to heart. She kept her head down and her mouth shut and continued her research. She obtained samples of the China Virus and soon discovered that its "backbone" was a bat coronavirus that had been isolated by the PLA, and that it had at least two artificial man-made "insertions" that make it particularly deadly to human beings.[26] The first insertion allows it to spread easily from person to person, while the second insertion allows the virus to infect different kinds of tissue once it is in the human body.

Those doing the splicing left "signatures" behind in the genome of the virus. To boost a virus's lethality, for example, gain-of-function researchers customarily insert a snippet of RNA that codes for two arginine amino acids. This snippet, called double CGG, has never been found in any other related coronaviruses, but it is present in the SARS-CoV-2 virus, which causes Covid-19.[27] Besides this damning evidence, there are other indications of tampering as well.

"Any scientist who has this knowledge [about the structure of viruses] will know that this coronavirus is not from nature," Dr. Yan told me. Her conclusion: China engineered the virus in the lab, deliberately making it more infectious and more deadly.

The dwindling ranks of lab-leak "deniers" continue to insist that the vast laboratory of nature is capable of infinite surprises. That's true, of course. And it's also theoretically true that if you have enough monkeys typing the four DNA bases A, C, G, and T on enough computer keyboards, they will eventually produce a complete and accurate copy of the human genome, which is 6.4 billion such bases long. But what are the odds?

Seriously, what are the odds that the virus passed naturally from animals to humans? Dr. David Asher, who headed the Trump administration's investigation into the origins of the China Virus, put that question to a biostatistician, who calculated the odds at roughly . . . one in 13 billion. Given that vanishingly small probability, Asher pointed out that "to say this came out of a zoonotic situation is sort of ridiculous."[28]

Dr. Yan and colleagues have published a series of scientific papers laying out precisely, in highly technical language, how the "unusual features of

Covid Truth and Consequences

In the early months of 2020 in Hong Kong, as Dr. Yan Li-Meng continued to gather evidence that Covid-19 had been created in the Wuhan lab, she became increasingly desperate to get the truth out. Lives were being lost every day she stayed silent. But to speak out in Hong Kong, which is now under the control of the Chinese Communist Party, would cost her life. It was with a heavy heart that she finally decided to defect to the United States. "I tried to persuade my husband, who worked in the same lab, to come with me," she told me. "But I failed."

On April 28, 2020, Dr. Yan went in secret to the Hong Kong airport and boarded a flight to Los Angeles. She spent her first two months in the United States being debriefed by U.S. intelligence officials in a safe house. But as China Virus cases began to spike dramatically all around the globe, she decided to go public.

When I interviewed her in July of 2020, Dr. Yan told me that the Chinese government knew the

coronavirus was man-made and that it could be transmitted from person to person. "It was made in their lab using a virus 'backbone' from the PLA," she said, pointing out that the "backbone" virus and the engineered virus were nearly identical—except for a few key modifications.

Dr. Yan has paid a heavy price for her honesty and integrity. She was fired by the University of Hong Kong, and the director of the lab she worked at has publicly dismissed her findings that the virus was man-made. Her husband has distanced himself from her, and her parents, who are still in China, have publicly called her a "traitor." Yan remains in hiding even today, and she told me that even in America, she fears for her life. All the same, she has no regrets.

"I do this because I am a scientist. I know the truth and I want to tell it to the world," she told me firmly. "But if they find me, they will kill me."[29]

the SARS-CoV-2 genome suggest . . . sophisticated laboratory modification rather than natural evolution."[30]

These were startling claims, but as virologists began to carry out their own detailed studies, many came to share Yan's view. Virology researchers outside the United States were the first to weigh in.

"The properties that we now see in the virus, we have yet to discover anywhere in nature," said Norwegian virologist Birger Sorensen in a July 13 interview with the scientific journal *Minerva*. "We know that these properties make the virus very infectious, so if it came from nature, there should also be many animals infected with this, but we have still not been able to trace the virus in nature." Sorensen, who works for Immunor AS, a Norwegian company that researches and develops vaccines, went on to say, "When we compare the novel coronavirus with the one that caused SARS, we see that there are altogether six inserts in this virus that stand out compared to other known SARS viruses."[31]

Australian Nikolai Petrokvsy, the director of endocrinology at Flinders University in Adelaide, also said that the virus could be man-made. "Our own research, which is currently under review and was based on rigorous molecular modeling, revealed some highly unexpected findings for a virus postulated to have recently crossed from animal to humans," he told me in an interview. "From the very earliest isolates it was uniquely adapted to infect humans above other species we tested."[32]

Another early supporter of the lab-leak theory of the virus's origins was Professor Joseph Tritto, the president of the Paris-based World Academy of Biomedical Sciences and Technologies (WABT). His book *Cina COVID 19: La Chimera che ha cambiato il Mondo*—which translated into English would be *China COVID 19: The Chimera That Changed the World*—argued persuasively that the China Virus was genetically engineered in the Wuhan Institute of Virology's P4 (high-containment) lab in a program supervised by the Chinese military.[33]

The U.S. virology establishment, dependent upon Anthony Fauci's National Institute of Allergies and Infectious Diseases (NIAID) for funding, was much more circumspect in the beginning. Its members were also heavily influenced by the story that a close natural analogue of the China Virus had been found in a Yunnan bat cave, especially because the Chinese researcher who reported it was someone many of them knew and several of them had trained. Her name was Shi Zhengli, and she just happened to be the director of the Wuhan Institute of Virology's P4 lab.

China's Batwoman: Dr. Shi Zhengli

By early January of 2020, following orders from China's National Health Commission, Dr. Shi Zhengli and her colleagues had undoubtedly destroyed any samples of the China Virus, along with any computerized record of its genetic sequence.[34] It was the equivalent of wiping the fingerprints from a gun that had just been used to commit murder

The "gun" itself couldn't be destroyed, however. In fact, the murder weapon used—the China Virus—was busy replicating itself by the billions within each and every person who came down with the disease.

Dr. Shi and her colleagues, including decorated military scientist Zhou Yusen, knew that the coronavirus they had assembled using recombinant technology was so different from known coronaviruses that it would raise suspicions.[35] No other beta-coronavirus—the family from which their "backbone" coronavirus came from—had anything resembling the genetic sequences they had inserted, including one used to make it more infectious to humans.

To reinforce the "wet market" cover story—namely, that this new pathogen had come from nature and not from her lab—something had to be done. And it had to be done quickly.[36] Anger against China for its lack of transparency about the origins and characteristics of the virus was growing.

Dr. Shi, who is known as China's Batwoman, decided to "discover" a new bat coronavirus very similar to the one she had engineered. That "discovery" would prove to the world that coronaviruses similar to the one that causes Covid were found in nature, and so deflect the growing suspicion that she had crafted the China Virus in her lab. The close relationship between the two coronaviruses—especially their shared ability to infect humans—would greatly reinforce China's story that SARS-CoV-2 had jumped from a bat to a human in a cave in Yunnan province.

Inventing a new coronavirus may sound complicated, but it's not. All Dr. Shi had to do was sit down in front of her computer keyboard, open a Word file, and begin to type in the genetic sequence of the China Virus she had already created. This would involve simply entering in a string of the letters A, G, C, and U, which stand for the four nucleotides, adenine, guanine, cytosine, and uracil, switching out one for another from time to time to mimic the "random mutations" that regularly occur in nature. She could easily have completed the "data entry" part of her task in a day, since coronaviruses contain fewer than thirty thousand different nucleotides.

And just like that, a natural analogue to the China Virus sprang into being. The missing link—proving that there was a bat coronavirus in nature that could easily mutate into one infecting humans—had been found, discrediting the suggestion that the China Virus had come from her Wuhan lab.[37]

On January 27, 2020, Dr. Shi registered her new virus with the National Center for Biotechnology Information (NCBI) of the U.S. National Institutes of Health, the customary repository for such information. She called it RaTG-13, Ra for *Rhinolophus affinis*, the Latin name of the intermediate horseshoe bat, and 13 for 2013, the year she had "discovered" it in a bat cave in Yunnan.[38]

★ ★ ★
Genetics 101

The genome of a cell contains the information that its machinery needs to make proteins. In the case of RNA, the "words" that make up the language of genetics consist of the four nucleotides, adenine, guanine, cytosine, and uracil, or A, G, C, and U for short. There are sixty-four "words" that can be spelled out using these four combinations, but only twenty different amino acids. That means that there is more than one combination of nucleotides for each amino acid. For example, there are no fewer than six different "words" for the amino acid arginine, which is the one used to supercharge viruses in gain-of-function research. Which combination is used can tell you a lot about whether the virus is natural or, as in the case of the China Virus, man-made.

In the years since, no one else has independently verified RaTG-13's existence. No other lab has a sample of this purported virus, and no one else has ever sequenced it. And no one ever will, of course, because it likely exists only as a string of letters on Dr. Shi's computer. But her misdirection worked, at least with some people.

The Chinese virology community—following new strict party guidelines—quickly signed on, publishing a flurry of studies suggesting that the existence of RaTG-13 proved that SARS-CoV-2 came from nature.[39] They did genomic analyses showing that RaTG-13 and SARS-CoV-2 were 96 percent identical throughout the whole sequence of the viral genome. They calculated that the two shared a common ancestor a few decades back. They claimed that other "first cousins" of the Covid-19 virus would soon be found in nature.[40] In fact, none has been found and none will, since the only thing the two virus genomes have in common is Dr. Shi herself, who engineered the one and appears to have fabricated the other.

Some Western virologists followed suit, suggesting that the existence of RaTG-13 called Chinese defector Dr. Yan Li-Meng's accusations of genetic engineering into question.

Virologist Jonathan Latham, a virologist and cofounder of the Bioscience Resource Project in Ithaca, New York, referred to RaTG-13 as evidence that the China Virus came from nature. Latham told me that his team of researchers believe that the Wuhan Institute of Virology studied tissue samples from miners who were infected with the virus in 2012 in the Yunnan bat caves, but said they don't know whether those samples were later manipulated in the lab. Of Dr. Yan's claim that the virus was actually created in the lab, he would only say, "We can't rule it out."[41]

Richard Ebright, a professor of chemistry and director of the Waksman Institute of Microbiology at Rutgers University in New Jersey, has indicated that he disagrees with Yan's theory of "insertions" because RaTG-13 has some of the same sequences. But he did grant that "this does not rule out the possibility the virus was laboratory constructed or laboratory-enhanced using methods that do not leave signatures.'[42]

Dr. Shi's scheme almost succeeded. As clever as China's Batwoman is, though, she did not commit the perfect deception. She left behind a few key clues that reveal what she was up to as clearly as fingerprints on a murder weapon.

A blogger writing at Nerd Has Power brilliantly teased these findings out of the data. Because he published his raw data, I and others have been able to check and verify his work. You can read the Nerd's efforts yourself if you have a free afternoon and a strong math background. Suffice it to say that Dr. Shi did not produce a truly random string of changes to her lab-engineered SARS-CoV-2 when she fabricated its "close cousin," RaTG-13.[43]

An Impossible Ratio

As viruses evolve, they mutate. That is to say, one of the four nucleotides is randomly replaced by another. Most of these random mutations do not produce changes in the amino acids that make up the protein, and so they are called "synonymous," since the three-nucleotide "codon" still codes for the same amino acid despite the change. Like a synonym in a thesaurus, it "looks" different but "means"—in terms of the amino acid and resulting protein—the same thing.

But then there are "non-synonymous" mutations—mutations that *do* change the resulting amino acid and hence the configuration of the resulting protein. In nature, the ratio of synonymous to non-synonymous is approximately 5:1.

Here's where Dr. Shi got into trouble. When typing in the genomic sequence of her "discovery," she made far too many non-synonymous changes at the beginning. Then, one-third of the way through the sequence, she apparently realized her error. After that, she made far too few non-synonymous changes.

So while the entire genome has the expected 5:1 ratio of synonymous to non-synonymous changes, there are stretches where the ratio is closer to 2:1 and other long stretches where it is as high as 44:1.

Nature's mutations are random. Dr. Shi's "mutations" are not. Dr. Lawrence Sellin has calculated that the odds that her "mutations" occurred naturally in just one area—the critical spike protein that makes Covid so infectious—are almost 10 million to one.[44]

Dr. Yan also rejects Dr. Shi's claim to have "found a close relative to the China Virus in nature" way back in 2013. Not only is RaTG-13 suspiciously similar to SARS-CoV-2, but a close study of its genome shows that it is a fabrication, according to defector Yan.[45]

If RaTG-13 is merely a strategic deception, then the trail leads back to the gain-of-function research that Dr. Shi was carrying out in her lab at the Wuhan Institute of Virology. How did she learn her trade, who funded her research, and finally, what coronavirus did she use as the "backbone" for the highly infectious SARS-CoV-2?

Taught and Funded by Us

Shi Zhengli received her master's degree from the Wuhan Institute of Virology in 1990. She earned her Ph.D. in France in 2000 and then returned to Wuhan to direct the institute's research into dangerous bat coronaviruses.[46] She collaborated extensively with several high-security biosafety level 4 (P4) research labs in the United States, including Ralph Baric's lab at the University of North Carolina and the Galveston National Laboratory run by the University of Texas Medical Branch, which specializes in exotic disease diagnosis and research.

Shi's research focused on naturally occurring SARS-like coronaviruses that, like the SARS virus itself, could infect human beings directly. Take, for example, her 2013 article in the scientific journal *Nature Medicine* entitled "Isolation and Characterization of a Bat SARS-like Coronavirus That Uses the ACE2 Receptor."[47] Shi Zhengli and her coauthor, Peter Daszak of EcoHealth Alliance, reported that "Chinese horseshoe bats are natural reservoirs of SARS-CoV, and that intermediate hosts may not be necessary for direct human infection by some bat SARS-like coronaviruses."[48]

But Dr. Shi and Peter Daszak were not content merely to study natural coronaviruses. They were also genetically engineering new ones. In a 2008 article in the *Journal of Virology*, Shi and her team described how they had engineered SARS-like coronaviruses from horseshoe bats to enable them to use angiotensin-converting enzyme 2 (ACE2) to gain entry into human cells.[49] In other words, more than ten years ago, Shi's team was already creating new and deadly coronaviruses. They did so by inserting that part of the dangerous SARS virus that allows it to infect people into a second bat coronavirus, which was then able to attack human cells just like the original SARS virus did.

But simply recreating a new SARS virus was only a first step. Shi and her team wanted to move beyond that to create completely new deadly and infectious coronaviruses. For that she needed a new, more advanced recombinant technique. And Professor Baric at the University of North Carolina, whose lab she was working with closely, had developed just such a technique for quickly and easily producing what he called "infectious clones." This involves taking coronaviruses from horseshoe bats and genetically engineering them to more easily infect human cells.[50]

Why would he—or anyone, for that matter—do such a thing?

Referring to the 2013 study by Shi and Daszak, Baric explained: "In 2013 preemergent SARS-like coronaviruses were identified in horseshoe bats and found to be poised for entry into the human population. . . . Preemergent coronaviruses (CoVs) pose a global threat that requires immediate intervention. Rapid intervention necessitates the capacity to generate, grow, and genetically manipulate infectious CoVs in order to rapidly

★ ★ ★
Reality Check

Celebrated evolutionary biologist Andrew Rambaut, who is not a fan of gain-of-function research, told Peter Daszak on Twitter in November of 2019, "The more we look, the more new viruses we find. The problem is we have no way of knowing which may be important or which may emerge [to cause a pandemic]. There is basically nothing we can do with that information to prevent or mitigate epidemics."

"Not true," Daszak shot back. "We've made great progress with bat SARS-related CoVs, ID'ing >50 novel strains, sequencing spike protein genes, ID'ing ones that bind to human cells, using recombinant viruses/humanized mice to see SARS-like signs, and showing some don't respond to MAbs, vaccines...."

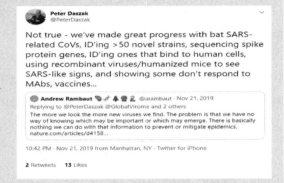

Even as Daszak was tweeting this on November 21, 2019, a deadly product of the Wuhan lab's gain-of-function research was indeed showing "SARS-like signs"—by killing people.[51]

evaluate pathogenic mechanisms, host and tissue permissibility, and candidate antiviral therapeutic efficacy."[52]

Now all of this—"preemergent coronaviruses," "poised for entry," "global threat," "requires immediate intervention"—sounds very ominous. But what people need to understand is that the good professor was not talking about coronaviruses that have actually infected even one single, living, breathing human being. It was all speculative. He was talking about coronaviruses that might, possibly, at some point in the future, make the leap from bats to humans. Or they might not. Ever.[53]

This means that the phrase "preemergent coronavirus" is at best misleading, at worst a fiction. Neither Professor Baric, Dr. Shi, Daszak, Fauci, nor anyone else can possibly know whether any one of these naturally occurring viruses will ever mutate into something capable of infecting people.

But rather than wait for the next coronavirus to make the leap from animal to human, these researchers decided to anticipate nature by creating such dangerous pathogens in the lab. That was what gain-of-function research was all about. Professor Baric, as we have seen, invented a quick and easy technique to construct unnatural coronaviruses in the lab, viruses that he could then test on mice to see if they would infect and kill them.[54] As he himself put it, "Much of the [coronavirus] research over the last 15 years has been possible because of the capacity to generate infectious clones using highly efficient reverse genetics platforms, coupled with robust small animal models of human disease."[55] Dr. Shi Zhengli learned these techniques from Baric and collaborated with him on research projects using them, as they revealed in a 2015 article in *Nature Medicine* where they discussed engineered bat coronaviruses that were potentially capable of infecting human beings.[56]

Now, a sane person might think that gain-of-function research—creating dangerous new pathogens for which humanity has no acquired immunity, no vaccines, and no drug therapies—might not be a good idea. If such a pathogen was released, either accidently or deliberately, it might well cause a pandemic. But Dr. Anthony Fauci was a big proponent of the research from its inception, and his National Allergy and Infectious Diseases Institute initially funded Professor Baric's research.

It wasn't long before people more prudent than Fauci had second thoughts, however, and on October 17, 2014, a moratorium on risky gain-of-function research on influenza, MERS, and SARS viruses was put in place for research funded by the U.S. government.[57] Not long thereafter Fauci himself—one can imagine with great reluctance—sent a letter notifying the University of North Carolina that Professor Baric's gain-of-function research on SARS-like coronaviruses might violate the new moratorium.

The letter ordered Baric to pause his gain-of-function research into SARS-like coronaviruses, referencing a new document from the "Public Health Emergency" office of the U.S. Department of Health and Human Services. This document defines gain-of-function research as "research that improves the ability of a pathogen to cause disease . . . [by] confer[ring] attributes to . . . SARS [coronaviruses] such that the virus would have enhanced pathogenicity and/or transmissibility (via the respiratory route) in mammals . . . [that] may entail biosafety and biosecurity risks."[58]

The original scientific rationale for "enhancing" the ability of certain coronaviruses to infect and kill human beings was to get one step ahead of the next pandemic. *We will create superbugs in the lab*, the scientists said to themselves, *and we will outsmart them by developing drug therapies and vaccines. Then, when the next superbug emerges from nature, we will be better prepared to outsmart it in turn.*

But what happens if you create a new superbug in the lab and, before you have devised a defense against it, it escapes from the lab?

Or, worse yet, what happens if you teach Communist China's leading virologist, Dr. Shi Zhengli, how to use gain-of-function techniques to engineer deadly viruses, and the CCP decides that she should use her newfound skills to create bioweapons?

We no longer have to guess what the cost on the world would be of unleashing such an "enhanced" coronavirus—a pathogen against which human beings had no natural defenses, and for which human science initially had no treatments or vaccines—because we are living through it. By mid-2022 the cost was over 6 million lives and $20 trillion—and counting.

Follow the Money

The U.S. pause on gain-of-function research was not lifted for three years, until December 29, 2017, when the National Institutes of Health put in place what it called "robust oversight," including a review of the "scientific merits and potential benefits of the research, as well as the potential to create, transfer, or use an enhanced potential pandemic pathogen."[59] But by that time, Peter Daszak of EcoHealth Alliance had moved his research on coronaviruses to the one country that was most interested in creating such a "potential pandemic pathogen": the People's Republic of China.

Fauci has hotly denied reports that he was funding the gain-of-function research at the Wuhan lab. In May of 2021, Senator Rand Paul of Kentucky confronted Fauci about funding of virus enhancement experiments at the Wuhan Institute of Virology, suggesting that Fauci was directly involved in the creation of SARS-CoV-2 and the subsequent outbreak. Fauci denied it.[60]

When Fauci was pressed again on this point by Senator Paul at a June 2021 congressional hearing, he insisted that the National Institutes of Health "has not ever and does not now fund gain-of-function research in the Wuhan Institute of Virology."[61]

But the paper trail says otherwise. We have long known that as head of NIAID, Fauci approved NIH grants to Peter Daszak's EcoHealth Alliance, which in turn subcontracted some of the work to Dr. Shi and the Wuhan Institute of Virology.[62] Shortly before the outbreak, Daszak said Shi's virology laboratory was a "world-class lab of the highest standards"[63] that was making "great progress."[64] Great progress towards what, exactly?

On December 9, 2019, just weeks before news of the Wuhan outbreak leaked out, Daszak gave an interview explaining that he had been funding research at the Wuhan Institute of Virology for fifteen years. The work involved collecting coronaviruses from nature and using gain-of-function techniques to make them more infectious and deadly. Coronaviruses were perfect for this work, he said enthusiastically: "You can manipulate them in the lab pretty easily. It's a spike protein. Spike protein drives a lot of what happens with the coronavirus, the zoonotic risk [to humans]. So you can get the sequence, build the protein. And we worked with Ralph Baric at the

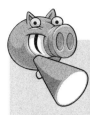

Then and Now: Conspiracy Theories

Peter Daszak's EcoHealth Alliance had worked closely with Dr. Shi and the Wuhan Institute of Virology,[65] which he called a "world-class lab of the highest standards." He and the Batwoman even authored research papers together. And right up to the eve of the pandemic, Daszak continued to brag about the "great progress" being made at the Wuhan Institute of Virology on the gain-of-function front.

As the China Virus began spreading around the world, however, the last thing Daszak wanted to talk about was his gain-of-function work with the Wuhan lab. He quickly endorsed the CCP's claim that it came from a wet market, and attacked anyone who said otherwise—including me—as an unhinged conspiracy theorist. In an April 2020 interview with Democracy Now he insisted, "The idea that this virus escaped from a lab is just pure baloney. It's simply not true. I've been working with that lab for 15 years. They're some of the best scientists in the world."

But Daszak had already gone even further. He had drafted a letter to the prestigious British medical journal *The Lancet* attacking the idea that the deadly virus could have been engineered in the Wuhan lab. The letter, which was published on February 19, 2020, under the signature of Daszak and twenty-six of his fellow virologists-apologists, declared in no uncertain terms, "We stand together to strongly condemn conspiracy theories suggesting that COVID-19 does not have a natural origin."[66]

The letter, followed by another by Kristian Andersen and other scientists in *Nature Medicine* the following month, had the desired effect.[67] Science journalists and others assumed the science was settled. Anyone who subsequently questioned the supposed "scientific consensus" that the virus came from nature was labeled a "fringe conspiracy theorist" to be mocked and censored.

Big Media and Big Tech both signed on. When they mentioned the Wuhan lab-leak theory at all, the major online, print, and broadcast media treated it as a paranoid fantasy, not all that different from the claim of CCP propagandists that the virus had originated in the U.S. Army's labs at Fort Detrick, Maryland, and been deliberately seeded in Wuhan.

No one was exempt from criticism. When no less a figure than Dr. Robert Redfield, the former director of the Centers for Disease Control and Prevention (CDC), came around to the view that the coronavirus came from the Wuhan lab, he was immediately attacked by the mainstream media. The *New York Times* published a hit piece entitled, "Ex-CDC Director Favors Debunked Covid-19 Origin Theory."[68]

Big Tech, as always, went even further, censoring any mention of the lab origins of the virus. Facebook and other media outlets had decided that even suggesting that the China Virus originated in the lab was a "conspiracy theory," so they banned discussion of the entire topic. I was among the banned.[69] Nevertheless, the investigation into Covid-19's origins continued to pick up steam into the first few weeks of the Biden administration. It took a year for cracks to emerge in Daszak's artificial consensus. On May 14, 2021, eighteen scientists wrote to *Science* magazine urging that "we must take hypotheses about both natural and laboratory spillovers seriously."[70] Facebook caved ten days later, announcing that it would "no longer take down posts claiming that Covid-19 was man-made or manufactured."[71] Even Dr. Anthony Fauci, ever alert to the shifting political winds, was forced to admit that he was "not convinced" that Covid-19 arose naturally.[72] The final blows to Daszak's effort to muzzle debate came that September. An investigation carried out by *The Telegraph* revealed that twenty-six of the twenty-seven *Lancet* letter scientists he had enlisted to trash the idea that the China Virus was a product of the Wuhan Institute of Virology had undisclosed conflicts of interest. They either had links to that same lab or were themselves engaged in gain-of-function research and risked losing their funding if it was banned.[73]

Even *The Lancet* finally reversed itself. On September 17, 2021, the journal published a letter from sixteen scientists chastising Daszak and his colleagues, saying that the pressure they had brought to bear against the lab-leak theory had had "a silencing effect on the wider scientific debate, including among science journalists." The letter, called "an appeal for an objective, open, and transparent scientific debate about the origin of SARS-CoV-2," urged scientific journals to "open their columns to in-depth analyses of all hypotheses." "As scientists, we need to evaluate all hypotheses on a rational basis, and to weigh their likelihood based on facts and evidence, devoid of speculation concerning possible political impacts," they wrote. "More importantly, science embraces alternative hypotheses, contradictory arguments, verification, refutability, and controversy. Departing from this principle risks establishing dogmas, abandoning the essence of science, and, even worse, paving the way for *conspiracy theories*" [emphasis added].[74]

The irony here is perhaps unintentional: the only "conspiracy theory" surrounding the origins of the China Virus was in fact organized and directed by the one person who had the most to lose if the lab origin of the virus was revealed—Peter Daszak himself. Although in the loser sweepstakes, the chief backer of gain-of-function research, Dr. Anthony Fauci, must be considered a close, close second.

University of North Carolina to do this. We insert the sequence into the backbone of another virus and then do some work in the lab."[75]

Baric's techniques had enabled Shi Zhengli to create killer coronaviruses. When questions about the prudence of such research were raised by evolutionary biologist Andrew Rambaut, Daszak tweeted back: "We've made great progress with bat SARS-related coronaviruses, identifying more than 50 novel strains, sequencing spike protein genes, identifying ones that bind to human cells, using recombinant viruses [and] humanized mice to see SARS-like signs, and showing some don't respond to MAbs [monoclonal antibodies], vaccines. . . ."[76]

Daszak claimed that the research he was carrying out with the Wuhan lab was necessary to create a vaccine to prevent the next global pandemic. In light of what has happened since, however, his December 9, 2019, interview almost reads like a confession. Apparently the man had no idea that the Chinese Communist Party might have other uses in mind for dangerous coronaviruses than the development of vaccines.[77]

By funding Daszak's EcoHealth Alliance, is Dr. Anthony Fauci linked to the gain-of-function research that Dr. Shi was doing at the Wuhan Institute of Virology? New documents obtained from the NIH in response to a FOIA request by The Intercept suggest that the answer is yes. After reviewing nine hundred pages of grant applications and progress reports, The Intercept reporters concluded:

> Scientists working under a 2014 NIH grant to the EcoHealth Alliance to study bat coronaviruses combined the genetic material from a "parent" coronavirus known as WIV1 with other viruses. They twice submitted summaries of their work that showed that, when in the lungs of genetically engineered mice, three altered bat coronaviruses at times reproduced far more quickly than the original virus on which they were based. The altered viruses

were also somewhat more pathogenic, with one causing the mice to lose significant weight. The researchers reported, "These results demonstrate varying pathogenicity of SARSr-CoVs with different spike proteins in humanized mice."[78]

Let's break this down into bite-size morsels. First, the EcoHealth Alliance grants—there were at least two—were intended to fund gain-of-function research, that is, the creation of new chimeric SARS-related coronaviruses that could more easily infect human cells and would be more deadly to human beings. And that's exactly what they did, as Daszak's progress reports back to the NIH make clear:

Increased Infectiousness: " … three altered bat coronaviruses at times reproduced far more quickly than the original virus."[79]

The faster the virus replicates, the faster you become ill.

Increased Pathogenicity: "The altered viruses were also somewhat more pathogenic, with one causing the mice to lose significant weight."[80]

This is not a Weight Watchers program for mice. The more weight the mice lose, the sicker they are, and the more dangerous the virus.

So if Dr. Shi and her research team succeeded in genetically engineering three viruses to be more infectious, one of which was more deadly as well, then it would seem that they met the gain-of-function goals. They certainly thought so: "These results demonstrate varying pathogenicity of SARS[-related-coronaviruses] with different spike proteins in humanized mice."

A number of American virologists agreed, including Dr. Vincent Racaniello, professor of microbiology and immunology at Columbia University, who told The Intercept: "There's no question . . . from the weight loss [of the mice], it's gain-of-function. Tony Fauci is wrong saying it's not."

Bear in mind that we are not talking about ordinary mice, but so-called "humanized" mice. These are mice that have been genetically engineered to resemble human beings in one very specific way: the mouse receptors on their lung cells have been replaced with human receptors.

Viruses make their way into cells by attempting to insert their spike protein "key" into the receptor's "lock." What Dr. Shi did in her Wuhan lab was attach various spike protein keys to the original coronavirus to see which one "fit" best. In three cases the new key worked so well on the human receptor that the virus was able to quickly gain entry and replicate that much faster.

If a chimeric virus can infect and kill a humanized mouse, it can also infect and kill a human being. That's what gain-of-function research is all about.

All the scientists interviewed by The Intercept insisted that the Fauci-funded research "could not have directly sparked the pandemic. None of the viruses listed in the write-ups of the experiment are related to the virus that causes Covid-19." But what if there was a secret military research program—run in parallel with the nominally civilian one—that Fauci and Daszak were unaware of and unwittingly supporting? What if the virus that causes Covid-19 came from that program?

CHAPTER 11

Bio War Games: How the Chinese People's Liberation Army Released a Bioweapon on the World

As we have seen, Dr. Anthony Fauci insists that the chimeric coronaviruses that were being created in the Wuhan lab had nothing to do with the SARS-CoV-2 virus. What Fauci's National Institute for Allergies and Infectious Diseases (NIAID) had funded through Peter Daszak's EcoHealth Alliance was, he has suggested, a purely civilian research program to advance the frontiers of knowledge about dangerous viruses that might one day emerge from nature to attack humanity.

The trouble is, there is no such thing as "pure science" in China. Under the principle of "Military-Civil Fusion," every possible technology—including biotechnology—is relentlessly being exploited for potential military uses.

Military-Civil Fusion and Fauci's Confusion

According to the U.S. State Department, "'Military-Civil Fusion,' or MCF, is an aggressive, national strategy of the Chinese Communist Party (CCP). Its goal is to enable the PRC to develop the most technologically advanced military in the world. . . . The CCP's MCF strategy allows a growing number of civilian enterprises and entities to undertake classified military R&D and weapons production. The CCP also exploits the open and transparent nature of the global research enterprise to bolster its own military capabilities . . . acquiring and diverting the world's cutting-edge technologies—including through theft—in order to achieve military dominance."[1]

The Wuhan Institute of Virology was one of those "civilian enterprises" undertaking classified military biotechnology research and development. The R&D in question involved, among other things, weaponizing coronaviruses.[2] Whether Fauci knew it or not, the American taxpayers' money he was sending to China helped to create a bioweapon called the China Virus that would come back to kill those same Americans.

Tricky Tony also claims that the SARS-CoV-2 virus was not one of the chimeric viruses created in the Wuhan lab's gain-of-function research program.[3]

Certainly, the Wuhan lab never reported the existence of the virus that would cause the pandemic, either in the published scientific literature or to NIAID, which was funding the lab's research through Peter Daszak's EcoHealth Alliance.[4]

But of course it wouldn't. If the China Virus was part of a parallel military research program run by the PLA in Wuhan using the same biotechnology that Fauci's NIAID was funding via Peter Daszak's EcoHealth Alliance, this PLA bioweapons program with genetically engineered viruses and humanized mice would naturally be top secret—the Chinese would hardly announce the bioweapons they were developing to the world. But all the evidence points to the fact that the China Virus was one of those bioweapons.

The first person to publicly suggest a connection between Covid-19 and the People's Liberation Army was Dr. Francis Boyle, an expert on biowarfare. As soon as the outbreak occurred, he suggested that "the coronavirus that we're dealing with here is an offensive biological warfare weapon." He added that there have been "previous reports of problems with that lab [the Wuhan Institute of Virology] and things leaking out of it."[5]

Defector Yan Li-Meng agrees. According to Yan, the Wuhan lab used a bat coronavirus registered under the name of ZC45 as the "backbone" of the virus, which was then reengineered using gain-of-function techniques to make it more infectious and deadly.[6] She explains, "The Wuhan lab was collecting hundreds of coronavirus from all over China. They claimed it was to better predict future coronavirus epidemics that might emerge from nature. But if they were worried about a coronavirus epidemic, why weren't they doing any vaccine research, as we were doing in our lab in Hong Kong?"[7]

David Asher, who led the State Department's 2020 task force investigating the origins of Covid-19, reached the same conclusion. Dr. Asher believes not only that the virus came from the Wuhan Institute of Virology but also that it was the result of bioweapons research. "The Wuhan Institute of Virology is not the National Institute of Health," he affirmed in March 2021. "It was operating a secret, classified program. In my view, and I'm just one person, my view is it was a biological weapons program."[8]

China has both the intention and the capability to develop offensive biological warfare weapons. The evidence is hiding in plain sight.

Despite being a signatory to the Biological Weapons Convention, the Chinese Communist regime has made no secret of the fact that it regards the development of bioweapons as a key part of achieving military dominance.[9] Since 2007, PLA researchers have been writing publicly about developing bioweapons using controversial gain-of-function research to make viruses more lethal.[10]

- In 2011, China informed the International Biological and Toxin Weapons Convention Review Conference that its military experts were working on the "creation of man-made pathogens," "genomics laying the foundation for pathogen transformation," "population-specific genetic markers," and "targeted drug-delivery technology making it easier to spread pathogens."[11]
- In 2015, He Fuchu (贺福初), the vice president of China's Academy of Military Medical Sciences, said that biomaterials were the new "strategic commanding heights" of warfare.[12]

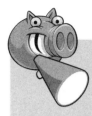

Then and Now: Investigations

In the fall of 2020, Secretary of State Mike Pompeo ordered investigators at the State Department to look into the origins of the China Virus. Pompeo was rightly concerned that the virus might have come from the Wuhan lab. Because of Chinese stonewalling and WHO complicity, direct evidence was hard to find, but the facts always led back to the lab. The preliminary results of the investigation were compelling. We know from the lead investigator, David Asher, that he was convinced that the virus was a bioweapon in development.[13]

But well before the investigators had completed their work—and just as the public narrative was shifting dramatically against China—the incoming president inexplicably called a halt to the investigation, in effect helping China to cover up its crimes.[14] Joe Biden did this without any public announcement, obviously hoping to keep his action secret.[15]

When news that the investigation had been cancelled leaked out on May 26, the White House engaged in a frantic effort at damage control. That very day, the president suddenly and very publicly announced that he was "ordering" U.S. intelligence agencies to conduct a ninety-day probe of the origins of the virus.[16] In announcing the probe, President Biden tried to frame the "origins" issue as a binary choice: the virus, he said, "either emerged from human contact with an infected animal or from a laboratory accident."

But it wasn't that simple. As we have seen, all the evidence points to the fact that the origin of the pandemic that shut down the world was in reality highly classified gain-of-function research carried out under the direction of the Chinese People's Liberation Army (PLA).

To confuse the matter further, as the new investigation got underway, Biden administration officials warned Americans that the origins of the Covid-19 virus might remain shrouded in mystery for all time. So it was no surprise when, three months later, "senior administration officials" leaked to sympathetic media outlets that the final report of the intelligence community[17] had been sent to Biden but was, sadly, "inconclusive."[18]

Of course, you can't read the report for yourself, because it is "classified." You must simply take these unnamed officials' word for it: we just don't know, and we may never know whether the novel coronavirus jumped from an animal to a human naturally, or if it was accidentally leaked from a lab in China.

But those same "senior administration officials" were all too eager to attack the idea that the

China Virus could have been a bioweapon in development. Because it has several naturally occurring features that are found in other coronaviruses, they insisted, it could not have been a product of genetic engineering. This is a non sequitur. The China Virus was engineered using the "backbone" of an existing coronavirus, so of course it shares some features in common with other coronaviruses. But it also has novel insertions—like the dropping of a bigger engine into an existing chassis—that make it more infectious and deadly. As I had explained the month before in the *New York Post*: "Those doing the splicing left 'signatures' behind in the genome itself. To boost a virus' lethality, for example, those doing gain-of-function research customarily insert a snippet of RNA that codes for two arginine amino acids. This snippet—called double CGG— has never been found in any other coronaviruses, but is present in CoV-2. Besides this damning evidence, there are other indications of tampering as well."[19]

But, no, a rushed investigation found that the evidence was all "inconclusive." Our intelligence analysts are utterly bamboozled about the origins of the disease that has killed more than 600,000 Americans. Yet they are absolutely certain that China did nothing nefarious. At worst, it was an "accident."

The meta-message from this mysterious report: Don't blame China. Don't demand reparations. Don't decouple our economies. Don't upset the geopolitical order in which China marches relentlessly on despite unleashing a devastating virus on the world. President Biden's behavior in covering up the crimes of the Chinese Communist Party is a disaster for America.

Matthew Pottinger, who served as a deputy national security advisor (DNSA) in the Trump administration, pointed out in a February 2021 interview that the PLA had been "doing secret classified animal experiments in that same laboratory [Wuhan Institute of Virology]" as early as 2017.[20] While the Wuhan lab poses as a "civilian institution," Pottinger said, U.S. intelligence has determined that the lab has collaborated with China's military on publications and secret bioweapons projects.[21]

- In 2017, China's top state television commentator revealed that biowarfare, using viruses, was a new priority under Xi Jinping's national security policy.[22]

A Chinese document that recently fell into the hands of the Australian Strategic Policy Institute (ASPI) confirms that China's military scientists have been focused on what they call the "new era of genetic weapons" since at least 2015.[23] The authors of the Chinese paper begin by asserting that World War III will be fought with biological weapons, and go on to describe how viruses can be collected from nature and "artificially manipulated into an emerging human disease virus, then weaponized and unleashed."[24] Sound familiar?

China's military scientists even singled out coronaviruses as a class of viruses that can be readily weaponized, and they suggest that the ideal candidate for a bioweapon would be something like the coronavirus that causes severe acute respiratory syndrome, or SARS. It is worth noting that the virus that causes Covid-19 is a type of SARS virus, which is why the World Health Organization insists that we call it SARS-CoV-2—as in, the second SARS virus.

Peter Jennings, the executive director of ASPI, said the new document "clearly shows that Chinese scientists were thinking about military application for different strains of the coronavirus and thinking about how it could be deployed. It begins to firm up the possibility that what we have here is the accidental release of a pathogen for military use." The Chinese paper, he said, is the closest thing to a "smoking gun as we've got."[25]

But perhaps the most chilling piece of evidence about China's bioweapons program comes from PLA general Zhang Shibo (张仕波). In his 2017 book *War's New High Ground*, General Zhang claimed that "modern biotechnology development is gradually showing strong signs characteristic of an offensive capability," including the potential for "specific ethnic genetic attacks" (特定种族基因攻击).[26]

General Zhang was referring to the development of bioweapons that would kill other races but for which Han Chinese would have a natural or acquired immunity. Such weapons would be designed to selectively target, say, Africans or Caucasians, or perhaps Japanese or Koreans, but leave the Han Chinese population of China unscathed. Those who might counter that one wild-eyed general does not necessarily speak for the Communist leadership should bear in mind that at the time he published this book Zhang was a full member of the 18th Central Committee (2012–2017) of the Chinese Communist Party and the president of China's National Defense University.[27]

According to David Asher, 2017 was the year that China shut down public discussion of research into coronavirus "disease vectors which could be used for weapons"—and, as it happened, the same year that its military began funding the research at the Wuhan Institute of Virology. "I doubt that's a coincidence," said Asher."[29]

In April of 2021, the month before the ASPI's revelations, I had laid out the case that both the express intentions and technical capabilities of the Chinese weighed in favor of a highly developed Chinese biowarfare program.[31] If the PLA's intentions with regard to bioweapons are clear, there are even fewer questions surrounding its scientific prowess. We know that China has mastered reverse genetics—the gene-splicing techniques that are needed to create a biological superweapon. As we saw in chapter 10, Dr. Shi Zhengli learned how to do

★ ★ ★

A Strange Coincidence

The final link in the chain of evidence that the Covid-19 virus was engineered in a lab came in early 2022, when scientists made a startling discovery. Covid's unique furin cleavage site on the spike protein—the key piece of genetic code that enables it to invade and infect human cells so effectively—is an exact match for a genetic sequence patented by Moderna in 2016.[28] So how did the snippet of code, which Moderna had patented for cancer research purposes, find its way into a bat coronavirus? It should be obvious by now that it was put there, inserted in gain-of-function research driven by the PLA's drive to develop bioweapons.

Dr. Fauci has claimed that it would be "molecularly impossible" for the Covid virus to have been created in a lab.[30] But what is truly "molecularly impossible" to believe is that such a homology occurred by random chance. Those who discovered it point out, "Conventional biostatistical analysis indicates that the probability of this sequence randomly being present in a 30,000-nucleotide viral genome is 3.21×10^{-11}."

That's 1 in 3 trillion.

research from Ralph Baric of the University of North Carolina, and American taxpayers actually funded her research[32]—you know, the gain-of-function research that created the China Virus that wreaked havoc on the world.

The bottom line is that China, thanks in part to training and funding it received from the United States, had everything it needed to create a deadly bioweapon: the facility, the technology, and the raw biomaterial.

Some have objected that the China Virus, with a case fatality rate of only 0.3 percent or so, does not fit the profile of a bioweapon. But defector Yan Li-Meng has pointed out that this virus is specifically an "unrestricted bioweapon" that has "relatively low lethality" but "spreads easily." Its "high rate of asymptomatic transmission . . . renders the control of SARS-CoV-2 extremely challenging." And its spread has "resulted in panic in the global community, disruption of social orders, and decimation of the world's economy." In fact, its "range and destructive powers" are "unprecedented."[33]

As research physiologist Dr. Lawrence Sellin, who has held positions at the Army Medical Research Institute of Infectious Diseases and at the biotechnology company AstraZeneca,[34] has pointed out, SARS-CoV-2 "was specifically designed to be highly contagious, but often asymptomatic, have low lethality, but produce uncontrollable variants and possessing characteristics providing plausible deniability as a bioweapon." Sellin explains, "According to Chinese military doctrine, such bioweapons are used prior to a declaration of war for political or international strategic needs, where the use of which can be denied."[35]

Dr. Sellin, who is also a retired U.S. Army colonel, spent much of 2020–2021 investigating the origins of the Covid virus, detailing the PLA's bioweapons program, and investigating the backgrounds of the PLA scientists involved. He was one of the first to point out that the China Virus contains a unique furin cleavage site on its spike protein.

If the China Virus is an "unrestricted bioweapon," this would go a long way towards explaining China's bizarre behavior—the secrecy, the serial lying, the brutal quarantine, the persecution of whistleblowers, the seeding of the virus around the world, and the furious rejection by Beijing of the idea of an international commission to investigate the origin and spread of the disease. It all seems wildly overwrought, even by the standards of a conspiratorial Communist Party whose leaders suffer from a pathological paranoia.

In the law, this is called "consciousness of guilt." It's like running out the back door of your house when the police show up at your front door. Or, in China's case, locking down the lab, destroying evidence, and blaming everything from innocent bats to your principal geostrategic adversary, the United States of America.

But if the China Virus is a bioweapon, whether accidentally or deliberately released on the world, it all makes sense.

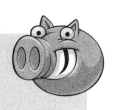

Then and Now: Biowarfare

Chinese strategic journals make it clear that anthrax, Ebola, and other pathogens obtained from nature are old-school. For the past decade or more, as Dr. Lawrence Sellin has documented, China has been determined to "use biotechnology to create new forms of designed 'biotechnological weapons' that would be 'controllable' and 'recoverable' for which China has sole possession of the vaccine or antidote. Such weapons would be highly contagious, but of low lethality and capable of being deployed under 'pre-war' conditions. Although artificially created, the new bioweapons would retain 'plausible deniability,' that is, could be attributed to a disease of natural origin."[36]
Sound familiar?

Leaky Lab or Sneaky Attack?

While there's compelling evidence that the China Virus was a lab-created bioweapon, it's not so clear how it made its way out of the Wuhan lab. On the one hand, it's easy to imagine a scientist accidentally being infected with the SARS-CoV-2 virus in the lab. After all, that's what happened—not once, but twice—with workers handling the original SARS virus in a Beijing P3 "medium containment" lab in 2004.[37] But the origin of the pandemic may not be as simple as the phrase "lab leak" implies. Dr.

Yan, who has spent years working in virology labs, told me in June of 2020 that it would be almost impossible for a virus to escape from a P4 "high containment" lab. "It was not an accident," she said. "No one in the lab got sick or died. There are always two people in the lab. No live virus would be able to escape."[38]

But in May of 2021, the U.S. State Department revealed that it had "reason to believe that several researchers inside the WIV became sick in autumn 2019, before the first identified case of the outbreak, with symptoms consistent with both COVID-19 and common seasonal illnesses."[39] If that is true—and there is no way to independently confirm it, since none of the workers has been identified—would this not prove that they were the victims of an accidental leak? Not necessarily. They could, for example, have been accidentally infected while serving as human guinea pigs in a vaccine trial.

This suggestion comes from well-known medical expert and bestselling author Steven Quay, the CEO of Atossa Therapeutics,[40] who believes that SARS-CoV-2 may have been a lab-made bioweapon. "But was SARS-CoV-2 more than just a gain-of-function experiment that escaped a laboratory?" Quay asks. "Could it have been one part of a two-part novel virus-vaccine bioweapons program?"[41] The first step in such a program would be to develop a viral bioweapon; the second would be develop a vaccine to protect your own people against it before you unleashed viral death upon the rest of the world.

Dr. Quay studied early viral samples taken from those who had fallen ill in Wuhan and noted that they contained engineered segments of a deadly avian flu virus. Was this contamination, he asked, or was it evidence that the Chinese were working on vaccines for this and other dangerous viruses—viruses they could use as bioweapons and vaccinate their own people against?[42]

Certainly the speed at which Chinese manufacturers developed a vaccine—the first was announced in June 24, 2020, six months ahead of

American manufacturers—suggests that they had a considerable head start.[43] And if the PLA was developing a vaccine to protect its own people against a bioweapon it had developed, this might explain how the virus "escaped" from the Wuhan lab. Lab workers who "volunteered" to be inoculated with a rushed vaccine against the China Virus may have come down with the disease itself, or they could have been deliberately exposed to the actual SARS-CoV-2 virus during "human challenge studies" to test the effectiveness of a vaccine, gotten infected, and ignited the Wuhan epidemic.

According to Dr. Sellin, sources in China have confirmed not only that the SARS-CoV-2 virus was a product of the lab, but also that by early 2019 it was ready to be deployed against human subjects—and that a parallel project to develop a vaccine was also well underway. Scientists from the Wuhan Institute of Virology were involved in testing the transmissibility of the China Virus in monkeys in a coronavirus

> ★ ★ ★
>
> ## Bioweapons: Virus Spears and Vaccine Shields
>
> Major General Chen Wei, who heads China's bioweapons program, alluded to the fact that the PLA's bioweapons program had two necessary and complementary parts in a classified speech she gave to the Academy of Military Medical Sciences.
>
> General Chen, who has specialized in vaccine research her entire military career, told the audience "只要有矛·才能研究盾," which means, "Only if you have a spear can you then research a shield."[44] The "spear" is the pandemic virus that you intend to release against your enemy; the shield is the vaccine that protects your own forces from being infected with it when you launch a bioweapons attack.

release-and-response drill at Wuhan's Tianhe airport in September 2019, and in an actual release of Covid-19 at the 2019 Military World Games from October 18 to October 27, 2019. According to Dr. Sellin's source, this was intended to be a small, short-term test release of Covid-19, and special health screenings of the athletes would be used to monitor the results.[45] Well-known Chinese dissident Wei Jingsheng has independently confirmed from his own sources in China that the China Virus was intentionally released on the athletes at the games.[46]

Some of the visiting athletes later recounted that they became ill in Wuhan and had to be quarantined during and after their return flights to their home countries. Canadian athletes were apparently especially hard-hit, with about one quarter of Canada's team falling so ill during their sojourn in Wuhan that they were quarantined in the back of the plane on their return flight to Canada.[47] Many other athletes from around the world—the games in Wuhan drew 9,308 athletes, representing 109 countries—developed symptoms that we now recognize as characteristic of Covid-19. It is strange that so many extremely fit young people would fall ill at once, unless they were deliberately infected.[48] Indeed, by blaming American athletes for bringing the virus to the Military World Games, the Chinese authorities themselves inadvertently confirmed that Covid was spread at the Wuhan event.[49]

Dr. Sellin's source explained, "The release of COVID-19 at the Military World Games was also a test of the longer-term effects of that type of bioweapon because foreign visitors to the Games would carry it back to their own countries and the consequences could be observed. . . . [T]he subsequent outbreak in Wuhan was entirely unexpected. That is, there was no laboratory leak, but the unintended spread among the Chinese population of Wuhan of a virus for which they had underestimated its transmissibility."[50]

These theories are not mutually exclusive. The PLA could have been carrying out community trials of a faulty vaccine for a newly developed bioweapon around the same time it deployed that virus in an attempt to infect the visiting athletes and turn them into superspreaders. In any case, one way or another the China Virus managed to escape into the general Wuhan population and spread from there.

However opaque the origin of the Covid outbreak remains, one thing is crystal clear: once China itself was unexpectedly in the grip of Covid, the CCP decided to use its own people as human disease vectors to deliberately spread the virus to the world.

The devastation that followed has few parallels in human history. Millions of people died. Nearly 20 percent of the world's GDP was destroyed. Democracies have been shaken. And all of this has happened without the PLA's having to fire a single shot.

The China Virus turned out to be the most effective weapon in history.

The Once and Future Bioweapon

From a bone-strewn hut in Hamin Mangha in 3000 BC through the SARS epidemic of AD 2002–2004, China has been plague central for millennia. Many of the most deadly pathogens that have afflicted humanity over the years first crossed from animal to man in China.

It is not difficult to understand why. Chinese dietary habits have long encouraged such zoonotic pathogens, and China's large population and robust commercial economy have allowed them to spread.

Famine has often forced the Chinese to eat anything that walks, crawls, swims, flies, or burrows. As recently as the Great Leap Forward famine (1960–1962), people were eating beetles and worms, peeling the bark off trees, and mixing sawdust with scarce cornmeal in a desperate effort to fill their empty bellies.[1] Some of these unconventional food choices have, over the course of centuries, become part of Chinese cuisine. Indeed, the Chinese have made a culinary virtue out of necessity—not a few of these dishes are considered great delicacies and command high prices. Think "bird's nest soup," which is made with dried avian saliva. Since almost any wild animal may be sold on the street or slaughtered in unsanitary wet markets and wind up on the dinner plate, it's easy to see how a novel virus might turn up from time to time.

China's Crimes against Humanity

A partial list of the Chinese Communist Party's crimes against humanity would include forced abortion and sterilization; mass famine; execution of political dissidents; ethnic genocide of Uyghurs, Kazakhs, and Tibetans; harvesting and selling organs from prisoners; kidnapping and holding hostages for diplomatic ransom; and the mass murder of American youth using fentanyl.

A list of the CCP's commercial crimes would include intellectual property theft, illegal trade practices, extortion, trafficking of people and weapons, and—what is truly China's largest industry—counterfeiting currency and products.

Releasing a dangerous bioweapon on the world may now be added to the CCP's crimes against the human race.

When a deadly pathogen does cross over the species barrier into the sea of Chinese humanity, it finds a steady supply of new hosts—hundreds of millions of them. An epidemic may recede only to have the disease that caused it become endemic in the population, and then be carried over time by warring armies or commercial traders to other lands, even to the far corners of the world.[2]

But what happened in Wuhan in 2019 was something different. Rather than a naturally occurring coronavirus leaping from animals to humans in an accidental encounter, what emerged from the Wuhan Institute of Virology was a man-made bioweapon—which, as we have seen, there is compelling evidence to believe was unleashed upon the world with malice aforethought.

The first salvo in the PLA's "war for biological dominance" has been fired. It will not be the last. The weaponization of viruses and other living organisms by the CCP is not going to stop.

More Labs for Bioweapons Research

Anyone who doubts that Beijing is moving ahead as rapidly as it can on the bioweapons front needs only to consider China's ambitious new plans to build more labs. Under the umbrella of a new CCP "biosecurity law" enacted in 2020, the country is moving forward as quickly as it can to greatly expand its capacity to carry out what it calls "biosecurity research."[3] Xiang Libin, China's deputy minister of science and technology, revealed in July 2021 that the ministry has already approved the construction of three more biosafety level-4 labs, that is, P4 labs modeled on the Wuhan Institute of Virology, along with eighty-eight biosafety level-3 labs, or P3 labs.[4]

The construction of these new labs will more than double China's existing inventory of labs. And like the Wuhan Institute of Virology, the new labs will "specialize in advanced pathogenic microbiology."[5] That means they will all probably have the capacity to engage in gain-of-function research of the kind that produced SARS-CoV-2. Chinese defector Yan Li-Meng, who worked in a P3 lab in Hong Kong, has said that it would have taken her lab, or any such lab, only six months to produce the coronavirus that caused Covid-19 or other dangerous pathogens.[6]

CCP officials claim the work is merely intended to combat future deadly diseases.[7] But the worry is that this is merely civilian cover for a further, and major, expansion of China's biological weapons program. To be sure, the People's Liberation Army operates its own networks of P3 labs. But it also collaborates extensively with supposedly civilian labs on research projects, including those involved in the production of bioweapons.[8] The CCP principle of civil-military fusion means that the distinction between the two kinds of labs is blurred in practice—if not, for all practical purposes, nonexistent.

The People's Liberation Army closely supervises two areas of research— research on gene modifications to create better soldiers, and research on microorganisms that can be gene-edited to make new biological weapons against which people have no defenses.[9]

Somewhere in China, perhaps even at the Wuhan Institute of Virology itself, they are even now genetically engineering new "unrestricted bioweapons." Anyone who thinks that the new P4 labs China is building are

★ ★ ★

The Zero-Covid Winter Olympics

China went all out to ensure that the 2022 Winter Olympics, held in Beijing from February 4 to February 20, 2022, did not turn into a Covid superspreader event. Or so CCP officials assured the world as they barred foreign visitors and kept the arriving athletes themselves in what has been described as the Olympic "superbubble."[10]

What these extraordinary precautions made clear to everyone was that the CCP is determined to continue its "Zero Covid" policy indefinitely, regardless of how many mild—and easily survivable—variants of Covid come along. The entire exercise, as the experience of Australia and New Zealand had long since demonstrated, made no sense in public health terms.

But as a mechanism of societal control, continually forcing people into isolation has no equal.

And, aside from regimentation, Zero Covid may serve one more purpose as well. If the Beijing regime is intent upon developing an arsenal of bioweapons—as its own strategic literature makes clear it is—then prudence dictates that it would want to train its population in how to respond to the release of a dangerous pathogen, whether accidental or deliberate. Viewed in this light, the lockdowns are a kind of civil defense exercise, not unlike setting off an air raid siren from time to time to see how fast everyone can run down to the shelter.

You've got sixty seconds to lock yourself into your apartment and put on your PPE, Comrade Wang. And don't forget your face diaper.

going to be used for noble scientific purposes is committing the same fatal error that Dr. Fauci did.[11] Another plague—again from China, and again deliberately released—is almost certain to hit us in our lifetimes. Indeed, the very bioweapon that will be used may already be lurking in a test tube somewhere.

Following the principle that General Chen Wei laid out—只要有矛.才能研究盾, "Only if you have a spear can you then research a shield"—the Chinese leadership will first, if they have not already done so, create the bioweapon, then make an effective vaccine for it, and only then release the virus on the world. Members of the CCP and the PLA will have priority for inoculations, followed by Han Chinese. As China's bioengineering capabilities grow more sophisticated, we may expect to see bioweapons designed to target specific non-Chinese ethnicities.

A Pandemic Dystopia of Our Own Making

Our experience of the Covid pandemic has made the threat of another bioweapons attack from China obvious. It also has revealed the threat to our liberties posed by our own elites. Lenin is often quoted as saying that the quickest way towards Communism is through the health care system. The quote may be apocryphal, but for those of us who lived through the Covid pandemic it has a certain ring of truth. If Lenin didn't say it, he should have.

The China Virus is not the worst disease that humanity has had to confront. It is not the bubonic plague. Unlike the citizens of sixth-century Constantinople, people were not jumping off the balconies of buildings or throwing themselves into the ocean to drown. Instead they died quietly—but in the worst way imaginable, totally isolated from family and friends, often with their mouths taped shut, sedated into near unconsciousness, with tubes stuck down their throats making it impossible for them even to talk.

★ ★ ★

"Now I Have Become Death, the Destroyer of Worlds"

When Robert Oppenheimer saw the first atomic bomb detonated in July of 1945, he quoted a line from the *Bhagavad-Gita*—"Now I have become Death, the destroyer of worlds." Within a month, 300,000 people died in those fiery blasts.

Six million people have been killed by the China Virus, and the death toll continues to rise. Nor are the deaths confined to a bomb's blast radius. They are spread out over the entire planet. From research stations in Antarctica to the tropical rainforest of the Amazon, no place is safe from viral attack. And genetically engineered viruses—not just coronaviruses, but all classes of viruses—offer endless possibilities for future weaponization.

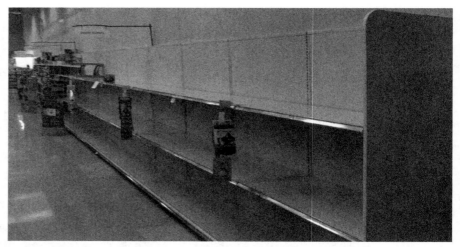

Empty shelves at a Walden, New York, grocery store, March 14, 2020. *Courtesy of Daniel Case*[12]

This is not to say that there are not parallels with past plagues. From time immemorial people have fled the plague for the countryside, and the same happened in 2020–2021. The Big Apple was hollowed out as people fled, voting with their feet against the city's harsh lockdowns. Some relocated to nearby Connecticut, but others kept moving until they reached the free states of Florida and Texas. Food shortages arose as panic buying set in and store shelves were emptied of bread, milk, and toilet paper.

Did we do a better job than the people in past pandemics—than, for example, the Americans who were confronted by the Spanish Flu a century ago? We should have. After all, we had all the tools of modern medicine at our disposal. But tools are only as good as the craftsmen wielding them. In many cases, the doctors on the front lines of our pandemic were denied the use of effective therapeutics.[13] Hospital administrators and public health officials seemed only too happy to run up the Covid count for profit and power.

In past public health emergencies, government officials from the president on down consistently tried to calm the public. During the Covid crisis, however, America's leading public health officials took the opposite tack. They did their best to stoke fear and panic. They projected wildly inflated death numbers, dissed drugs that were producing credible results, and chattered on endlessly about high numbers of "cases" resulting from widespread testing of people with no symptoms—a meaningless statistic used to justify onerous public health measures. They forced us to wear masks to signal our servility before their dictates. When President Trump tried to calm the public, a passive-aggressive Anthony Fauci undermined him at every opportunity, and Biden's election was followed by even more hysterical rhetoric and the imposition of vaccine mandates.

In past pandemics, those who survived the disease and had natural immunity were often recruited—or volunteered—to take care of others who had fallen ill. They were regarded as heroes by the wider society. But not during the last days of Covid, when a mania for vaccine mandates took hold. Nurses, truck drivers, and others who had acquired immunity by working tirelessly on the front lines for a year were fired for refusing a vaccine that

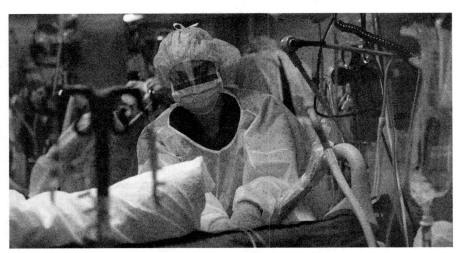

An intensive care nurse with a Covid patient. *U.S. Navy Mass Communication Specialist 2nd Class Sara Eshleman*

offered them zero benefit.[14] Compounding the irrationality, these coura-geous workers were often replaced by workers whose mandatory vaccina-tions turned out not to provide them with permanent protection or stop them from spreading the disease.[15]

Tens of millions of Americans, worried not only about their own health but the health of others, had dutifully lined up for multiple doses of an experimental vaccine on the promise that it was highly effective. After all, President Biden himself had assured them, "You're not going to get Covid if you have these vaccinations."[16] But that claim was falsified by the data. As the *Washington Examiner* reported, "Fully vaccinated adults are testing positive for Covid-19 at about the same rate as unvaccinated people, regard-less of how many booster shot they've gotten."[17] On January 10, 2022, even CDC director Rochelle Walensky was finally forced to admit that the vax "can't prevent transmission."

But at that point vax advocates simply retreated to their second line of defense. As Walensky put it, "Our vaccines are working exceptionally well. They continue to work well for Delta with regard to severe illness and death. They prevent it . . . what they can't do anymore is prevent transmission."[18] If the vaccine didn't keep people from getting sick but still kept people out of the hospital and, more important, out of a coffin, that would have been a reason for at least the elderly and those at high risk to get vaccinated. That was the narrative. But was it true? It was hard to prove or disprove this claim, since the health data released by the United States and other coun-tries was being presented in a way that made direct comparisons between the vaxxed and the unvaxxed difficult, if not impossible.[19] In fact, it eventu-ally came out that crucial data was not being released at all. The *New York Times* revealed on February 20, 2022, that the CDC was withholding much of the data it had collected surrounding the vaccines from the public for fear it would be "misinterpreted by anti-vaccine groups."[20]

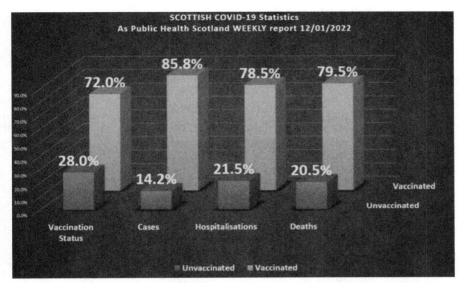

Scottish public health statistics showing that the vaccinated were at greater risk from Covid than the unvaccinated. *Public Health Scotland*

There were a few countries, such as Scotland, whose health agencies were more transparent with the data. And instead of supporting the claim of vax advocates that the mRNA vaccines protected against hospitalizations and deaths, those statistics began to move in the opposite direction. By January 12, 2022, the Scottish Covid-19 statistics were showing that those who had received two doses of the vaccine were at greater risk of infection, hospitalization, and even death than those who were not vaccinated.

Now I suppose that Public Health Scotland could have claimed that these numbers were a statistical anomaly resulting from relatively small sample size. Or it could have reissued them in another format, effectively obscuring the results. Or, best of all, it could have announced that it was pausing the vaccination campaign while it took another look at their safety and efficacy.

But the Scottish authorities did none of these things. Instead, they elected to join the CDC in playing "hide the data." As the *Glasgow Times* reported on February 17, 2022, "Covid data will not be published [from now on] over concerns it's misrepresented by anti-vaxxers."[21]

As Alex Berenson wryly pointed out at the time, "It's not clear how sharing screenshots of publicly available data on social media is 'misrepresenting' it."[22] What is clear in retrospect is that nothing encouraged "vaccine hesitancy" more than acts of censorship like this.

The efforts of public health authorities to hide the raw data did not save the mandates. And in the absence of a government diktat, demand for the mRNA vaccines evaporated.[23] The number of those injured and killed by the vax was simply too large to be missed.

None of what happened—the masks, the school closures and the business lockdowns, the social distancing and quarantines, the vaccines and the vaccine mandates—was preordained. The decision to impose these controls was made by a small group of health bureaucrats led by Anthony Fauci, whose clout was amplified by his nearly $6 billion annual budget.[24] They were aided by Big Tech monopolies that censored any dissent from the official Covid narrative.[25] Not to mention that almost the entire corporate ruling class, which had its own interests and not ours in mind, came together in support of it.

This oligarchy told us that the pandemic could only be ended if we followed their instructions to the letter. We did, and yet it didn't—for a very long time. All too many of us willingly abandoned freedom for the false promise of security.

The politicians (including the kind who wear white lab coats) who approved and mandated the jab clearly hope that members of the public quickly forget that they were ever ordered to take an experimental vaccine, and that every last claim made about its "safety and efficacy" turned out to be untrue.

One other curious fact about the mRNA vaccines: China has decided not to use them, defaulting instead to the use of a traditional attenuated, or weakened, version of the coronavirus to induce immunity. And, perhaps to no one's surprise, it turns out that such a vaccine is much better at creating long-term immunity than the supposedly more advanced Pfizer and Moderna versions.[26]

One of the clearest voices throughout the pandemic has been that of former Harvard professor Martin Kulldorff. Kulldorff, who is one of America's leading epidemiologists, discovered early on that the China Virus disproportionately targeted the elderly. He joined with others in the Great Barrington Declaration to argue in favor of "focused protection" to protect these and other high-risk individuals.[27] It didn't take long for Fauci to go on NBC to denounce the declaration as "ridiculous."[28] Around the same time, Google began to censor search results for "Great Barrington Declaration."[29]

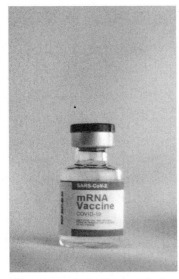

The mRNA vaccinations against Covid proved to be both dangerous and ineffective. *Courtesy of Spencerbdavis*[30]

Not surprisingly, Kulldorff lays much of the blame for the distorted response to the pandemic on Fauci. As Kulldorff explains, many of his colleagues have been intimidated into silence. "If you dare speak out against [Fauci's] views on the pandemic, you can lose funding. And if you agree with him and support him, you can gain funding."

Fauci's acolytes in academe and the medical establishment repeated ad nauseam that they were merely "following the science." But one of America's leading epidemiologists says no—what they were really doing was following the money, and they needed Fauci's approval to get it. In the aftermath of the pandemic, Kulldorff says sadly, "Science and public health are broken."[31]

In the end, Americans were saved by the two things over which the politicians not only had no control, but which they actively disparaged for most of the two years of the pandemic: natural immunity and herd immunity.

★ ★ ★

Herd Immunity über Alles

In the end it was herd immunity that ended the pandemic. That and the inevitable emergence of milder variants that allowed the virus to live with us and forced us to learn to live with it. It was the Spanish Flu story all over again.

Sweden had proven to be a beacon of sanity in a Covid-crazed world. It refused to impose brutal lockdowns or close its schools. Because of that, it reached herd immunity early and was the first to exit the Covid nightmare. On February 9, 2022, Sweden scrapped all remaining restrictions and declared the pandemic "over."[32]

Iceland had taken the opposite approach. It quickly became one of the most highly vaccinated countries on the planet and then, as the vaccines failed and the Omicron variant hit, quickly one of the most infected. But on February 23, 2022, Iceland's health ministry announced that all pandemic restrictions, including border controls, would be lifted two days later. Iceland had belatedly decided that the way out of the pandemic was by infecting as many people as possible to achieve widespread societal resistance.[33] Otherwise known as herd immunity.

The Covid pandemic of 2020–2021 showed that we face two threats—one from without and one from within. The external threat is obvious. It comes from Communist China, whose leaders, pursuing their ambitions for world domination, unleashed the China Virus on the world. To defend against that threat we must decouple our economy from China's and guard against future bioweapons attacks.

The other threat, much more insidious, comes from within. Our corporate ruling elite—Washington, Wall Street, and Big Tech—profited from the Covid pandemic both politically and economically. While the "public health" measures that they imposed on the rest of us damaged the mental and physical health of many, they also enabled the biggest transfer of wealth from the middle class to the elite in American history.

The predatory behavior of this new American oligarchy is a disease of the heart—and heart disease can kill you just as surely as a virus can.

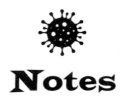

Notes

Introduction: The Plague Village of Hamin Mangha, China (circa 3000 BC)

1. Yonggang Zhu and Ping Ji, "Investigation on the Mass Graves Found in House Foundations at the Hamin Mangha Site, Inner Mongolia: Exploration and Reflection on Prehistoric Catastrophic Events," *Archaeology and Cultural Relics* 5 (2016), 5, https://en.cnki.com.cn/Article_en/CJFDTotal-KGYW201605005.htm. For a summary of the article in English, see "Prehistoric Mass Grave Excavated in China," Archaeology, July 31, 2015, https://www.archaeology.org/news/3530-150731-china-prehistoric-mass-grave; "The Discovery and Cognition of the Haminmangha Prehistoric Settlement Site," Kaogu, October 25, 2012, http://www.kaogu.cn/en/News/New_discoveries/2013/1026/43062.html.
2. Francis Aidan Gasquet, *The Black Death of 1348 and 1349*, 2nd ed. (London: Bell, 1908), vii.
3. Zhu and Ji, "Investigation on the Mass Graves."
4. Variolation was known in China as early as 1122 BC.
5. A. S. Benenson, "Smallpox," in Richard A. Kaslow and Alfred S. Evans, eds., *Viral Infections of Humans* (New York: Plenum Publishing Corporation, 1997).
6. Liang Huigang et al., "A Brief History of the Development of Infectious Disease Prevention, Control, and Biosafety Programs in China," *Journal of Biosafety and Biosecurity* 2, no. 1 (March 2020): 23–26.
7. Nectar Gan and Jessica Yeung, "China Seals Off Village after Bubonic Plague Death in Inner Mongolia," CNN, August 7, 2020, https://www.cnn.com/2020/08/07/asia/china-mongolia-bubonic-plague-death-intl-hnk-scli-scn/index.html.
8. Iain Meiklejohn, "Manchurian Plague, 1910–11," Disaster History, https://disasterhistory.org/the-manchurian-plague-1910-11.
9. I say this as an anthropologist who lived in China, Taiwan, and Hong Kong for ten years and, for the most part, happily ate everything that was put in front of me.

10. I am counting here not only the 100 million or so born Chinese who have perished, one way or another, at the hands of the Chinese Communist Party, but also the roughly 400 million tiny victims of the CCP's misguided "one-child policy," which resulted in many millions of forced abortions each year for three and a half long decades. See my *Population Control: Real Costs and Illusory Benefits* (New Brunswick, New Jersey: Transaction Press, 2008).

Chapter 1: Who Conquered Whom? The Antonine Plague (165–180)

1. See the Introduction.
2. Cassius Dio, *Roman History* (Loeb Classical Library, 1927), chapter 71, section 3, https://penelope.uchicago.edu/Thayer/E/Roman/Texts/Cassius_Dio/71*.html#2.
3. Martin Sicker, "The Struggle over the Euphrates Frontier" in *The Pre-Islamic Middle East* (Santa Barbara, California: Greenwood Publishing Group, 2000), 169.
4. The epidemic is sometimes also called the "Plague of Galen," after the Roman physician who recorded the symptoms of the disease.
5. Dio, *Roman History*, chapter 73, section 14.
6. R. J. Littman and M. L. Littman, "Galen and the Antonine Plague," *American Journal of Philology* 94 (1973): 243–255, at 255.
7. A. S. Benenson, "Smallpox" in A. S. Evans and R. A. Kaslow, eds., *Viral Infections of Humans* (Boston: Springer, 1976), 429–55, https://doi.org/10.1007/978-1-4613-3988-5_20.
8. A. W. Downie, "Smallpox" in S. Mudd, ed., *Infectious Agents and Host Reactions* (Philadelphia: Saunders, 1970), 487–518.
9. I offer a population figure with some trepidation. As the eminent Israeli ancient historian Ben Isaac wrote, "Demography is one of those topics which are as important as they are frustrating to those interested in the ancient world. The absence of information is such that modern specialists consider any effort at serious study an idle undertaking." Ben Isaac, "Jews, Christians and Others in Palestine: The Evidence from Eusebius," in *Jews in a Graeco-Roman World*, ed. M. Goodman (Oxford: Clarendon Press, 1998), 65. Some scholars have, nevertheless, attempted to estimate the size of the empire's population, and occasionally a figure of 60 million is mentioned. Professor Ian Haynes of Newcastle University has written, "I am pretty convinced that this is too low. What makes such estimates so doubtful is the basis on which they are calculated and the way in which local studies repeatedly suggest higher population levels than those once suspected. Britain, one of the most intensely studied provinces, offers an example of this phenomenon. Up until recently, scholars tended to imagine that the population stood at around 2 million (approximately twice the generally accepted estimate for the Iron Age population at

the beginning of the 1st millennium BC). Now scholars talk of figures of 6 to 8 million, after field survey and aerial reconnaissance reveal the existence of much denser settlement patterns. At the same time, prehistorians have started to question their earlier estimates, observing not only much denser settlement, but also that far higher agricultural yields were possible with Iron Age farming methods than was hitherto believed." Ian Haynes in personal correspondence with the author, February 29, 2000.

10. See Littman and Littman, "Galen," at 255. April Pudsey, a senior lecturer in Roman History at Manchester Metropolitan University, gives the lower estimate of 5 million dead. April Pudsey, "Disability and Infirmitas in the Ancient World: Demographic and Biological facts in the *Longue Durée*," in *Disability in Antiquity*, ed. Christian Laes (London, New York: Routledge, 2017), 22–34.

11. James H. Oliver, *Greek Constitutions of Early Roman Emperors from Inscriptions to Papyri* (Philadelphia: American Philosophical Society, 1989), 366–88.

12. R. P. Duncan-Jones, "The Impact of the Antonine Plague," *Journal of Roman Archaeology* 9 (1996): 108–36; R. S. Bagnall, "*P.Oxy.* 4527 and the Antonine Plague in Egypt: Death or Flight?" *Journal of Roman Archaeology* 13 (2000): 288–292, https://doi.org/10.1017/S1047759400018936.

13. Dominic Perring, "Two Studies on Roman London. A: London's Military Origins; B: Population Decline and Ritual Landscapes in Antonine London," *Journal of Roman Archaeology* 24 (2011): 249–268, https://doi.org/10.1017/S1047759400003378.

14. William Foege, "This image depicts a patient with smallpox . . . ," Centers for Disease Control, image ID# 2003, https://phil.cdc.gov/details.aspx?pid=2003.

15. Sarah Yeomans, "Classical Corner: The Antonine Plague and the Spread of Christianity," Biblical Archaeology Society, May 12, 2021, http://www.biblicalarchaeology.org/daily/ancient-cultures/daily-life-and-practice/the-antonine-plague-and-the-spread-of-christianity/.

16. Julio Rodríguez González, *Historia de las legiones Romanas* (Madrid: Almena Ediciones, 2003), especially 203–9.

17. Duncan-Jones, "The Impact of the Antonine Plague," 124.

18. Galen's theory, which derived from Hippocrates, was that human health was regulated by the four "humors": black bile, yellow bile, phlegm, and blood. When these humors were in balance, people remained in good health, but if they fell out of balance or were vitiated in some way, disease took over.

19. The Sarmatians were a large Iranian confederation whose tribes ranged from the Vistula River to the mouth of the Danube and eastward to the Volga, bordering the shores of the Black and Caspian seas as well as the Caucasus to the south. In the first century AD, the Sarmatians, in alliance with Germanic tribes, began encroaching upon the Roman Empire.

20. Abu Bakr Al Razi (AD 865–925) is the most famous physician of the Islamic world. While serving as the chief physician in Baghdad, he was the first to describe smallpox and to differentiate it from measles. Samir S. Amr and Abdulghani Tbakhi, "Abu Bakr Muhammad Ibn Zakariya Al Razi (Rhazes): Philosopher, Physician and Alchemist," *Annals of Saudi Medicine* 27, no. 4 (2007): 305–7, https://doi.org/10.5144/0256-4947.2007.241.

21. See Yuki Furuse et al., "Origin of Measles Virus: Divergence from Rinderpest Virus between the 11th and 12th Centuries," *Virology Journal* 7, article 52 (2010), https://virologyj.biomedcentral.com/articles/10.1186/1743-422X-7-52.

22. James Hicks, "This image was captured in 1973 . . . ," Centers for Disease Control, image ID# 3265, https://phil.cdc.gov/details.aspx?pid=3265.

23. Genomic analysis places the evolution of smallpox at sixteen thousand to sixty-eight thousand years before the present. See Yu Li et al., "On the Origin of Smallpox: Correlating Variola Phylogenics with Historical Smallpox Records," *Proceedings of the National Academy of Sciences of the United States of America* 104, no. 40 (2007): 15787–92, doi:10.1073/pnas.0609268104.

24. "History of Smallpox," Centers for Disease Control and Prevention, February 20, 2021, https://www.cdc.gov/smallpox/history/history.html.

25. The Egyptian-Hittite Wars that began in the mid-fourteenth century BC marked the high tide of the Hittite Empire, which was so weakened by this great scourge of mankind that by a century later it had ceased to exist. See Oliver Robert Gurney, *The Hittites* (Middlesex: Penguin, 1952).

26. Robert J. Littman, "The Plague of Athens: Epidemiology and Paleopathology," *Mount Sinai Journal of Medicine* 76, no. 5 (2009): 456–67, doi:10.1002/msj.20137.

27. G. Elliot Smith, "Head of Mummy of Pharaoh Ramesses V," February 22, 2010, https://commons.wikimedia.org/wiki/File:Ramses_V_mummy_head.png.

28. Wen W. Shen, "State and Federal Authority to Mandate COVID-19 Vaccination," Congressional Research Service, April 2, 2021, https://crsreports.congress.gov/product/pdf/R/R46745/3; *Jacobson v. Massachusetts*, February 20, 1905, Oyez, https://www.oyez.org/cases/1900-1940/197us11.

29. John Ioannidis et al., "Covid-19 Antibody Seroprevalence in Santa Clara County, California" (version 2), MedRxiv, April 27, 2020, https://www.medrxiv.org/content/medrxiv/early/2020/04/30/2020.04.14.20062463.full.pdf.

30. Li et al., "On the Origin of Smallpox."

31. C. W. Dixon, *Smallpox* (London: Churchill, 1962).

32. It was known in China as early as AD 1122.

33. Wellcome Library, "Figures Showing Vaccination Pustules: From a Chinese Work on Vaccination," XVIIth International Congress of Medicine, London, 1913, https://uplo

ad.wikimedia.org/wikipedia/commons/5/5c/Figures_showing_vaccination_pustu
les._Wellcome_L0017918.jpg.

34. Rafe de Crespigny, *A Biographical Dictionary of Later Han to the Three Kingdoms
(23–220 AD)* (Leiden: Brill, 2007), 514. The plagues that afflicted the Eastern Han
Empire during the reigns of Emperor Huan of Han (r. 146–168) and Emperor Ling of
Han (r. 168–189) were just as devastating to China as the Antonine Plague was to
Rome. De Crespigny lists outbreaks in AD 151, 161, 171, 173, 179, 182, and 185.

35. See John E. Hill, *Through the Jade Gate to Rome: A Study of the Silk Routes during the
Later Han Dynasty, First to Second Centuries CE* (BookSurge, 2009), 27.

36. China Sage, "Silk Road: Han Dynasty," https://chinasage.info/maps/SilkRoad.jpg.

37. De Crespigny, *A Biographical Dictionary*, 60. The Chinese records note that the
embassy claimed to represent "Andun" (安敦), a transliteration of the name of Marcus
Aurelius Antoninus, or possibly his predecessor Antoninus Pius.

38. Thucydides, *The History of the Peloponnesian Wars*, book 2, chapter 7, "Second Year
of the War—The Plague of Athens . . . ," https://www.gutenberg.org/files/7142/7142
-h/7142-h.htm.

39. Ibid., 514–15.

Chapter 2: The Rats and the Roman Empire: The Plague of Justinian (541–750)

1. "Maps and Statistics: Plague in the United States," Centers for Disease Control and
Prevention, https://www.cdc.gov/plague/maps/index.html.

2. "This disease always took its start from the coast, and then went up to the interior."
Procopius, *History of the Wars*, book 2, section 22, line 10.

3. Lester K. Little, *Plague and the End of Antiquity: The Pandemic of 541–750*
(Cambridge: Cambridge University Press, 2007), 63.

4. R. S. Bray differentiated this mechanism from "a human consciously clearing his
throat," explaining that it involves "the relaxation of pumping muscles which suck
up the blood when the flea senses a lack of success followed by a clearing of the
obstruction due to the back flow consequent on the sudden cessation of pumping."
R. S. Bray, *Armies of Pestilence: The Impact of Disease on History* (Cambridge:
Lutterworth Press, 1996), 20.

5. Procopius, *History of the Wars*, book 2, section 22, lines 1–7, https://www.gutenberg
.org/files/16764/16764-h/16764-h.htm.

6. Ibid., lines 19–24.

7. Ibid., line 15.

8. John Malalas, *Chronographia*, cited in Little, *Plague*, 109.

9. Little, *Plague*, 78.

10. J. N. Biraben and Jacques Le Goff, "The Plague in the Early Middle Age" in *Biology of Man in History*, ed. Robert Forster and Orest Ranum, trans. Elborg Forster and Patricia M. Ranum (Baltimore: Johns Hopkins University Press, 1975).

11. "As he passed by he saw a man blind from birth. His disciples asked him, 'Rabbi, who sinned, this man or his parents, that he was born blind?' Jesus answered, 'Neither he nor his parents sinned; it is so that the works of God might be made visible through him.'" John 9:1–3 (New American Bible).

12. Timothy S. Miller, "Symposium on Byzantine Medicine: Byzantine Hospitals," *Dumbarton Oaks Papers*, 38 (1984): 53–63, https://doi.org/10.2307/1291494.

13. Warren Treadgold, *A History of the Byzantine State and Society* (Stanford: Stanford University Press, 1997). See chapter 6, "Reconquests and the Arrival of the Plague."

14. "Now the disease in Byzantium ran a course of four months, and its greatest virulence lasted about three. And at first the deaths were a little more than the normal, then the mortality rose still higher, and afterwards the tale of dead reached five thousand each day, and again it even came to ten thousand and still more than that." Procopius, *History of the Wars*, book 2, section 13, lines 4–10, https://www.gutenberg.org/files/16764/16764-h/16764-h.htm.

15. T. H. Hollingsworth, *Historical Demography*, cited in Dionysios Stathakopoulos, *Famine and Pestilence in the Late Roman and Early Byzantine Empire: A Systematic Survey of Subsistence Crises and Epidemics,* Birmingham Byzantine and Ottoman Monographs, vol. 9 (London: Ashgate Publishing, 2004).

16. John Scarborough, "Symposium on Byzantine Medicine: Early Byzantine Pharmacology," *Dumbarton Oaks Papers* 38 (1984): 213–32, https://doi.org/10.2307/1291507.

17. The World Health Organization says that, today, "Plague can be a very severe disease in people, with a case-fatality ratio of 30% to 60% for the bubonic type, and is always fatal for the pneumonic kind when left untreated." In late antiquity, given the poor nutrition and lack of medical care, the mortality rate of those who contracted it would be even higher. See "Plague," World Health Organization, October 31, 2017, https://www.who.int/en/news-room/fact-sheets/detail/plague.

18. "The first epidemic lasted from the end of 541 for about three years, and then, after an eight- or twelve-year period, tended to recur at intervals of slightly less than four years—at Constantinople in 556–8, 561, 567–8, 573, 577, 586, 618, and 622–4 and in Gaul 552–4, 571, 583–4, and 588." Josiah C. Russell, "That Earlier Plague," *Demography* 72, no. 3 (1968): 174–184, at 179. According to Lester Little, "In a total of 210 years from 541 to 750, there were about eighteen outbreaks of the plague. This amounts to an average of one outbreak about every 11.6 years" (Little, *Plague*, 105).

19. "First, the loss of so many productive lives had a crippling impact on the economy. Second, this near-collapse of the empire's economic base triggered a financial crisis of the imperial state." Andrew Latham, "Justinian's Plague and the Birth of the Medieval World," Medievalists.net, November 27, 2020, www.medievalists.net/2020 /11/justinian-plague-medieval-world/#:~:text=At%20one%20level%2C%20this%20p lague,devotion%20to%20the%20Virgin%20Mary. See also Russell, "That Earlier Plague," at 181.

20. Lester Little gives an example of this economic collapse. Before the Justinian Plague, the city of Scythopolis (Beit She'an in modern Israel) had seen major growth, with "the persistence of a tradition of public civic architecture into the sixth century." In the fifth century and into the sixth, streets were paved, public baths were constructed, and a great basilica was built. Justin I had seen that the city walls were fortified, and his successor Justinian had improved upon the existing buildings and ordered that more be built. But when the plague arrived in AD 541, public works stopped. As Little remarks, "It is clear that the level of new building activity, especially secular building, had declined markedly [throughout the empire] by the end of the sixth century" (Little, *Plague*, 92).

21. John W. Barker, *Justinian and the Later Roman Empire* (Madison: University of Wisconsin Press, 1966), 191–92.

Chapter 3: The Greatest Public Health Disaster in History: The Black Death (1347–1351)

1. In England, "the economy supported a population of over 17,000 men and women living under rule in religious houses, and possibly twice that number of ordained priests in the parishes. . . . These are impressive numbers. They seem to tell of a countryside crowded with farms." A. R. Bridbury, "Before the Black Death," *Economic History Review* 30, no. 3 (August 1977): 393-410, at 399, https://doi. org/10.2307/2594875.

2. Beginning around the year 1300, the Little Ice Age brought decades of unseasonable cold, hail, and rainstorms. The Baltic Sea froze over in 1303, 1306, and 1307.

3. The Italian chronicler Gabriele de' Mussi, in his *Istoria de Morbo sive Mortalitate quae fuit Anno Domini 1348*, describes in detail how the Mongols threw their dead into the besieged city, and how ships transporting Genovese soldiers, rats, and fleas brought the plague to Mediterranean ports. See Mark Wheelis, "Biological Warfare at the 1346 Siege of Caffa," *Emerging Infectious Diseases* 8, no. 9 (September 2002), https://doi.org/10.3201/eid0809.010536.

4. David Herlihy and Samuel Kline Cohn, *The Black Death and the Transformation of the West* (Cambridge: Harvard University Press, 1997), 5.

5. Wheelis, "Biological Warfare," *Emerging Infectious Diseases,* 971–75, at 973. The "stench" was a reference to the disease, not to its smell per se, as the two were thought to be identical. See also Herlihy and Cohn, *The Black Death,* 59.

6. John Kelly says the ships out of Caffa were probably "costeggiare," meaning they "would inch along a coastline like rock climbers on a ledge, stopping every third or fourth day to trade and buy supplies. The practice . . . would have allowed Y. pestis to proceed to Europe in a step-wise fashion, moving from port to port and fleet to fleet, allowing it to kill crews at will." John Kelly, *The Great Mortality: An Intimate History of the Black Death, the Most Devastating Plague of All Time* (New York: HarperCollins, 2005), 85.

7. Johannes Nohl, *The Black Death: A Chronicle of the Plague* (New York: Harper & Row, 1969), 36.

8. Roger Zenner, "Spread of the Bubonic Plague in Europe 1347–1351," enlarged, translated, and edited by Jaybear, https://commons.wikimedia.org/w/index.php?curid=142219.

9. Francis Aidan Gasquet, *The Black Death of 1348 and 1349*, 2nd ed. (London: G. Bell, 1908), 227.

10. Marchionne di Coppo di Stefano Buonaiuti, *Florentine Chronicle of Marchionne di Coppo di Stefano Buonaiuti (1327–1385)*, trans. Jonathan Usher, https://www.brown.edu/Departments/Italian_Studies/dweb/plague/perspectives/marchionne.php.

11. Samuel K. Cohn, "The Black Death and the Burning of Jews," *Past & Present* 196 (August 2007): 3–36, at 8, https://doi.org/10.1093/pastj/gtm005.

12. Buonaiuti, *Florentine Chronicle*.

13. Nohl, *The Black Death,* 46. This quotation appears in Nohl's book underneath a section titled "Circumstantial Narrative of the Plague at Vienna and of the Distressful Time," taken from Abraham of Santa-Clara, *Merk's Wien* [Take Notice, Vienna] (Frankfort, 1681).

14. Herlihy and Cohn, *The Black Death,* 59.

15. Buonaiuti, *Florentine Chronicle*.

16. Nohl, *The Black Death,* 32–33.

17. Daniel Defoe, *A Journal of the Plague Year* (New York: The Floating Press, 2009), 92.

18. Ibid., 102.

19. Ibid., 44.

20. R. S. Bray, *Armies of Pestilence: The Impact of Disease on History* (New York: Barnes & Noble, 2000), 77.

21. Sigrid Undset, *Catherine of Siena* (San Francisco: Ignatius Press edition, 2009).

22. James Westfall Thompson, "The Aftermath of the Black Death and the Aftermath of the Great War," *American Journal of Sociology* 26, no. 5 (1921): 565–72, at 567, https://www.journals.uchicago.edu/doi/pdf/10.1086/213206.

23. "Pieter Brueghel, Detail of *Triumph of Death*," Wellcome Images no. L0005002, https://commons.wikimedia.org/wiki/File:Pieter_Brueghel,_detail_of_Triumph_of _Death_Wellcome_L0005002.jpg, Creative Commons license, https://creativecommo ns.org/licenses/by/4.0/legalcode.

24. Kelly, *The Great Mortality,* 93–94; Nohl, *The Black Death*, 109.

25. Giovanni Boccaccio, *The Decameron* (London: Folio Society, 1966). The complete text of *The Decameron* is online at https://www.brown.edu/Departments/Italian_Studies /dweb/texts/DecShowText.php?myID=d01intro&expand=empty&lang=eng. Boccaccio (1313–1375) invented the art of keeping yourself entertained while quarantined. In 1349, as the Black Death was raging in his native Florence, he wrote *The Decameron*. As the story goes, a group of seven young women and three young men have fled the plague and taken up residence in a secluded villa, and to pass the time they take turns telling each other tales. The *Decameron* is a collection of the stories they tell.

26. Kelly, *The Great Mortality*, 22.

27. The quotation is from paragraph 13 of the section entitled "Day the First" of Boccaccio's *The Decameron*. The complete text is available online at https://www.gu tenberg.org/files/23700/23700-h/23700-h.htm.

28. Robert W. Malone, "Mass Formation Psychosis, or . . . Mass Hypnosis—the Madness of Crowds," Robert W. Malone MD (Substack), December 9, 2021, https://rwmalon emd.substack.com/p/mass-formation-psychosis.

29. Defoe, *A Journal of the Plague Year*, 122.

30. Kelly, *The Great Mortality*, 112.

31. Nohl, *The Black Death*, 72.

32. Ibid., 95.

33. Cohn, *The Black Death*, 10.

34. Arlene Weintraub, "COVID-19 Vaccine Players Will Split $100B in Sales and $40B in Profits, with Moderna Leading the Way: Analyst," Fierce Pharma, August 13, 2020, https://www.fiercepharma.com/pharma/lead-covid-19-vaccine-players-will-split-10 0b-sales-and-40b-profits-analyst.

35. Cited in Nohl, *The Black Death*, 87.

36. Ann Shively and Jim Shively, "A Change Born of Death," *Calliope* 11, no. 7 (March 2001): 24–25, at 1.

37. Bray, *Armies of Pestilence*, 57.

38. Thomas Malthus famously argued that plagues and epidemics were cyclic events that occurred whenever population had outstripped food supply. Thomas Malthus, *Essay on the Principle of Population* (1798), https:// www.gutenberg.org/files/4239/4239-h/4239-h.htm. See especially chapter 7, "A Probable Cause of Epidemics."

39. Adam Jezard, "Even as Birth Rates Decline Overpopulation Remains a Global Challenge," World Economic Forum, April 5, 2018, https://www.weforum.org/agenda /2018/04/almost-everywhere-people-are-having-fewer-children-so-do-we-still-need -to-worry-about-overpopulation/. See also William Roper, "COVID-19 Could See US Population Shrink Faster," World Economic Forum, October 6, 2020, https://www.we forum.org/agenda/2020/10/united-states-population-predictions-graph-millions-ch ange/.

40. Kelly, *The Great Mortality*, 285.

41. Sharon DeWitte, "Mortality Risk and Survival in the Aftermath of the Medieval Black Death," *PLOS ONE* 9, no. 5 (May 7, 2014), https://doi.org/10.1371/journal. pone.0096513.

42. Sean Martin, *The Black Death* (Harpenden: Oldcastle Books, 2001), 14.

43. Kelly, *The Great Mortality*, 6. See also William Hardy McNeill, *Plagues and Peoples* (New York: Anchor, 1977).

44. As I will discuss in more detail in the next chapter, a team of medical geneticists collected data on all the known strains of *Yersinia pestis* and constructed a family tree of the bacteria. The major branches of the tree can all be traced back to China, where the root of their phylogenetic tree is located. They concluded that "*Y. pestis* evolved in or near China, and has been transmitted via multiple epidemics that followed various routes, probably including transmissions to West Asia via the Silk Road and to Africa by Chinese marine voyages." G. Morelli et al., "*Yersinia Pestis* Genome Sequencing Identifies Patterns of Global Phylogenetic Diversity," *Nature Genetics* 42 (October 31, 2010): 1140–43, https://doi.org/10.1038/ng .705.

Chapter 4: Shipping Routes: The Yunnan Plague (1772–1960)

1. Carol Benedict, *Bubonic Plague in Nineteenth-Century China* (Stanford, California: Stanford University Press, 1996), 23. Chinese researcher Xu Lei and his co-authors date the beginning of the Yunnan Plague even earlier, from 1772. Xu Lei et al., "Wet Climate and Transportation Routes Accelerate Spread of Human Plague," *Proceedings of the Royal Society B* 281, no. 1780 (April 7, 2014), http:// dx.doi.org/10.1098/rspb.2013.3159.

2. John Kelly, *The Great Mortality: An Intimate History of the Black Death, the Most Devastating Plague of All Time* (New York: HarperCollins, 2005), 112.

3. Shi Daonan, "The Death of Rats," translation into English by the author. Benedict, *Bubonic Plague in Nineteenth-Century China*, 23.

4. Francis Aidan Gasquet, *The Black Death of 1348 and 1349*, 2nd ed. (London: Bell, 1908), vii.

5.   Myron Echenberg, "Pestis Redux: The Initial Years of the Third Bubonic Plague
     Pandemic, 1894–1901," *Journal of World History* 13, no. 2 (2002): 429–49, at 431,
     http://www.jstor.org/stable/20078978.

6.   Ibid., 448.

7.   Samuel Kline Cohn, *The Black Death Transformed: Disease and Culture in Early
     Renaissance Europe* (London, New York: Arnold, 2003), 9.

8.   Lars Walløe, "Medieval and Modern Bubonic Plague: Some Clinical Continuities,"
     Medical History 27, supplement (2008), 59–73, https://www.ncbi.nlm.nih.gov/labs
     /pmc/articles/PMC2632865/. Walløe notes: "It is difficult to identify the conditions
     under which a person who has been exposed to *Yersinia pestis* acquires immunity
     and for how long acquired immunity lasts. This issue has been under discussion for
     at least eighty years. One fact is certain: vaccination with killed bacteria gives only
     short-lived protection. . . . One reason why the long-lasting immunity in humans
     observed during medieval epidemics has not been confirmed in modern epidemics
     is, of course, that in modern times very few people have been exposed to plague
     infection more than once. However, immunity acquired from vaccination cannot be
     compared to immunity acquired from surviving a fulminate infection."

9.   Xu Lei et al., "Wet Climate."

10. According to the Yunnan authorities, the registered population of the province—and
     many were not registered—was 7,522,00 in 1855, but by 1884 had fallen to only
     2,982,664. Plague, rebellion, and emigration all played a significant role in the
     depopulation of the province. Benedict, *Bubonic Plague in Nineteenth-Century
     China*, 123.

11. On February 10, 2022, China's government was reporting 5,703 Covid deaths to the
     World Health Organization. See "Global: China," World Health Organization, https://
     covid19.who.int/region/wpro/country/cn for the latest figures. For the evidence from
     the Wuhan crematoria see my article, "Evidence from Wuhan's Morgues,
     Crematoriums Suggests Covid-19 Deaths 20 Times Higher than Official Count,"
     LifeSiteNews, April 6, 2020, https://www.lifesitenews.com/blogs/evidence-from-wu
     hans-morgues-crematoriums-suggests-covid-19-deaths-20-times-higher-than-official
     -count/.

12. Benedict, *Bubonic Plague in Nineteenth-Century China*, 131 passim. See also Carol
     Benedict, "Bubonic Plague in Nineteenth-Century China," *Modern China* 14, no. 2
     (April 1988): 107–55, 136, http://www.jstor.org/stable/189268. Canton's population at
     the time was estimated to be roughly 400,000. If the French doctor cited by Benedict
     is correct and "2.6% of that city's population died in the first four months of the 1894
     epidemic," that would work out to be 10,400 fatalities.

13. Ibid.

14. Echenberg, "Pestis Redux," 440.

15. Guenther B. Risse, *Plague, Fear, and Politics in San Francisco's Chinatown* (Baltimore: Johns Hopkins University Press, 2012), 118. The objections of the Chinese-American community were also mentioned in Joan B. Trauner, "The Chinese as Medical Scapegoats in San Francisco, 1870–1905," *California History* 57, no. 1 (1978): 70–87, at 78, doi:10.2307/25157817.

16. Echenberg, "Pestis Redux," 440.

17. Shi Daonan, "The Death of Rats."

18. Benedict, "Bubonic Plague in Nineteenth-Century China," 119.

19. Alice Salles, "Bubonic Plague May Join Homelessness, Rats among Crises in Los Angeles," *Epoch Times*, August 14, 2019, https://www.theepochtimes.com/bubonic-plague-may-join-homelessness-rats-on-list-of-crises-in-los-angeles_3035204.html.

20. Edward G. Pryor, "The Great Plague of Hong Kong," *Journal of the Hong Kong Branch of the Royal Asiatic Society* 15 (1975): 61–70, at 63.

21. Cohn, *The Black Death Transformed*, 3.

22. "1925 Geneva Protocol," United Nations, https://www.un.org/disarmament/wmd/bio/1925-geneva-protocol. The Geneva Protocol was signed by nearly every nation in the world.

23. See Daniel Barenblatt, *A Plague upon Humanity: The Secret Genocide of Axis Japan's Germ Warfare Operation* (New York: HarperCollins, 2004).

24. Kathy Glatter and Paul Finkelman, "History of the Plague: An Ancient Pandemic for the Age of Covid-19," *American Journal of Medicine* 134, no. 2 (February 21, 2021): 176–81, at 179. Originally published September 23, 2020, https://www.amjmed.com/article/S0002-9343(20)30792-0/fulltext.

25. Barenblatt, *A Plague upon Humanity*, 143.

26. Ibid.

27. Ibid., 173.

28. Ibid.

29. Liang Huigang, "A Brief History of the Development of Infectious Disease Prevention, Control, and Biosafety Programs in China," *Journal of Biosafety and Biosecurity* 2, no. 1 (March 2020): 23–26.

30. Nectar Gan and Jessica Yeung, "China Seals off Village after Bubonic Plague Death in Inner Mongolia" CNN, August 7, 2020, https://www.cnn.com/2020/08/07/asia/china-mongolia-bubonic-plague-death-intl-hnk-scli-scn/index.html.

31. I myself have been treated to mole, snake, sparrow, silkworm pupae, and, sadly, dog while traveling in China. And these are just the ones I care to recall. My hosts would often not tell me what I was eating until after I took the first bite. Once I learned what it was, that sometimes proved to be the last bite as well.

32. Benedict, "Bubonic Plague in Nineteenth-Century China," 109.

33. R. Devignat, "Varietes de l'espece Pasteurella pestis: Nouvelle hypothese," *Bulletin of the World Health Organization* 4, no. 2 (1951): 247–63, https://www.ncbi.nlm.nih.gov/pmc/articles/PMC2554099/.

34. Michel Drancourt et al., "Genotyping, Orientalis-Like Yersinia Pestis, and Plague Pandemics," *Emerging Infectious Disease* 10, no. 9 (September 2004). Drancourt's findings have been verified by others. See M. Harbeck et al., "*Yersinia Pestis* DNA from Skeletal Remains from the 6th Century AD Reveals Insights into Justinianic Plague," *PLOS Pathogens* 9, no. 5, e1003349 (May 2, 2013), https://doi.org/10.1371/journal.ppat.1003349.

35. "Our observations thus suggest that Y. pestis evolved in China and spread to other areas on multiple occasions." G. Morelli et al., "*Yersinia Pestis* Genome Sequencing Identifies Patterns of Global Phylogenetic Diversity," *Nature Genetics* 42 (October 31, 2010): 1140–43, https://doi.org/10.1038/ng.705.

36. Gasquet, *The Black Death*, vii.

37. Morelli et al., "Yersinia Pestis," 4.

38. Chuck DeVore, "Official Lies, Bubonic Plague, and California's Homeless Challenge," *Forbes*, August 19, 2019, https://www.forbes.com/sites/chuckdevore/2019/08/19/official-lies-bubonic-plague-and-californias-homeless-challenge/.

39. "Plague Vaccine," *MMWR Weekly* 31, no. 22 (June 11, 1982): 301–4, https://www.cdc.gov/mmwr/preview/mmwrhtml/00041848.htm.

40. Jeffrey E. Harris, "The Repeated Setbacks of HIV Vaccine Development Laid the Groundwork for SARS-CoV-2 Vaccines (Working Paper 28587)," National Bureau of Economic Research, March 2021, https://www.nber.org/papers/w28587.

41. "Recommended Antibiotic Treatment for Plague," Centers for Disease Control, August 2015, https://www.cdc.gov/plague/resources/Recommended-antibiotics-for-plague_revision-Aug-2015_Final-(00000002).pdf.

42. Gan and Yeung, "China Seals Off Village."

43. Paul S. Mead, "Yersinia Species (Including Plague)," in John E. Bennett, Raphael Dolin, and Martin J. Blaser, eds., *Mandell, Douglas, and Bennett's Principles and Practice of Infectious Diseases*, 8th ed. (W. B. Saunders, 2015): 2607–18, at 2607, https://doi.org/10.1016/B978-1-4557-4801-3.00231-9.

44. Liyuan Shi et al., "Reemergence of Human Plague in Yunnan, China in 2016," *PLOS One* 13, no. 6 (June 13, 2018), https://doi.org/10.1371/journal.pone.0198067.

45. Gan and Yeung, "China Seals Off Village."

46. E. Tikhomirov, "Epidemiology and Distribution of Plague," *Plague Manual: Epidemiology, Distribution, Surveillance and Control*, World Health Organization, 2011, http://www.who.int/csr/resources/publications/plague/whocdscsredc992a.pdf.

47. Jonathan Watts, "'Rats' on the Menu after China Swamped by 2 Billion Rodents," *The Guardian*, July 16, 2007, https://www.theguardian.com/world/2007/jul/17/natural

disasters.china. See also Lia Eustachewich, "Chinese Market at Center of Coronavirus Outbreak Sold Wolves, Rats to Eat," *New York Post*, January 23, 2020, https://nypost.com/2020/01/23/chinese-market-at-center-of-coronavirus-outbreak-sold-wolves-rats-to-eat/.

48. John Ellis Van Courtland Moon, "Biological Warfare Allegations: The Korean War Case," *Annals of the New York Academy of Sciences* 666 (1992): 55. Cited in Eric Croddy, "China's Role in the Chemical and Biological Disarmament Regimes," *Nonproliferation Review* 9, no. 1 (Spring 2002): 16–47, at 25, http://www.nonproliferation.org/wp-content/uploads/npr/91crod.pdf.

Chapter 5: The First (and Worst) Truly Global Pandemic: The Spanish Flu (1918–1920)

1. Ailan Evans, "Here Are All the Times the Biden Administration Has Called for Tech Censorship," The Daily Caller, February 6, 2022,https://dailycaller.com/2022/02/06/joe-biden-big-tech-jen-psaki-misinformation/. On July 16, 2021, Biden himself demanded that Facebook "do something" about the misinformation on its platform. "They're killing people," Biden claimed. "I mean, they're really—look, the only pandemic we have is among the unvaccinated. And they're killing people." Shelby Talcott, "Biden Says 'Facebook Isn't Killing People' Days after Appearing to Accuse Company of Doing Just That," The Daily Caller, July 19, 2021, https://dailycaller.com/2021/07/19/joe-biden-facebook-isnt-killing-people-coronavirus-misinformation-disinformation/.

2. As the Covid epidemic spread throughout Wuhan and neighboring Chinese cities, Chinese Communist officials censored anyone who mentioned the burgeoning threat or criticized the government's response. See Bradford Betz, "China Has Arrested Hundreds for Speaking Out about Coronavirus, Reports Show," Fox News, May 13, 2020, https://www.foxnews.com/world/china-arrested-hundreds-speaking-out-coronavirus.

3. Milorad Radusin, "The Spanish Flu, Part II: The Second and Third Wave," *Vojnosanitetski pregled* 69, no. 10 (2012): 917–27, at 920.

4. Carol R. Byerly, "The U.S. Military and the Influenza Pandemic of 1918–1919," *Public Health Reports* 125, supplement 3 (2010): 82–91.

5. Sandra M. Tomkins, "The Influenza Epidemic of 1918–19 in Western Samoa," *Journal of Pacific History* 27, no. 2 (December 1992): 181–97, at 181.

6. Eric Felten, "Woodrow Wilson's Strange Silence on Flu Epidemic during Great War," The Daily Signal, April 15, 2020, https://www.dailysignal.com/2020/04/15/woodrow-wilsons-strange-silence-on-flu-epidemic-during-great-war/.

7. John M. Barry, "Pandemics: Avoiding the Mistakes of 1918," *Nature* 459, no. 7245 (2009): 324–25, https://doi.org/10.1038/459324a.

8. David Rosner, "'Spanish Flu, or Whatever It Is. . . .': The Paradox of Public Health in a Time of Crisis," *Public Health Reports* 125, supplement 3, (April 2010): 38–47, at 44.

9. The Italian government forced the largest and most influential newspaper in the country, *Corriere della Sera*, to stop reporting the number of deaths in Milan when they rose to over 160 deaths a day on the grounds that "the reports caused great anxiety among the citizenry." Because of this censorship, the public in combatant countries like Italy often had no idea why they were being asked to, for example, wear masks. It did not help that Italians referred to face masks as "muzzles." Eugenia Tognotti, "Lessons from the History of Quarantine, from Plague to Influenza A," *Emerging Infectious Diseases* 19, no. 2 (2013): 254–59, at 257.

10. Barry, "Pandemics."

11. Arnstein Aassve et al., "Epidemics and Trust: The Case of the Spanish Flu," *Health Economics* 30, no. 4 (2021): 840–57, at 842–43.

12. Becky Little, "When Mask-Wearing Rules in the 1918 Pandemic Faced Resistance," History, May 6, 2020, https://www.history.com/news/1918-spanish-flu-mask-wearing -resistance.

13. Radusin, "The Spanish Flu, Part II," 921.

14. Ryan M. Alexander, "The Spanish Flu and the Sanitary Dictatorship: Mexico's Response to the 1918 Influenza Pandemic," *The Americas* 76, no. 3 (2019): 443–65, at 453–54.

15. Ibid.

16. "Coronavirus: How They Tried to Curb Spanish Flu Pandemic in 1918," BBC, May 10, 2020, https://www.bbc.com/news/in-pictures-52564371.

17. Tognotti, "Lessons from the History of Quarantine," 257.

18. James Bishop, "Economic Effects of the Spanish Flu," *Reserve Bank of Australia Bulletin* (June 2020): 8–17, at 10, https://www.rba.gov.au/publications/bulletin/2020 /jun/pdf/economic-effects-of-the-spanish-flu.pdf.

19. Alexander, "The Spanish Flu," 451–53.

20. Martin C. J. Bootsma and Neil M. Ferguson, "The Effect of Public Health Measures on the 1918 Influenza Pandemic in U.S. Cities," *Proceedings of the National Academy of Sciences, U.S.A.* 104, no. 18 (May 1, 2007): 7588–93, doi: 10.1073/pnas.0611071104, originally published online April 6, 2007.

21. Svenn-Erik Mamelund, "Profiling a Pandemic. Who Were the Victims of the Spanish Flu?" *Natural History Magazine*, September 2017, 6, https://oda.oslomet.no/oda-xml ui/bitstream/handle/10642/5480/Pages+6-10+from+Sep17+iPad+edition.pdf?sequen ce=1.

22. Arthur Newsholme, "Discussion on Influenza," *Proceedings of the Royal Society of Medicine* 12 (November 1919): 1–18, at 14, https://doi.org/10.1177/003591571901200502.

23. Henry Wood, "Can't Catch the Real Flu Twice," *Monrovia Daily News*, November 26, 1920.

24. See, for instance, Irma R. Latarissa et al., "Potential of Quinine Sulfate for COVID-19 Treatment and Its Safety Profile: Review," *Clinical Pharmacology* 13 (December 6, 2021), 225–34, doi: 10.2147/CPAA.S331660.

25. Andrea Savarino et al., "Effects of Chloroquine on Viral Infections: An Old Drug against Today's Diseases," *The Lancet* 3, no. 11 (November 1, 2003): 722–27, https://doi.org/10.1016/S1473-3099(03)00806-5.

26. "Quinine: The Tonic for COVID-19," Penn Medicine: Department of Otorhinolaryngology, https://www.pennmedicine.org/departments-and-centers/otorhinolaryngology/about-us/newsletters/latest-newsletter/quinine-the-tonic-for-covid19.

27. David Jones and Stefan Helmreich, "A History of Herd Immunity," *The Lancet* 396, no. 10254 (September 19, 2020): 810–11, https://www.thelancet.com/journals/lancet/article/PIIS0140-6736(20)31924-3/fulltext.

28. Vinay Prasad, "Why Did Dr. Fauci Move the Herd Immunity Goalposts," December 29, 2020, Medpage Today, https://www.medpagetoday.com/opinion/vinay-prasad/90445.

29. The Cytokine Storm is also known as "cytokine release syndrome," or CRS, and is also observed in severe cases of SARS, MERS, and Covid-19. See Dounia Darif et al., "The Pro-inflammatory Cytokines in COVID-19 Pathogenesis: What Goes Wrong?," *Microbial Pathogenesis* 153, no. 104799 (April 2021), https://pubmed.ncbi.nlm.nih.gov/33609650/.

30. Jeffery K. Taubenberger et al., "Characterization of the 1918 Influenza Virus Polymerase Genes," *Nature* 437, no. 6 (October 2005): 889–93, https://www.researchgate.net/publication/7557897_Characterization_of_the_1918_influenza_virus_polymerase_genes.

31. N. Johnson and J. Mueller, "Updating the Accounts: Global Mortality of the 1918–1920 'Spanish' Influenza Pandemic," *Bulletin of the History of Medicine* 76, no. 1 (2002): 105–15. The authors of this widely cited study give the estimate of 50 million global deaths and suggest that even that may be an underestimation—and that the true death toll could have been as high as 100 million. The paper includes detailed breakdowns of mortality estimates by world region and country.

32. Ibid.

33. See K. D. Patterson and G. F. Pyle, "The Geography and Mortality of the 1918 Influenza Pandemic," *Bulletin of the History of Medicine* 65, no. 1 (Spring 1991): 4–21.

Patterson and Pyle wrote, "We believe that approximately 30 million is the best estimate for the terrible demographic toll of the influenza pandemic of 1918," and gave a range of 24.7–39.3 million deaths. See also Peter Spreeuwenberg et al., "Reassessing the Global Mortality Burden of the 1918 Influenza Pandemic," *American Journal of Epidemiology* 187, no. 12 (December 2018): 2561–67, https://doi .org/10.1093/aje/kwy191. These authors estimate global mortality as 17.4 million based on mortality counts from "national registries." The problem is, as they acknowledge, that only "13 countries had sufficient data for our study period (1916– 1921)" and that "most countries in the data set are in Europe." Clearly, the mortality rate in much of Asia, Africa, and Latin America from the Spanish Flu was much larger than that experienced by Europe and North America, and the authors' addition of some data from India does not begin to account for this.

34. By way of comparison, the worst famine in human history occurred in China from 1960 to 1962, in the aftermath of the failure of the Great Leap Forward. The most astute observer of China at the time, a Jesuit priest by the name of Laszlo Ladany who served as the editor of the Hong Kong–based *China News Analysis*, wrote in the August 10, 1962, issue that China had suffered a "real, black famine." His "realistic estimate" of the number of lives lost to starvation and disease during this period was 50 million. Skeptics scoffed at Father Ladany's estimate, dismissing it as wildly inflated. It wasn't until the 1980s that we learned the real number of victims was 42.5 million. Entire villages had been annihilated, and no one outside of China had had the slightest inkling. See Steven Mosher, *China Misperceived: American Illusions and Chinese Reality* (New York: New Republic, 1990), especially chapter 5.

35. Early on in the pandemic, Dr. Deborah Birx confirmed that the federal government was classifying all deaths of people who tested positive for the novel coronavirus as Covid-19 deaths, regardless of the actual cause of death. Louis Casiano, "Birx Says Government Is Classifying All Deaths of Patients with Coronavirus as 'Covid-19' Deaths, Regardless of Cause," Fox News, April 7, 2020, https://www.foxnews.com/po litics/birx-says-government-is-classifying-all-deaths-of-patients-with-coronavirus-as -covid-19-deaths-regardless-of-cause. Normally, autopsies of the deceased would be used to make the final determination of cause of death, but autopsies were halted for fear of contagion, so the inflated numbers stood unchallenged.

36. John M. Barry, *The Great Influenza: The Story of the Deadliest Pandemic in History* (New York: Penguin Books, 2004).

37. Cited in Mark Osborne Humphries, "Paths of Infection: The First World War and the Origins of the 1918 Influenza Pandemic," *War in History* 21, no. 1 (2014): 55–81, at 56, https://doi.org/10.1177/0968344513504525.

38. D. R. Olson et al., "Epidemiological Evidence of an Early Wave of the 1918 Influenza Pandemic in New York City," *Proceedings of the National Academy of Sciences* 102,

no. 31 (August 2, 2005): 11059–63, at 11062, https://www.pnas.org/content/pnas/102/31/11059.full.pdf.

39. G. Dennis Shanks et al., "Relationship between 'Purulent Bronchitis' in Military Populations in Europe prior to 1918 and the 1918–1919 Influenza Pandemic," *Influenza and Other Respiratory Viruses* 6, no. 4 (July 2012): 235–39.

40. J. S. Oxford et al., "Early Herald Wave Outbreaks of Influenza in 1916 prior to the Pandemic of 1918," *International Congress Series* 1219 (2001): 155–61, https://doi.org/10.1016/S0531-5131(01)00336-3.

41. Paul Fussell, *The Great War and Modern Memory* (New York: Oxford University Press, 1975), 9.

42. Xu Guoqi, *Strangers on the Western Front: Chinese Workers in the Great War* (Cambridge, Massachusetts: Harvard University Press, 2011).

43. Mark Osborne Humphries, "Paths of Infection," 55–81, at 73.

44. Ibid., 74.

45. Xu Guoqi, *Strangers*, 21.

46. Humphries, "Paths of Infection," 81.

47. G. Dennis Shanks. "No Evidence of 1918 Influenze Pandemic Origin in Chinese Laborers/Soldiers in France," *Journal of the Chinese Medical Association* 79, no. 1 (January 2016): 46–48, doi:10.1016/j.jcma.2015.08.009.

48. Michael Worobey et al., "The Origins of the Great Pandemic," *Evolution, Medicine, and Public Health* 2019, no. 1 (January 2019): 18–25, at 21, doi:10.1093/emph/eoz001.

49. Humphries, "Paths of Infection," 75.

50. G. D. Shanks, "No Evidence of 1918 Influenza Pandemic Origin in Chinese Laborers/Soldiers in France," *Journal of the Chinese Medical Association* 79, no. 1 (January 2016): 46–48, doi: 10.1016/j.jcma.2015.08.009.

51. Christopher Langford, "Did the 1918–19 Influenza Pandemic Originate in China?" *Population and Development Review* 3, no. 3 (2005): 473–505, http://www.jstor.org/stable/3401475.

Chapter 6: Flu in the Time of Air Travel: The Asian Flu (1957–1958) and Hong Kong Flu (1968–1969)

1. Douglas Jordan, "The Deadliest Flu: The Complete History of the Discovery and Reconstruction of the 1918 Pandemic Virus," Centers for Disease Control and Prevention, December 17, 2019, https://www.cdc.gov/flu/pandemic-resources/reconstruction-1918-virus.html.

2. "1957–1958 Pandemic (H2N2 virus)," Centers for Disease Control and Prevention, https://www.cdc.gov/flu/pandemic-resources/1957-1958-pandemic.html. The H2N2 virus started out as the Spanish Flu, which is an H1N1 virus, but swapped out three

of its genes with an avian influenza A virus, giving us a new virus and sparking the Asian Flu.

3. Jeffery Taubenberger and David Morens, "1918 Influenza: The Mother of All Pandemics," *Emerging Infectious Diseases* 12, no. 1 (2006): 15–22, https://wwwnc.cdc .gov/eid/article/12/1/05-0979_article.

4. Ibid. A "drifted" virus is one that has mutated under selection pressure to be less lethal in order to persist in a human population. A "reassorted" virus is composed of genes from two different viruses that combine into a new and sometimes highly infectious and deadly version to plague humanity.

5. Donald A. Henderson et al, "Public Health and Medical Responses to the 1957–58 Influenza Pandemic," *Biosecurity and Bioterrorism: Biodefense Strategy, Practice, and Science* 7, no. 3 (2009): 265–73, http://www.upmc-biosecurity.org/website/resour ces/publications/2009/2009-08-05-public_health_medical_responses_1957.html.

6. Qin Ying et al., "中国流感大流行的百年历史" ["History of Influenza Pandemics in China during the past century"], 中华流行病学杂志 [*Chinese Journal of Epidemiology*] 39, no. 8 (2018): 1028–31, http://html.rhhz.net/zhlxbx/20180803.htm. People's Republic of China researchers openly acknowledge that the Asian Flu and the Hong Kong Flu originated in China.

7. "Hong Kong Battling Influenza Epidemic," *New York Times*, April 17, 1957, https:// www.nytimes.com/1957/04/17/archives/hong-kong-battling-influenza-epidemic .html.

8. Claire Jackson, "History Lessons: The Asian Flu Pandemic," *British Journal of General Practice* 59, no. 565 (2009): 622–23, doi:10.3399/bjgp09X453882.

9. Ibid.

10. Donald A. Henderson et al., "Public Health and Medical Responses to the 1957–58 Influenza Pandemic," *Biosecurity and Bioterrorism: Biodefense Strategy, Practice, and Science* 7, no. 3 (2009): 265–73, https://www.liebertpub.com/doi/10.1089/bsp.20 09.0729.

11. Associated Press, "'Planting' of Flu Germs by Reds Held Impossible," *Evening Star*, August 26, 1957, A9, https://chroniclingamerica.loc.gov/lccn/sn83045462/1957-08-26 /ed-1/seq-9/.

12. "Symposium on the Asian Influenza Epidemic, 1957," *Proceedings of the Royal Society of Medicine* 51, no. 12 (May 16, 1958): 100918, doi:10.1177/00359157580510 1205.

13. Associated Press, "'Planting' of Flu Germs by Reds Held Impossible."

14. Henderson et al., "Public Health and Medical Responses."

15. Ibid.

16. Cécile Viboud et al., "Global Mortality Impact of the 1957–1959 Influenza Pandemic," *Journal of Infectious Diseases* 213, no. 5 (March 1, 2016): 738–45, doi:10.1093/infdis

/jiv534. Viboud and her co-authors write, "The age patterns of the 1957 pandemic have been well described in the United States and Canada and align well with our findings in a larger set of countries. We found a sharp elevation of excess mortality rates among school-aged groups at the time of the pandemic, with a consistent signature even in countries mildly affected by the pandemic overall. The impact on school-aged children was particularly pronounced in the first year of influenza A (H2N2) virus circulation, while the impact on older adults was stronger in subsequent years" (744). Most authorities assert that the Asian Flu ended in 1958, but Viboud was able to track a small effect into the following year.

17. Jackson, "History Lessons."

18. Henderson et al., "Public Health and Medical Responses."

19. Yu-Chia Hsieh et al., "Influenza Pandemics: Past, Present and Future," *Journal of the Formosan Medical Association* 105, no. 1 (2006): 1–6, at 2.

20. Edwin D. Kilbourne, "Influenza Pandemics of the 20th Century," *Emerging Infectious Diseases* 12, no. 1 (2006): 9–14, doi:10.3201/eid1201.051254. See also Donald B. Louria et al., "Studies on Influenza in the Pandemic of 1957–1958. II. Pulmonary Complications," *Journal of Clinical Investigation* 38, no. 1 (1959): 213–65, https://doi.org/10.1172/JCI103791. Louria and his co-authors reported on thirty-three patients with acute Asian influenza A infection during the pandemic of 1957–1958, of whom 72.7 percent had chronic diseases or were pregnant and 21.2 percent had leukopenia (low white blood cell counts). The death rate related to acute illness was 27.3 percent. Some rapidly progressive cases presented with symptoms such as cyanosis and shortness of breath resembling those observed in the Spanish Flu pandemic.

21. Robert Oseasohn et al., "Clinicopathologic Study of Thirty-Three Fatal Cases of Asian Influenza," *New England Journal of Medicine* 260 (1959): 509–18, doi:10.1056/NEJM195903122601101. Oseasohn and his co-authors reported "the clinicopathologic study of thirty-three fatal cases caused by Asian influenza, mostly focusing on previously healthy young individuals dying rapidly during the course of the disease. Postmortem examination showed pulmonary congestion, edema, intra-alveolar hemorrhage, varying degrees of consolidation and hyaline membrane formation indistinguishable from the pathologic findings of the 1918 pandemic."

22. Henderson et al., "Public Health and Medical Responses."

23. E. Kaitlynn Allen et al., "The Asian Flu: The H2N2 Influenza Outbreak (1957)," *Opinions throughout History: Diseases & Epidemics*, ed. Micah L. Issit (New York: Grey House Publishing, 2020), 261–70.

24. Max Skidmore, *Presidents, Pandemics, and Politics* (New York: MacMillan, 2016), 25 passim.

25. "Health Officers' Meeting on Asian Influenza," *Public Health Reports (1896–1970)* 72, no. 11 (1957): 998–1000.

26. Henderson et al., "Public Health and Medical Responses."

27. Ibid.

28. G. E. R. Hamilton, "Influenza Publicity," *British Medical Journal* 2, no. 5047 (1957): 763.

29. Ibid.

30. Allen et al., "The Asian Flu," *Opinions throughout History*, 261–70.

31. Mark Honigsbaum, "Revisiting the 1957 and 1968 Influenza Pandemics," *The Lancet* 395, no. 10240 (2020): 1824–26, doi:10.1016/S0140-6736(20)31201-0.

32. Honigsbaum, "Revisiting the 1957 and 1968 Influenza."

33. Skidmore, *Presidents, Pandemics, and Politics*, 25 passim.

34. "Hong Kong Battling Influenza Epidemic," *New York Times*.

35. Theodore H. Tulchinsky, "Maurice Hilleman: Creator of Vaccines That Changed the World," *Case Studies in Public Health* (March 30, 2018): 443–70, doi:10.1016/B978-0-12-804571-8.00003-2.

36. The College of Physicians of Philadelphia, "1957 Asian Flu Pandemic," History of Vaccines, https://www.historyofvaccines.org/content/1957-asian-flu-pandemic.

37. Jackson, "History Lessons."

38. Henderson et al., "Public Health and Medical Responses."

39. Rob Volansky, "Revisiting 1957–1958 Influenza Pandemic May Provide Clues to Combating H1N1," *Infectious Diseases in Children*, September 1, 2009, https://www.healio.com/news/pediatrics/20120325/revisiting-1957-1958-influenza-pandemic-may-provide-clues-to-combating-h1n1.

40. Henderson et al., "Public Health and Medical Responses."

41. K. E. Jensen, F. L. Dunn, and R. Q. Robinson, "Influenza, 1957: A Variant and the Pandemic," *Progress in Medical Virology* 1 (1958): 165–209.

42. Henderson et al., "Public Health and Medical Responses."

Chapter 7: "Fiasco": The Great Swine Flu Hoax of 1976 (1976–1977)

1. The College of Physicians of Philadelphia, "Timeline," History of Vaccines, https://www.historyofvaccines.org/timeline#EVT_102235.

2. "History of Smallpox," Centers for Disease Control and Prevention, https://www.cdc.gov/smallpox/history/history.html.

3. My account of the swine flu draws heavily on the chronology laid out in R. E. Neustadt and H. V. Fineberg, *The Swine Flu Affair: Decision-Making on a Slippery Disease* (Washington, D.C.: National Academies Press, 1978).

4. Ibid.

5. Harold M. Schmeck Jr., "U.S. Calls Flu Alert on Possible Return Of Epidemic's Virus," *New York Times,* February 20, 1976, 1, https://www.nytimes.com/1976/02/20/arch ives/us-calls-flu-alert-on-possible-return-of-epidemics-virus-us-flu.html.

6. Ibid.

7. Harvey V. Fineberg, "Preparing for Avian Influenza: Lessons from the 'Swine Flu Affair,'" *Journal of Infectious Diseases* 197, supplement 1: "Avian and Pandemic Influenza" (February 15, 2008): S14–S18, http://www.jstor.org/stable/30086987.

8. Anthony S. Fauci, "Research on Highly Pathogenic H5N1 Influenza Virus: The Way Forward," *mBio*, October 9, 2012, https://www.ncbi.nlm.nih.gov/pmc/articles/PMC3 484390/.

9. Philip M. Boffey, "Soft Evidence and Hard Sell," *New York Times,* September 5, 1976, 137, https://www.nytimes.com/1976/09/05/archives/soft-evidence-and-hard-sell-in -the-next-few-months-the-government.html.

10. Richard Krause, "The Swine Flu Episode and the Fog of Epidemics," *Emerging Infectious Disease* 12, no. 1(2006): 40–43, doi: 10.3201/eid1201.051132.

11. The four manufacturers of swine flu vaccine were Merck, Merrell, Parke-David, and Wyeth. All were notified by their insurance companies that their casualty coverage would not cover liabilities arising from the Fort Dix swine flu vaccines, and the manufacturers then demanded that the government indemnify them from all lawsuits arising from the vaccine. It seems that everyone, with the exception of too many members of the public, was aware that the rushed vaccine might well harm some of those who received it.

12. R. E. Neustadt and H. V. Fineberg, "Swine Flu Chronology January 1976–March 1977," in *The Swine Flu Affair: Decision-Making on a Slippery Disease* (Washington, D.C.: National Academies Press, 1978), doi:10.17226/12660.

13. Albert B. Sabin, "Washington and the Flu," *New York Times*, November 5, 1976, https://www.nytimes.com/1976/11/05/archives/washington-and-the-flu.html.

14. "Guillain-Barré Syndrome Fact Sheet," National Institute of Neurological Disorders and Stroke, https://www.ninds.nih.gov/Disorders/Patient-Caregiver-Education/Fact -Sheets/Guillain-Barré-Syndrome-Fact-Sheet.

15. Neustadt and Fineberg, "Swine Flu Chronology."

16. Kenrad E. Nelson, "Invited Commentary: Influenza Vaccine and Guillain-Barré Syndrome—Is There a Risk?," *American Journal of Epidemiology* 175, no. 11 (June 1, 2012): 1129–32, doi: 10.1093/aje/kws194.

17. George Dehner, "WHO Knows Best? National and International Responses to Pandemic Threats and the 'Lessons' of 1976," *Journal of the History of Medicine and Allied Sciences* 65, no. 4 (October 2010): 478–513, https://doi.org/10.1093/jhmas/jr q002.

18.	Ashley Sadler, "It's Happened Before: Gov't Launched Dangerous Mass Immunization Program during 1976 Swine Flu 'Pandemic,'" LifeSiteNews, September 10, 2021, https://www.lifesitenews.com/blogs/739968/.

Chapter 8: A Pandemic Unlike Any Other: The China Virus (2019–2022)

1.	Russell J. Westergard, "Surviving the Outbreak," *State Magazine*, April 2020, https://statemag.state.gov/2020/04/0420feat05/.

2.	Josh Margolin and James Gordon Meek, "Intelligence Report Warned of Coronavirus Crisis as Early as November: Sources," ABC News, April 9, 2020, https://abcnews.go.com/Politics/intelligence-report-warned-coronavirus-crisis-early-november-sources/story?id=70031273. The Pentagon later denied the existence of such a report, but ABC stood by its sources.

3.	武汉市卫健委[Wuhan Municipal Health Commission], "武汉市卫健委关于当前我市肺炎疫情的情况通报 " [Wuhan Municipal Health Department's Message about Our City's Present Pneumonia Situation], wjw.wuhan.gov.cn (in Chinese), https://web.archive.org/web/20200418182736/http://tv.cctv.com/2019/12/31/VIDE9N8qRty36PkLirFVxMW6191231.shtml.

4.	"CDC Implements Extra Inspection Measures for Wuhan Flights," Taiwan Today, January 2, 2020, https://taiwantoday.tw/news.php?unit=2,6,10,15,18&post=168773.

5.	Henry Holloway, "Alarm Bell: Taiwan's Coronavirus December Warning to WHO about Person-to-Person Spreading Went Unheeded, Bombshell Email Reveals," *The Sun*, April 14, 2020, https://www.thesun.co.uk/news/11395934/taiwan-coronavirus-warning-who-human-transmission-china/. See also Keoni Everington, "Early Screenings of China Arrivals Key to Taiwan's Success: CECC Head," *Taiwan News*, March 13, 2020, https://www.taiwannews.com.tw/en/news/3896475.

6.	Zachary Evans, "Taiwan Accuses WHO of Failing to Heed Warning of Coronavirus Human-to-Human Transmission," *National Review*, March 20, 2020, https://www.nationalreview.com/news/taiwan-accuses-who-of-failing-to-heed-warning-of-coronavirus-human-to-human-transmission/.

7.	"CDC Confirms Person-to-Person Spread of New Coronavirus in the United States," Centers for Disease Control, January 30, 2020, https://www.cdc.gov/media/releases/2020/p0130-coronavirus-spread.html; World Health Organization (@WHO), "To date, new #coronavirus (2019-nCoV) person-to-person transmission . . . ," Twitter, January 30, 2020, 1:07 p.m., https://twitter.com/who/status/1222944438181335040?lang=en.

8. Amy Qin, Steven Lee Myers, and Elaine Yu, "China Tightens Wuhan Lockdown in 'Wartime' Battle with Coronavirus," *New York Times*, February 6, 2020, https://www.nytimes.com/2020/02/06/world/asia/coronavirus-china-wuhan-quarantine.html.

9. Shan Li, Brianna Abbott, and Joyu Wang, "Major Test of China's System, Says Xi Jinping," *Wall Street Journal*, February 3, 2020, https://www.wsj.com/articles/new-coronavirus-hospital-is-completed-as-cases-deaths-keep-climbing-11580720077?mod=article_inline.

10. Minyvonne Burke, Suzanne Ciechalski, and Dawn Liu, "Video Appears to Show People in China Forcibly Taken for Quarantine over Coronavirus," NBC News, February 9, 2020, https://www.nbcnews.com/news/world/video-appears-show-people-china-forcibly-taken-quarantine-over-coronavirus-n1133096.

11. Steven Mosher, "Evidence from Wuhan's Morgues, Crematoriums Suggests COVID-19 Deaths 20 Times Higher than Official Count," LifeSiteNews, April 6, 2020, https://www.lifesitenews.com/blogs/evidence-from-wuhans-morgues-crematoriums-suggests-covid-19-deaths-20-times-higher-than-official-count/. The Wuhan authorities claimed that only 170 people had died in Wuhan and the surrounding area by January 30. Yet two days before, on January 28, they had announced that they were "dispatching extra vehicles, staff, and protective gear to all of the local mortuaries to improve the capacity of transporting and dealing with corpses." They also suddenly offered "free cremation for the corpses of coronavirus victims who died on January 26 or later." Why? Obviously because the bodies were piling up.

12. Liza Lin, "China Marshals Its Surveillance Powers against Coronavirus," *Wall Street Journal*, February 4, 2020, https://www.wsj.com/articles/china-marshals-the-power-of-its-surveillance-state-in-fight-against-coronavirus-11580831633?mod=article_inline.

13. James Griffiths and Amy Woodyatt, "China Goes into Emergency Mode as Number of Confirmed Wuhan Coronavirus Cases Reaches 2,700," CNN, January 27, 2020, https://www.cnn.com/2020/01/26/asia/wuhan-coronavirus-update-intl-hnk/index.html.

14. Cassidy Morrison, "Trump Declares Coronavirus Outbreak a Public Emergency, Will Ban Foreign Travel from China and Quarantine US Citizens," *Washington Examiner*, January 31, 2020, https://www.washingtonexaminer.com/news/trump-administration-declares-coronavirus-outbreak-a-public-health-emergency.

15. Becket Adams, "Yes, Biden Absolutely Did Oppose the China Travel Restrictions and Call Them 'Xenophobic,'" *Washington Examiner*, October 8, 2020, https://www.washingtonexaminer.com/opinion/yes-biden-absolutely-did-oppose-the-china-travel-restrictions-and-call-them-xenophobic; Stephen Sorace, "Fauci, Who Opposed China Travel Ban and Praised Their Transparency, Criticizes Trump Response," Fox News, March 11, 2021, https://www.foxnews.com/politics/fauci-china-travel-ban-coronavirus-transparency-criticizes-trump-response.

16. Rose Tennent, "Fauci's Biggest Lie: 'Lie of Omission Committed on January 28th, 2020' with Peter Navarro," Rumble, November 1, 2021, https://rumble.com/vojscp-fau cis-biggest-lie-lie-of-omission-committed-on-january-28th-2020-with-pete.html.

17. Joe Biden (@JoeBiden), "We are in the midst of a crisis with the coronavirus . . . ," Twitter, February 2, 2020, 5:01 p.m., https://twitter.com/JoeBiden/status/12237279773 61338370.

18. Yuliya Talmazan, "China Criticizes U.S. Border Closure as Coronavirus Death Toll Rises," NBC News, February 1, 2020, https://www.nbcnews.com/news/world/china -criticizes-u-s-border-closure-coronavirus-death-toll-rises-n1128161.

19. Yaron Steinbuch, "China Accuses US of Spreading 'Panic' over Coronavirus Outbreak," *New York Post*, February 3, 2020, https://nypost.com/2020/02/03/china-ac cuses-us-of-spreading-panic-over-coronavirus-outbreak/.

20. Ibid.

21. Steven Lee Myers, "China Pushes Back as Coronavirus Crisis Damages Its Image," *New York Times*, March 6, 2020, https://www.nytimes.com/2020/03/06/world/asia /china-coronavirus-image.html.

22. Steve Eder et al., "430,00 People Have Traveled from China to U.S. Since Coronavirus Surfaced," *New York Times*, April 4, 2020, https://www.nytimes.com/2020/04/04/us /coronavirus-china-travel-restrictions.html.

23. Miles Maochun Yu, "Big Lies That Won't Die: Chinese Communist Party Propaganda about Korea and COVID-19," Hoover Institution, September 13, 2021, https://www.ho over.org/research/big-lies-wont-die-chinese-communist-party-propaganda-about-ko rea-and-covid-19. As Yu writes, "[T]he Party has called up the ghost of the Korean war bacterial weapons hoax. In their coverage of the pandemic, state media outlets are resurrecting the now demonstrably false accusations that the U.S. military used biological weapons during the Korean War. Some lies never die."

24. WHO (@WHO), "'The speed with which #China detected the outbreak . . . ,'" Twitter, January 30, 2020, 2:41 p.m., https://twitter.com/who/status/1222968207524450308.

25. TomoNews US, "Coronavirus Has People Keeling Over in Streets—TomoNews," YouTube, February 3, 2020, https://www.youtube.com/watch?v=Uf4-Vzf1CyM.

26. Edward Wong, Matthew Rosenberg, and Julian E. Barnes, "Chinese Agents Helped Spread Messages That Sowed Virus Panic in U.S., Official Say," *New York Times*, January 5, 2021, https://www.nytimes.com/2020/04/22/us/politics/coronavirus-ch ina-disinformation.html.

27. In fact the official death toll from Wuhan is a tiny fraction of the true casualty rate, which is at least twenty-five times higher. The official death toll from New York City, on the other hand, undoubtedly exaggerates the number of Covid deaths, as we will see. For the Wuhan casualty rate, see Mosher, "Evidence from Wuhan's Morgues." Also see Alex Lo, "Lies, Damned Lies, and Statistics about China's Covid-19 Death

Toll," *South China Morning Post*, January 13, 2022, https://www.scmp.com/comment/opinion/article/3163283/lies-damned-lies-and-statistics-about-chinas-covid-19-death-toll.

28. Steven Mosher, "Did China's Leaders Deliberately 'Seed' Coronavirus around the World?," LifeSiteNews, April 20, 2020, https://www.lifesitenews.com/opinion/chinas-communist-govt-forcibly-rounds-up-coronavirus-victims-treats-them-like-animals/.

29. TomoNews US, "Coronavirus Has People Keeling Over."

30. Global Preparedness Monitoring Board (GPM Board), "Executive Summary," *A World at Risk: Annual Report on Global Preparedness for Health Emergencies* (Geneva: World Health Organization, September 18, 2019), 3, 8, 15, https://www.gpmb.org/annual-reports/annual-report-2019.

31. Alan J. Stein, "First Confirmed Case of COVID-19 in the United States Is Diagnosed in Snohomish County on January 20, 2020," HistoryLink.org, April 20, 2020, https://historylink.org/File/21018.

32. "CDC, Washington State Report First COVID-19 Death," Centers for Disease Control and Prevention, February 29, 2020, https://www.cdc.gov/media/releases/2020/s0229-COVID-19-first-death.html.

33. "Chinese Migration to Europe: Challenges and Opportunities," Parliamentary Assembly, Council of Europe, June 24, 2013, http://www.assembly.coe.int/LifeRay/MIG/pdf/TextesProvisoires/2015/20150000-ChineseMigration-EN.pdf.

34. "Italy Coronavirus (COVID-19) Statistics. Total and Daily Confirmed Cases and Deaths," World Health Organization, November 14, 2021, https://covid19.who.int/region/euro/country/it. The number at the link is a running total.

35. "Iran Coronavirus (COVID-19) Statistics. Total and Daily Confirmed Cases and Deaths," World Health Organization, November 14, 2021, https://covid19.who.int/region/emro/country/ir; Secretariat of the National Council of Resistance of Iran (NCRI), "Iran: The Staggering COVID-19 Death Toll Exceeds 469,700," National Council of Resistance of Iran, November 3, 2021, https://www.ncr-iran.org/en/ncri-statements/iran-the-staggering-covid-19-death-toll-exceeds-469700/. The numbers at the links are running totals.

36. Rosie Rossi, "Chinese Girl: Please..'Hug Me I'm Not a Virus,'" YouTube, February 22, 2020, https://www.youtube.com/watch?v=-IK2v897J7A; CGTN, "Italian Residents Hug Chinese People to Encourage Them in Coronavirus Fight," YouTube, February 4, 2020, https://www.youtube.com/watch?v=mNMdg4morQs.

37. "Cultural Etiquette: China," eDiplomat, http://www.ediplomat.com/np/cultural_etiquette/ce_cn.htm. Under the section entitled "Body Language," the visitor is advised, "The Chinese dislike being touched by strangers. Do not touch, hug, lock arms, slap or make any body contact."

38. John Gage, "Fauci: 'Not Ruling Out' Aerosol Transmission of Coronavirus," *Washington Examiner*, March 20, 2020, https://www.washingtonexaminer.com/news /fauci-not-ruling-out-aerosol-transmission-of-coronavirus.

39. Peter Navarro, *In Trump Time: A Journal of America's Plague Year* (St. Petersburg, Florida: All Seasons Press, 2021). See especially chapter 2, "Fear, Loathing, and Saint Fauci in the Situation Room."

40. "Dr. Fauci: 'Possible' That Millions Could Die in US," CNN, March 15, 2020, https:// www.cnn.com/videos/politics/2020/03/15/sotu-fauci-millions.cnn.

41. Berkeley Lovelace Jr., "Dr. Fauci Says All the 'Valid' Scientific Data Shows Hydroxychloroquine Isn't Effective in Treating Coronavirus," CNBC, July 29, 2020, https://www.cnbc.com/2020/07/29/dr-fauci-says-all-the-valid-scientific-data-shows -hydroxychloroquine-isnt-effective-in-treating-coronavirus.html; "'Don't Do It': Dr. Fauci Warns against Taking Ivermectin to Fight Covid-19," CNN, August 29, 2021, https://www.cnn.com/videos/health/2021/08/29/dr-anthony-fauci-ivermectin-covid -19-sotu-vpx.cnn.

42. Gabriella Muñoz, "Anthony Fauci Urges Coronavirus 'National Shutdown,'" *Washington Times*, March 15, 2020, https://www.washingtontimes.com/news/2020 /mar/15/anthony-fauci-urges-coronavirus-national-shutdown/.

43. Paul Joseph Watson, "Fauci Says Lockdown Will Continue until There Are No 'New Cases' of Coronavirus," SummitNews, April 2, 2020, https://summit.news/2020/04 /02/fauci-says-lockdown-will-continue-until-there-are-no-new-cases-of-coronavi rus/.

44. The Associated Press, "Dr. Fauci Warns of 'Suffering and Death' If US Reopens Too Soon during Coronavirus Pandemic," *The Oregonian*, May 12, 2020, https://www.ore gonlive.com/coronavirus/2020/05/dr-fauci-warns-of-suffering-and-death-if-us-reo pens-too-soon-during-coronavirus-pandemic.html.

45. Lee Brown, "Fauci Doubles Down on Claim That Attacks on Him Are 'Actually Criticizing Science,'" *New York Post*, June 21, 2021, https://nypost.com/2021/06/21/fa uci-attacks-on-him-are-actually-criticizing-science/.

46. Billy Perrigo, "President Trump's Advisors 'Argued Strongly' against Easing Coronavirus Measures Too Early, Anthony Fauci Says," *Time*, March 30, 2020, https://time.com/5812439/trump-coronavirus-measures-fauci/.

47. Brown, "Fauci Doubles Down."

48. "Timeline: Owosso Barber Karl Manke Defies State Orders and Is Issued an Injunction to Stop Operating," WLNS6, May 30, 2020, https://www.wlns.com/news /timeline-owosso-barber-karl-manke-defies-state-orders-and-is-issued-an-injunction -to-stop-operating/.

49. Lee Brown, "Texas Salon Owner Chooses Jail over Coronavirus Lockdown," *New York Post*, April 30, 2020, https://nypost.com/2020/04/30/texas-salon-owner-chooses-jail-over-coronavirus-lockdown/.

50. "Maine Restaurant Owner Defies State Stay-at-Home Order, Loses Health License," WMTW News (ABC), May 2, 2020, https://www.wmtw.com/article/maine-restaurant-owner-to-open-friday-to-dine-in-customers-defying-state-order/32343952.

51. Amanda Mull, "Georgia's Experiment in Human Sacrifice," *The Atlantic*, April 29, 2020, https://www.theatlantic.com/health/archive/2020/04/why-georgia-reopening-coronavirus-pandemic/610882/.

52. Joshua Berlinger et al., "April 3 Coronavirus News," CNN, April 4, 2020, https://edition.cnn.com/world/live-news/coronavirus-pandemic-04-03-20-intl/h_6a6afd8d891d8655fcfbc9e7e9c71491.

53. Jack Hadfield, "Michigan Gov Whitmer Wants to Extend Lockdown to Punish Protestors," The Political Insider, April 20, 2020, https://thepoliticalinsider.com/michigan-gov-whitmer-wants-to-extend-lockdown-to-punish-protestors/.

54. Jon Dougherty, "Mich Gov Whitmer Blows Off Her Own Extended Lockdown Order to March with George Floyd Protesters," BizPac Review, June 5, 2020, https://www.bizpacreview.com/2020/06/05/mich-gov-whitmer-defies-her-own-extended-lockdown-order-to-march-with-george-floyd-protesters-930388/.

55. "Timeline: Owosso Barber."

56. Craig Mauger and James David Dickson, "With Little Social Distancing, Whitmer Marches with Protesters," Detroit News, https://www.detroitnews.com/story/news/local/michigan/2020/06/04/whitmer-appears-break-social-distance-rules-highland-park-march/3146244001/.

57. Quint Forgey, "Trump Breaks with His Own Guidelines to Back Conservative Anti-Quarantine Protesters," *Politico*, April 17, 2020, https://www.politico.com/news/2020/04/17/trump-states-stay-at-home-orders-192386.

58. Carlie Porter, "Dr. Fauci on GOP Criticism: 'Attacks on Me, Quite Frankly, Are Attacks on Science,'" *Forbes*, June 9, 2021, https://www.forbes.com/sites/carlieporterfield/2021/06/09/fauci-on-gop-criticism-attacks-on-me-quite-frankly-are-attacks-on-science/?sh=834ef6845429.

59. PBS NewsHour, "Watch: Rep. Jim Jordan Asks Dr. Fauci If Nationwide Protests Helped Spread the Coronavirus," YouTube, July 31, 2020, https://youtu.be/Kd_99cRfoTU.

60. Brain Kilmeade, "Senator Tom Cotton: Dr. Fauci Is a Democrat Activist in a White Lab Coat," Fox News, June 22, 2021, https://radio.foxnews.com/2021/06/22/senator-tom-cotton-dr-fauci-is-a-democrat-activist-in-a-white-lab-coat/.

61. Betsy McCaughey, "Public Health 'Professionals' Keep Showing How Unprofessional They Really Are," *New York Post*, June 8, 2020, https://nypost.com/2020/06/08/public

-health-professionals-keep-showing-how-unprofessional-they-really-are/.
McCaughey did not mention Fauci by name, but he certainly fits the description here.

62. John Fund, "'Professor Lockdown' Modeler Resigns in Disgrace," *National Review*, May 6, 2020, https://www.nationalreview.com/corner/professor-lockdown-modeler -resigns-in-disgrace/. See also Kevin Dayaratna, "Failures of an Influential COVID-19 Model Used to Justify Lockdowns," Heritage Foundation, May 18, 2020, https://www .heritage.org/public-health/commentary/failures-influential-covid-19-model-used -justify-lockdowns.

63. Emma Colton, "Here Are Fauci's Biggest Flip-Flops and Backtracks amid the Coronavirus Pandemic," *Washington Examiner*, December 1, 2020, https://www.was hingtonexaminer.com/news/here-are-faucis-biggest-flip-flops-and-backtracks-amid -the-coronavirus-pandemic. Colton wrote, "Fauci, the leading White House coronavirus task force member, has changed positions or faced scientific data proving his stances are flawed on issues ranging from mask wearing to the severity of the virus and from asymptomatic spread to effective treatments for patients, among other issues, since January."

64. Natalie Bettendorf and Jason Leopold, "Anthony Fauci's Emails Reveal the Pressure That Fell on One Man," BuzzFeed News, June 1, 2021, https://www.buzzfeednews .com/article/nataliebettendorf/fauci-emails-covid-response.

65. Brown, "Fauci Doubles Down."

66. "Fact Check: Outdated Video of Fauci Saying 'There's No Reason to Be Walking Around with a Mask,'" Reuters, October 8, 2020, https://www.reuters.com/article/uk -factcheck-fauci-outdated-video-masks/fact-checkoutdated-video-of-fauci-saying-the res-no-reason-to-be-walking-around-with-a-mask-idUSKBN26T2TR.

67. Tamar Lapin, "Fauci Defends Mixed Messaging on Masks in Early Days of Pandemic," *New York Post*, April 11, 2021, https://nypost.com/2021/04/11/fauci- defends-mixed-messaging-on-masks-in-early-days-of-pandemic/.

68. Scott Johnson, "Would You Wear 2 Masks? Dr. Fauci Says It 'Likely Would Be More Effective,'" ClickOrlando, January 25, 2021, https://www.clickorlando.com/news/lo cal/2021/01/25/dr-fauci-says-double-masking-likely-would-be-more-effective/.

69. Carolyn Crist, "Fauci: Americans May Need to Wear Masks through 2022," WebMD, February 23, 2021, https://www.webmd.com/lung/news/20210223/fauc—says-amer icans-may-need-to-wear-masks-through-2022.

70. "Fauci's Agency Admits It Funded Gain-of-Function Work in Wuhan: What Else Are They Keeping from Us?," *New York Post*, October 21, 2021, https://nypost.com/2021 /10/21/faucis-agency-admits-it-funded-gain-of-function-work-in-wuhan-what-else -are-they-keeping-from-us/.

71. Kaylee McGhee White, "Do Masks Actually Work? The Best Studies Suggest They Don't," MSN, August 12, 2021, https://www.msn.com/en-us/health/medical/do-mas

ks-actually-work-the-best-studies-suggest-they-don-t/ar-AANfurl; Jim Meehan, "Surgeon Destroys Myth: 'If Masks Don't Work, Why Do Surgeons Wear Them?,'" CNSNews, March 10, 2021, https://cnsnews.com/commentary/dr-jim-meehan/surge on-destroys-myth-if-masks-dont-work-why-do-surgeons-wear-them.

72. Elizabeth Cohen and John Bonifield, "People Vaccinated against Covid-19 Can Go without Masks Indoors and Outdoors, CDC Says," CNN, May 13, 2021, https://edition .cnn.com/2021/05/13/health/cdc-mask-guidance-vaccinated/index.html.

73. Tucker Carlson, "Tucker: Fauci Deserves to Be under 'Criminal Investigation,'" Fox News, June 3, 2021, https://www.foxnews.com/transcript/tucker-fauci-deserves-to-be -under-criminal-investigation.

74. Michael Wilner, "Take the Vaccine Even If You've Already Had Coronavirus, Fauci Says," McClatchyDC, November 27, 2020, https://www.mcclatchydc.com/news/polit ics-government/white-house/article247454710.html.

75. Jackie Salo, "People Who Had COVID-19 May Only Need One Vaccine Dose, Fauci Says," *New York Post*, February 21, 2021, https://nypost.com/2021/02/21/people-who -had-covid-19-may-only-need-one-vaccine-dose-fauci/.

76. Berkeley Lovelace Jr., "Fauci Says Studies Show People Who Have Had Covid and Get Vaccinated May Have More Protection against Variants," CNBC, May 5, 2021, https:// www.cnbc.com/2021/05/05/fauci-says-studies-show-people-whove-had-covid-and -get-vaccinated-may-have-more-protection-against-variants.html.

77. Paul Elias Alexander, "128 Research Studies Affirm Naturally Acquired Immunity to Covid-19: Documented, Linked, and Quoted," Brownstone Institute, October 17, 2021, https://brownstone.org/articles/79-research-studies-affirm-naturally-acquired-im munity-to-covid-19-documented-linked-and-quoted/. This is a case where the science really *is* settled. The Brownstone Institute has compiled a list of 128 scientific studies, evidence reports, and position statements that affirm that natural immunity to Covid-19 is equal to or more robust than vaccine-induced immunity.

78. Calvin Freiburger, "CDC Admits It Has No Evidence That People with Natural Immunity Spread COVID," LifeSiteNews, November 12, 2021, https://www.lifesitene ws.com/news/cdc-admits-it-has-no-evidence-that-the-naturally-immune-can-spread -covid-19/. Natural immunity was one of the most important public health questions in America during the pandemic. The CDC did its best to ignore it out of existence. But my guess is that if those who had recovered from the China Virus were even occasionally infectious the CDC would have reams of data to share with us about how natural immunity is unreliable and how vaccination offers the only true protection against spreading the virus. This is a case where absence of evidence is tantamount to evidence of absence.

79. "Contact Tracing for COVID-19," Centers for Disease Control, February 25, 2021, https://www.cdc.gov/coronavirus/2019-ncov/php/contact-tracing/contact-tracing-pl an/contact-tracing.html.

80. Emma Betuel, "Exclusive: Watch Dr. Anthony Fauci Explain Why Contact Tracing Is So Critical," Inverse, August 15, 2020, https://www.inverse.com/mind-body/anthony -fauci-motivates-contact-tracers.

81. Betsy McCaughey, "Sorry: Contact Tracing Isn't the Answer to Ending Lockdowns," New York Post, April 22, 2020, https://nypost.com/2020/04/22/sorry-contact-tracing -isnt-the-answer-to-ending-lockdowns/.

82. Janice Dean, "Janice Dean: COVID-19 Killed My In-Laws after Cuomo's Reckless New York Nursing Home Policy," USA Today, July 22, 2020, https://www.usatoday.com/sto ry/opinion/voices/2020/07/22/andrew-cuomo-nursing-homes-coronavirus-janice-de an-new-york-column/5472713002/.

83. Martin Kulldorff, Sunetra Gupta, and Jay Bhattacharya, "The Great Barrington Declaration," Great Barrington Declaration, October 4, 2020, https://gbdeclaration .org/. The declaration, published on October 4, 2020, had been signed by 860,000 public health scientists, medical practitioners, and concerned citizens by November 4, 2021.

84. Kayla Rivas, "Fauci Calls Coronavirus Herd Immunity Approach 'Nonsense, Very Dangerous,'" Fox News, October 15, 2020, https://www.foxnews.com/health/fauci-co ronavirus-herd-immunity-great-barrington-declaration-nonsense.

85. Martin Kulldorff, Sunetra Gupta, and Jay Bhattacharya, "We Should Focus on Protecting the Vulnerable from COVID Infection," Newsweek, October 30, 2020, https://www.newsweek.com/we-should-focus-protecting-vulnerable-covid-infection -opinion-1543225.

86. Jay Bhattacharya and Sunetra Gupta, "How to End Lockdowns Next Month," Wall Street Journal, December 17, 2020, https://www.wsj.com/articles/how-to-end-lockdo wns-next-month-11608230214?page=1.

87. Henning Bundgaard et al., "Effectiveness of Adding a Mask Recommendation to Other Public Health Measures to Prevent SARS-CoV-2 Infection in Danish Mask Wearers," Annals of Internal Medicine 174, no. 3 (March 2021), https://doi. org/10.7326/M20-6817.

88. Jordan Schachtel, "Dr. Flip Flop: A Timeline of Fauci's School Reopening Positions," The Dossier, November 30, 2020, https://dossier.substack.com/p/dr-flip-flop-a-timel ine-of-faucis.

89. "Dr. Fauci Press Briefing on Coronavirus Outbreak," CSPAN, March 12, 2020, https:// www.c-span.org/video/?470338-1/dr-fauci-press-briefing-coronavirus-outbreak.

90. Matt Dixon, "Fauci: Kids Could Get 'Infected' If Florida Reopens Schools," *Politico*, April 10, 2020, https://www.politico.com/states/florida/story/2020/04/10/fauci-kids -could-get-infected-if-florida-reopens-schools-1274822.

91. Jon Miltimore, "8 Things Children Are More Likely to Die from Than COVID-19, according to the CDC," Foundation for Economic Education, August 9, 2021, https:// fee.org/articles/8-things-children-are-more-likely-to-die-from-than-covid-19-accordi ng-to-the-cdc/.

92. Public Health Agency of Sweden, "Covid-19 in Schoolchildren: A Comparison between Finland and Sweden," *Folkhälsomyndigheten*, no. 20108-1 (2020), https:// www.folkhalsomyndigheten.se/contentassets/c1b78bffbfde4a7899eb0d8ffdb57b09 /covid-19-school-aged-children.pdf; also see the Swedish researchers' summary of the report in the *New England Journal of Medicine*: J. F. Ludvigsson et al., "Open Schools, Covid-19, and Child and Teacher Morbidity in Sweden," *New England Journal of Medicine* 384, no. 7 (February 18, 2021): 669–71, https://www.nejm.org/doi /full/10.1056/NEJMc2026670.

93. Public Health Agency of Sweden, "Covid-19 in Schoolchildren."

94. Bethany Mandel, "Lockdowns Are Breaking Our Kids—and the Damage May Be Permanent," *New York Post*, February 8, 2021, https://nypost.com/2021/02/08/lockdo wns-are-breaking-our-kids-and-the-damage-may-be-permanent/.

95. Martin Kulldorff and Jay Bhattacharya, "How Fauci Fooled America," *Newsweek*, November 1, 2021, https://www.newsweek.com/how-fauci-fooled-america-opinion -1643839. Martin Kulldorff is an epidemiologist, biostatistician, and professor of medicine at Harvard Medical School, while Jay Bhattacharya is a professor of health policy at Stanford University School of Medicine. Their highly critical essay is called "How Fauci Fooled America," but in my opinion "How Fauci Killed Americans" would have been closer to the mark.

96. Ellen Sauerbrey, "Wrecking the Economy with Discredited Computer Models," American Thinker, May 13, 2020, https://www.americanthinker.com/blog/2020/05 /wrecking_the_economy_with_discredited_computer_models.html.

97. Hannah Ritchie et al., "Taiwan: Coronavirus Pandemic Country Profile," OurWorldinData, May 26, 2020, https://ourworldindata.org/coronavirus/country/tai wan#citation.

98. Steven Mosher, "The World Has a Lot to Learn from Taiwan's Hugely Successful Response to Chinese Coronavirus," LifeSiteNews, March 19, 2020, https://www.lifes itenews.com/blogs/the-world-has-a-lot-to-learn-from-taiwans-hugely-successful- response-to-chinese-coronavirus/.

99. On March 2, 2021, a World Health Organization panel strongly advised against using hydroxychloroquine to prevent Covid-19. They based their conclusion, published in the British Medical Journal as well as on the WHO's website, on a review of only six

randomized controlled trials that included a mere six thousand participants. François Lamontagne et al, "A Living WHO Guideline on Drugs to Prevent Covid-19," British Medical Journal 372, no. 526 (March 2, 2021), https://www.bmj.com/content/372/bmj.n526.long. A much broader, more sophisticated study called "HCQ for COVID-19: Real-Time Meta Analysis of 312 Studies" reached the opposite conclusion, namely, that "94.3% of early treatment studies report a positive effect [from HCQ], with an estimated reduction of 64% in the effect measured (death, hospitalization, etc.) from the random effects meta-analysis." "HCQ for COVID-19: Real-Time Meta Analysis of 312 Studies," Covid Analysis, February 23, 2022, https://hcqmeta.com/.

100. Philip Charlier, "Taiwan FDA Distributing Hydroxychloroquine for Free after WHO Declares It Ineffective for COVID Treatment," Taiwan News, April 4, 2021, https://taiwanenglishnews.com/taiwan-fda-distributing-hydroxychloroquine-for-free-after-who-declares-it-ineffective-for-covid-treatment/.

101. "Taiwan Death from COVID-19 Vaccination Exceeds Death from COVID-19 for the First Time," MedicalTrend, October 10, 2021, https://medicaltrend.org/2021/10/10/taiwan-death-from-covid-19-vaccination-exceeds-death-from-covid-19/.

102. Tiffany Meier, "More Die after Vaccination than from COVID-19 in Taiwan," NTD, October 13, 2021, https://news.ntd.com/more-die-after-vaccination-than-from-covid-19-in-taiwan_688004.html. Looking at the data from Taiwan, Robert Malone, who invented the mRNA technology that the major vaccines use, predicted, "Vaccinating low death rate countries (such as much of Africa) will elicit more deaths from the jab than from disease." Dr. Malone's tweet, formerly available at this url, disappeared when Twitter suspended his account: https://twitter.com/RWMaloneMD/status/1447909123505463296?ref_src=twsrc%5Etfw%7Ctwcamp%5Etweetembed%7Ctwterm%5E1447909123505463296%7Ctwgr%5E%7Ctwcon%5Es1_&ref_url=https%3A%2F%2Fwww.polygraph.info%2Fa%2Ffact-check-taiwan-covid-vaccine-death%2F31521527.html.

103. Brie Stimson, "California's Newsom Ordered to Pay $1.35M in Settlement with LA-Area Church over Coronavirus Restrictions," Fox News, Mary 26, 2021, https:// www.foxnews.com/politics/gavin-newsom-to-pay-1-35-million-in-settlement-with-la -church-over-coronavirus-restrictions.

104. Sheri Fink, "White House Takes New Line after Dire Report on Death Toll," New York Times, March 3,2020, https://www.nytimes.com/2020/03/16/us/coronavirus-fatality-rate-white-house.html.

105. Kulldorff and Bhattacharya, "How Fauci Fooled America."

106. "HIV Surveillance Reports," Centers for Disease Control, June 24, 2021, https://www.cdc.gov/hiv/library/reports/hiv-surveillance.html.

107. Nadia Whitehead, "A $100 Million HIV Vaccine Project Failed. But All Hope Is Not Lost," NPR, March 2, 2020, https://www.npr.org/sections/goatsandsoda/2020/03/02/809729417/a-100-million-hiv-vaccine-project-failed-but-all-hope-is-not-lost.

108. Adrian Horton, "'You Are Not Absolutely Invulnerable': Fauci Talks to Trevor Noah about Coronavirus," The Guardian, March 27, 2020, https://www.theguardian.com/culture/2020/mar/27/trevor-noah-fauci-interview-coronavirus-daily-show-recap.

109. Sivan Gazit et al., "Comparing SARS-CoV-2 Natural Immunity to Vaccine-Induced Immunity: Reinfections versus Breakthrough Infections," MedRxiv, August 25, 2021, https://www.medrxiv.org/content/10.1101/2021.08.24.21262415v1. The CDC quickly produced a study of its own based on U.S. data on hospitalizations that purported to show that natural immunity offers relatively less protection that the vaccine does. The structure of the study enabled it to reach the authors' preferred conclusion, which was naturally strongly in favor of vaccine mandates, to wit: "All eligible persons should be vaccinated against Covid-19 as soon as possible, including unvaccinated persons previously infected with SARS-Cov-2." Catherine H. Bozzio et al., "Laboratory-Confirmed COVID-19 among Adults Hospitalized with COVID-19–Like Illness with Infection-Induced or mRNA Vaccine-Induced SARS-CoV-2 Immunity—Nine States, January–September 2021," *Morbidity and Mortality Weekly Report* (MMWR) 70, no. 44 (November 5, 2021): 1539–44, https://www.cdc.gov/mmwr/volumes/70/wr/mm7044e1.htm. For a critique of the study, see Martin Kulldorff, "A Review and Autopsy of Two Covid Immunity Studies," Brownstone, November 2, 2021, https://brownstone.org/articles/a-review-and-autopsy-of-two-covid-immunity-studies/. For a more irreverent take, see Alex Berenson, "The CDC Hits a New Low," Unreported Truths (Substack), October 30, 2021, https://alexberenson.substack.com/p/the-cdc-hits-a-new-low/comments.

Chapter 9: A Pandemonium of Errors

1. "Transcript: Coronavirus: Leadership during Crisis with Anthony S. Fauci, MD," *Washington Post*, May 20, 2021, https://www.washingtonpost.com/washington-post-live/2021/05/20/transcript-coronavirus-leadership-during-crisis-with-anthony-s-fauci-md/. Fauci often used "eliminate" in describing his approach to the pandemic. For example, he told the press that "the delta variant is currently the greatest threat in the US to our attempt to eliminate COVID-19. Good news our vaccines are effective against the Delta Variant. Conclusion: we have the tools so let's use them to crush the outbreak." Berkeley Lovelace Jr., "Fauci Declares Delta Variant 'Greatest Threat' to the Nation's Efforts to Eliminate Covid," CNBC, June 22, 2021, https://www.cnbc.com/2021/06/22/fauci-declares-delta-variant-greatest-threat-to-the-nations-efforts-to-eliminate-covid.html.

2.   "Dr. Fauci: U.S. Needs 'People to Step Up and Get Vaccinated' to End Covid Pandemic," NBC
      News, September 10, 2021, https://www.nbcnews.com/now/video/dr-fauci-on-biden-s-plan-to
      -end-the-covid-pandemic-120566341802, at 2:00.

3.   The phrase comes from the October 2020 presidential debate, in which Biden promised to "shut
      down the virus, not the country," a line that he has used repeatedly. Spencer Brown, "12+ Times
      Biden Promised He had a Plan to 'Shut Down the Virus,'" Townhall, December 28, 2021, https://to
      wnhall.com/tipsheet/spencerbrown/2021/12/28/12-times-biden-promised-he-had-a-plan-to-shut
      -down-the-virus-n2601143.

4.   Joe DePaola, "Fauci Says Covid Zero Is a Pipe Dream: 'We Certainly Are Not Going to Eradicate
      It,'" Mediaite, November 29, 2021, https://www.mediaite.com/news/fauci-says-covid-zero-is-a-pi
      pe-dream-we-certainly-are-not-going-to-eradicate-it/.

5.   England, Germany, and a handful of other nations came out in favor of an annual COVID shot.
      On England, for example, see Gareth Iacobucci, "Covid-19: England Is Preparing to Offer Annual
      Booster Vaccination, Says NHS Boss," *British Medical Journal* 375, no. 2824 (November 17, 2021),
      https://www.bmj.com/content/375/bmj.n2824. German health officials were, if anything, even
      more determined to give everyone the booster. See Jenipher Camino Gonzalez, "Germany:
      Doctors' Association Says Fourth Booster needed," DW, November 12, 2021, https://www.dw.com
      /en/germany-doctors-association-says-fourth-booster-needed/a-60088867. Fauci, as usual,
      danced around the issue. See Phil Shiver, "Fauci Doesn't Rule Out Boosters Every Year to Stop
      COVID: 'We Don't Know What's Going to Be Required,'" The Blaze, December 2, 2021, https://
      www.theblaze.com/news/fauci-doesnt-rule-out-annual-boosters; and also Sophie Mellor,
      "Scientists Said We'd Take Annual COVID Jabs like Flu Shots. Now Fauci Says It Might Be Only
      Every 5 Years," Fortune, February 9, 2022, https://fortune.com/2022/02/09/scientists-said-wed-ta
      ke-annual-covid-jabs-like-flu-shots-now-fauci-says-it-might-be-only-every-5-years/.

6.   Tim Hains, "CDC Director: Vaccines No Longer Prevent You from Spreading COVID,"
      RealClearPolitics, August 6, 2021, https://www.realclearpolitics.com/video/2021/08/06/cdc_direc
      tor_vaccines_no_longer_prevent_you_from_spreading_covid.html#.

7.   The infection fatality rate (IFR) is simply the number of deaths divided by the number of
      infections. Based on sixty-one studies and eight preliminary national estimates, Stanford
      researcher John Ioannidis suggests a median IFR of 0.05 percent and an upper-bound IFR of 0.3
      percent for ages below seventy. See John P. A. Ioannidis, "Infection Fatality Rate of COVID-19
      Inferred from Seroprevalence Data," *Bulletin of the World Health Organization* 99, no. 1 (2021):
      19–33F, doi:10.2471/BLT.20.265892; Michael S. Rosenwald, "History's Deadliest Pandemics, from
      Ancient Rome to Modern America," *Washington Post*, October 3, 2021, https://www.washington
      post.com/graphics/2020/local/retropolis/coronavirus-deadliest-pandemics/.

8.   Henrik Pettersson, Byron Manley, and Sergio Hernandez, "Tracking Covid-19's Global Spread,"
      CNN, November 20, 2021, https://www.cnn.com/interactive/2020/health/coronavirus-maps-and
      -cases/.

9. Charlie Bradley, "China's 40 Million Deaths Cover-Up Exposed amid Coronavirus Controversy," *Daily Express*, September 1, 2021, https://www.express.co.uk/news/world/1329961/china-news-deaths-cover-up-coronavirus-controversy-spt.

10. Steven Mosher, "Evidence from Wuhan's Morgues, Crematoriums Suggests COVID-19 Deaths 20 Times Higher than Official Count," LifeSiteNews, April 6, 2020, https://www.lifesitenews.com/blogs/evidence-from-wuhans-morgues-crematoriums-suggests-covid-19-deaths-20-times-higher-than-official-count/.

11. See Steven Mosher, *China Misperceived: American Illusions and Chinese Reality* (New York: Harper Collins, 1990), for past examples of how alienated Western intellectuals have romanticized China and looked the other way when the Chinese Communist Party, like all Communist dictatorships, set about liquidating its political opponents.

12. Helen Davidson and Vincent Ni, "'People Are Starting to Wane': China's Zero-Covid Policy Takes Toll," *The Guardian*, October 30, 2021, https://www.theguardian.com/world/2021/oct/30/people-are-starting-to-wane-china-zero-covid-policy-takes-toll.

13. Reuters, "Mainland China Sees Imported Coronavirus Cases Exceed New Local Infections for First Time," *Straits Times*, March 14, 2020, https://www.straitstimes.com/asia/east-asia/mainland-china-reports-11-new-coronavirus-cases-on-march-13.

14. Ben Westcott and Shanshan Wang, "The Coronavirus Pandemic Began in China. Today, It Reported No New Local Infections for the First time," CNN, March 19, 2020, https://www.cnn.com/2020/03/19/asia/coronavirus-covid-19-update-china-intl-hnk/index.html.

15. Mosher, "Evidence from Wuhan's Morgues, Crematoriums."

16. Luke Hawker, "Jacinda Ardern Fury as NZ in Lockdown after One Covid Case: 'Never-Ending Nightmare,'" *Daily Express*, August 17, 2021, https://www.express.co.uk/news/world/1477950/Jacinda-ardern-news-new-zealand-lockdown-covid-strategy-Auckland. See also Pettersson, Manley, and Hernandez, "Tracking Covid-19's Global Spread."

17. Yilin Yang, "WHO Congratulates China on 20 Days of Zero Local COVID-19 Cases in Many Provinces (Video)," *China Daily* (Global Edition), September 8, 2020, https://global.chinadaily.com.cn/a/202009/08/WS5f56a57ea310675eafc580a4.html.

18. Amelia Wade, "Covid-19 Coronavirus: Controversial Bill Passed to Enforce Alert Level 2 Powers," *New Zealand Herald*, May 13, 2020, https://web.archive.org/web/20200513223302/https://www.nzherald.co.nz/nz/news/article.cfm?c_id=1&objectid=12331547.

19. Peter Dutton, "Australian Health Management Plan for Pandemic Influenza," Australian Government Department of Health, August 2019, https://www1.health.gov.au/internet/main/publishing.nsf/Content/519F9392797E2DDCCA257D47001B9948/$File/w-AHMPPI-2019.PDF. In their panic, Australian authorities completely ignored the pandemic influenza plan they had drawn up in August 2019, just months before the arrival of China Virus. The 232-page white paper defined a mild pandemic as one where "the majority of cases are likely to experience mild to moderate clinical features. People in at-risk groups may experience more severe illness" (p. 22). That seems an apt description of the Covid pandemic. The report argued against internal border

closures and school closures on the sensible grounds that "[t]he level of disruption is likely to outweigh the benefits." The authorities' use of the army to enforce lockdowns of entire cities for months on end was never part of the plan. It was simply inconceivable that a Western country would ever adopt such draconian policies—until it did.

20.   Scott Morrison, "Media Statement," Prime Minister of Australia Press Release, March 29, 2020, https://www.pm.gov.au/media/national-cabinet-statement.

21.   Dave Urbanski, "Australian Health Officer Tells Citizens Not to Talk to Each Other—'Even . . . Your Next-Door Neighbor in the Shopping Center'—to Prevent COVID Spread," The Blaze, July 20, 2021, https://www.theblaze.com/news/australian-health-officer-do-not-talk-to-each-other. "Whilst it's human nature to engage in conversation with others—to be friendly—unfortunately this is not the time to do that. So even if you run into your next-door neighbor in the shopping center . . . don't start up a conversation."

22.   "Coronavirus Update for Victoria," Victoria State Government Health and Human Services, June 6, 2020, https://www.dhhs.vic.gov.au/coronavirus-update-victoria-06-june-2020.

23.   Julia Hollingsworth and Chandler Thornton, "New Zealand Announces It's Locking Down the Entire Country . . . over One Covid Case," CNN, August 17, 2021, https://www.cnn.com/2021/08/17/asia/new-zealand-lockdown-one-case-intl-hnk/index.html. See also Praveen Menon, "New Zealand Thrown into Lockdown over Single Suspected Delta Case," Reuters, August 17, 2021, https://www.reuters.com/world/asia-pacific/virus-free-new-zealand-investigating-new-community-covid-19-case-2021-08-17/.

24.   Jack Newman, "New Zealand Finally Abandons 'Covid Zero' Strategy after Jacinda Ardern Admits Delta Variant Is a 'Game-Changer'—with 40% of the Population Now Double-Jabbed after Slow Roll-Out," Daily Mail, October 4, 2021, https://www.dailymail.co.uk/news/article-10056295/New-Zealand-finally-abandons-Covid-zero-strategy-Jacinda-Ardern-admits-Delta-game-changer.html.

25.   Caitlin Cassidy, "Victoria Covid Update: Police Arrest 44 People and Fire Rubber Pellets during Melbourne Construction Protests," The Guardian, September 21, 2021, https://www.theguardian.com/australia-news/2021/sep/21/victoria-covid-update-rubber-bullets-fired-on-second-day-of-construction-protests-which-block-freeway. Victoria's police chief commissioner, Shane Patton, was quoted as saying officers used pepper balls, foam baton rounds, smoke bombs, and stinger grenades which deploy rubber pellets.

26.   Angus Thompson, "Rescue Dogs Shot Dead by NSW Council due to COVID-19 Restrictions," Sydney Morning Herald, August 22, 2021, https://www.smh.com.au/national/nsw/rescue-dogs-shot-dead-by-nsw-council-due-to-covid-19-restrictions-20210821-p58ksh.html#comments.

27. Adrian Zorzut, "Australia's Brutal Lockdown Sees Protesters Covered in Pepper Spray and Pinned to the Ground in Clashes with Cops," *The Sun*, September 18, 2021, https://www.the-sun.com/news/3685424/covid-anti-lockdown-protesters-confronted-by-cops-australia/.

28. Jake Massey, "Police in Australia Shake Coffee Cup to Check Covid-19 Rules Being Followed," LADbible, October 18, 2021, https://www.ladbible.com/news/news-austra lia-police-shake-coffee-cup-to-check-covid-19-rules-20211018.

29. Francis Mao, "Why Has Australia Switched Tack on Covid Zero?," BBC News, September 3, 2021, https://www.bbc.com/news/world-australia-58406526.

30. Jay Bhattacharya and Donald J. Boudreaux, "Eradication of Covid Is a Dangerous and Expensive Fantasy," *Wall Street Journal*, August 4, 2021, https://www.wsj.com/articl es/zero-covid-coronavirus-pandemic-lockdowns-china-australia-new-zealand-11628 101945?page=1.

31. Sen Pei et al., "Burden and Characteristics of COVID-19 in the United States during 2020," *Nature* 598 (August 26, 2021), https://www.nature.com/articles/s41586-021-03914-4.

32. As John Ioannidis has written, "Early data from China suggested a 3.4% case fatality rate and that asymptomatic infections were uncommon, thus the case fatality rate and the infection fatality rate would be about the same." See Ioannidis, "Infection Fatality Rate of COVID-19." In other words, the Chinese data suggested that everyone who tested positive for Covid would come down with the disease, and three or four out of every hundred would die, a terrifying prospect.

33. Ibid.

34. Bloomberg Markets and Finance, "Coronavirus Is 10 Times More Lethal than Seasonal Flu, Fauci Says," YouTube, March 11, 2020, https://www.youtube.com/wat ch?v=2DekzGCJhJw.

35. Bruce Haring, "White House Experts Offer Grim Coronavirus Predictions on Sunday Talk Shows: '100,000 to 200,000 Deaths,' Says Dr. Anthony Fauci," Yahoo, March 29, 2020, https://www.yahoo.com/entertainment/white-house-experts-offer-grim-165014 937.html.

36. Adrian Horton, "'You Are Not Absolutely Invulnerable': Fauci Talks to Trevor Noah about Coronavirus," *The Guardian*, March 27, 2020, https://www.theguardian.com /culture/2020/mar/27/trevor-noah-fauci-interview-coronavirus-daily-show-recap.

37. Anthony S. Fauci, H. Clifford Lane, and Robert R. Redfield, "Covid-19—Navigating the Uncharted," *New England Journal of Medicine* no. 382 (March 26, 2020): 1268–69, https://www.nejm.org/doi/full/10.1056/NEJMe2002387?fbclid=IwAR3psHRYCZL1uI MKU2cJuSrpcc7SCs7kAIjjfDCmXqG_bOjcWd2Li-xXZHs.

38. K. D. Patterson and G. F. Pyle, "The Geography and Mortality of the 1918 Influenza Pandemic," *Bulletin of the History of Medicine* 65, no. 1 (1991), 4, https://www.jstor.

org/stable/44447656. Patterson and Pyle wrote, "We believe that approximately 30 million is the best estimate for the terrible demographic toll of the influenza pandemic of 1918," and gave a range from 24.7 to 39.3 million deaths.

39. N. Johnson and J. Mueller, "Updating the Accounts: Global Mortality of the 1918–1920 'Spanish' Influenza Pandemic," *Bulletin of the History of Medicine* 76, no. 1 (2002): 105–15, https://doi.org/10.1353/bhm.2002.0022. This widely cited study by Johnson and Mueller estimates 50 million global deaths, but the authors suggest that this could be an underestimate; the true death toll may have been as high as 100 million, they say.

40. The CDC has given widely varying estimates of mortality from the Hong Kong Flu over time, from the 100,000 figure found in the CDC publication "1968 Pandemic (H3N2)," https://www.cdc.gov/flu/pandemic-resources/1968-pandemic.html, down to the 33,800 figure found in an earlier publication, "Pandemics and Pandemic Threats since 1900," https://web.archive.org/web/20090331065518/http://www.pan demicflu.gov/general/historicaloverview.html.

41. "GLOBAL WHO Coronavirus (COVID-19) Dashboard," World Health Organization, November 22, 2021, https://covid19.who.int/. The page updates daily.

42. "Italy Coronavirus (COVID-19) Statistics. Total and Daily Confirmed Cases and Deaths," World Health Organization, November 14, 2021, https://covid19.who.int/re gion/euro/country/it. The page updates daily.

43. "Comunicati Stampa," Istituto Superiore di Sanità, fall 2021, https://www.iss.it/web /guest//comunicati-stampa/-/asset_publisher/fjTKmjJgSgdK/content/id/5868665.

44. For the United States, see for example, Blake Fussell, "CDC Director Agrees Hospitals Have Monetary Incentive to Inflate Covid-19 Data," Christian Post, August 4, 2020, https://www.christianpost.com/news/cdc-director-agrees-that-hospitals-have-monet ary-incentive-to-inflate-covid-19-data.html. For Italy, see Sarah Newey, "Why Have So Many Coronavirus Patients Died in Italy?" *The Telegraph*, March 23, 2020, https:// www.telegraph.co.uk/global-health/science-and-disease/have-many-coronavirus-pa tients-died-italy/. See also Tommaso Ebhardt, Chiara Remondini, and Marco Bertacche, "99% of Those Who Died from Virus Had Other Illness, Italy Says," Bloomberg, March 18, 2020, https://www.bloomberg.com/news/articles/2020-03-18 /99-of-those-who-died-from-virus-had-other-illness-italy-says.

45. "Comunicati Stampa."

46. "Provisional Death Counts for Coronavirus Disease 2019 (COVID-19)," Centers for Disease Control and Prevention, November 22, 2021. The CDC updates the "death counts" weekly.

47. Rebecca Wright, "There's an Unlikely Beneficiary of Coronavirus: The Planet," CNN, March 17, 2020, https://www.cnn.com/2020/03/16/asia/china-pollution-coronavirus -hnk-intl/index.html.

48. Bertrand Russell, *The Impact of Science Upon Society* (New York: Simon and Schuster, 1953), 102–4.

49. As reported by Deutsche Press Agentur (DPA), August 1988. Also in Prince Philip's "Foreword" to *People as Animals*, a strange anthology compiled by Fleur Cowles (London: R. Clark, 1986).

50. National Vital Statistics System, "Guidance for Certifying Deaths due to Coronavirus Disease 2019 (COVID-19)," Centers for Disease Control and Prevention, April 2020, https://www.cdc.gov/nchs/data/nvss/vsrg/vsrg03-508.pdf.

51. The CDC has an interactive page which perfectly illustrates the inverse relationship between Covid and the flu that materialized in the 2020–21 flu season. See FluViewInteractive, "Pneumonia and Influenza Mortality Surveillance from the National Center for Health Statistics Mortality Surveillance System," Centers for Disease Control and Prevention, https://gis.cdc.gov/grasp/fluview/mortality.html. The same pattern was observed in Australia. While eight hundred flu deaths were recorded Down Under in 2019, the number dropped to below forty in 2020 and stood at zero halfway through the 2021 season. Aisha Dow, "Seasonal Flu 'Nowhere to Be Seen' in Australia," *Sydney Morning Herald*, June 13, 2021, https://www.smh.com.au/national/seasonal-flu-nowhere-to-be-seen-in-australia-20210612-p580gk.html. The CDC said that masking and social distancing were responsible for the flu's taking a year off, but it seems more likely that flu deaths were being misclassified as Covid deaths to help the hospital industry's bottom line. See Michelle Rogers, "Fact Check: Hospitals Get Paid More If Patients Listed as Covid-19, on Ventilators," *USA Today*, April 24, 2020, https://www.usatoday.com/story/news/factcheck/2020/04/24/fact-check-medicare-hospitals-paid-more-covid-19-patients-coronavirus/3000638001/.

52. Danielle Lama, "Fox 35 Investigates: Questions Raised after Fatal Motorcycle Crash Listed as COVID-19 Death," Fox 35 Orlando, July 16, 2020, https://www.fox35orlando.com/news/fox-35-investigates-questions-raised-after-fatal-motorcycle-crash-listed-as-covid-19-death.

53. "Excess Deaths Associated with COVID-19. Provisional Death Counts for Coronavirus Disease (COVID-19)," Centers for Disease Control and Prevention, https://www.cdc.gov/nchs/nvss/vsrr/covid19/excess_deaths.htm.

54. Michael Austin, "MN Senator/Physician Blows Whistle: The Bizarre, Non-Covid Types of Deaths Being Blamed on Covid," Western Journal, December 21, 2020, https://www.westernjournal.com/mn-senator-physician-blows-whistle-bizarre-non-covid-types-deaths-blamed-covid/?utm_source=facebook&utm_medium=westernjournalism&utm_content=2020-12-21&utm_campaign=manualpost.

55. Jensen and a Minnesota state senate colleague reviewed thousands of death certificates and concluded that Covid deaths in their state might be inflated by 40 percent. Emma Colton, "Minnesota Lawmakers Say Coronavirus Deaths Could Be

Inflated by 40% after Reviewing Death Certificates," *Washington Examiner*, December 22, 2020, https://www.washingtonexaminer.com/news/coronavirus-death -certificates-minnesota-inflated.

56. Tim Hains, "CDC Director Walensky Estimates up to 40% of Hospitalizations 'with' Covid Are Not 'because of' Covid," RealClearPolitics, January 9, 2022, https://www.re alclearpolitics.com/video/2022/01/09/cdc_director_walensky_estimates_40_of_hos pitalizations_with_covid_are_not_because_of_covid.html.

57. Joel Achenbach, "US 'Excess Deaths' during the Pandemic Surpassed 1 Million, with Covid Killing Most but Other Diseases Adding to the Toll," Yahoo, February 15, 2022, https://www.yahoo.com/news/us-excess-deaths-during-pandemic-215337856.html.

58. "Influenza (Flu) 1918 Pandemic," Centers for Disease Control and Prevention, 2019, https://www.cdc.gov/flu/pandemic-resources/1918-pandemic-h1n1.html.

59. Elizabeth Arias et al., "Provisional Life Expectancy Estimates for 2020," *Vital Statistics Rapid Release Report* no. 015 (July 2021), National Center for Health Statistics, Centers for Disease Control and Prevention, https://www.cdc.gov/nchs/da ta/vsrr/vsrr015-508.pdf. According to this CDC report, life expectancy declined from 78.8 years in 2019 to 77.3 years in 2020. While three-fourths of the decline came from COVID deaths, the rest came from increases in accidents, drug overdoses, homicide, diabetes, and chronic liver disease—which is to say, from the unintended consequences of the lockdowns and social isolation.

60. Kyle Becker, "The CDC Finally Admits a Massive Number of Americans Have 'Natural Immunity,'" Becker News, November 13, 2021, https://beckernews.com/22 -new-cdc-natural-immunity-42976/. In October 2021, the CDC stealthily admitted that 146.6 million Americans have already had and recovered from the China Virus. Kyle Becker believes this to be an underestimate; given the large numbers of unreported cases, the actual number could be as high as 187.6 million. That is to say, over half of the U.S. population may already have had natural immunity by the end of 2021. Not everyone had symptomatic illnesses, but of the 124 million who did, only 1 in 4 sought medical treatment. (That would include me and several members of my family, who took only vitamins and aspirin.) You have to dig, and I mean really dig, into the CDC's website to find these buried numbers, but Becker does an excellent job in uncovering them. Post-Omicron, of course, the number of Americans with natural immunity is even higher.

61. Achenbach, "US 'Excess Deaths' during the Pandemic."

62. Margaret Menge, "Indiana Life Insurance CEO Says Deaths Are Up 40% among People ages 18–64," The Center Square, January 1, 2022, https://www.thecentersqua re.com/indiana/indiana-life-insurance-ceo-says-deaths-are-up-40-among-people -ages-18-64/article_71473b12-6b1e-11ec-8641-5b2c06725e2c.html.

63. "2020 Annual Report," OneAmerica, April 26, 2021, https://oasf.my.salesforce.com /sfc/p/#50000000bbUu/a/2J000000FAPH/rGTCw.REDLHs6acxN2G41z2iCmvyeBbY WBk8RWAIkCM.

64. The numbers are from Prudential's "Quarterly Financial Supplement, Third Quarter 2021," https://s22.q4cdn.com/600663696/files/doc_financials/2021/q3/3Q21-QFS .pdf; Pacific Life's "Quarterly Statement as of September 30, 2021," https://www.pacif iclife.com/content/dam/paclife/crp/public/financials/statutory-statements/PLA_Q3 _2021_Statutory_Statement.pdf; and New York Life's "Quarterly Statement as of September 30, 2021," https://www.newyorklife.com/assets/docs/pdfs/financial-info /2021/NYLIC-3rd-Qtr-2021-Statement.pdf.

65. Menge, "Indiana Life Insurance CEO Says Deaths Are Up."

66. VAERS is an acronym for Vaccine Adverse Event Reporting System. This system is co-maintained by the U.S. Centers for Disease Control and Prevention (CDC) and the Food and Drug Administration (FDA). The CDC describes VAERS as "an early warning system used to monitor events that happen after vaccination. VAERS is the frontline system of a comprehensive vaccine safely monitoring program in the United States. . . . VAERS gives vaccine safety experts valuable information so they can assess possible vaccine safety concerns, including the new Covid-19 vaccines. . . . 'Adverse events' . . . might indicate a possible safety problem with a vaccine." "Vaccine Adverse Event Reporting System (VAERS)," Centers for Disease Control and Prevention, https://www.cdc.gov/coronavirus/2019-ncov/vaccines/safety/vaers .html.

67. Spiro Pantazatos and Hervé Seligmann, "Covid Vaccination and Age-Stratified All-Cause Mortality Risk," ResearchGate, October 2021, https://www.researchgate.net /publication/355581860_COVID_vaccination_and_age-stratified_all-cause_mortality _risk. The authors note, accurately, that "existing surveillance studies are not designed to reliably estimate life-threatening events or vaccine-induced fatality rates (VFR)." Instead, those pushing mRNA vaccines for funding and profit blame Covid, Long Covid, or pandemic-related delays in medical care for nearly all deaths and injuries.

68. Pantazatos and Seligmann note that another recent study, whose findings were derived independently from VAERS and other data sources, comports well with their findings. Jessica Rose and Matthew Crawford estimated "over 150,000" vaccine-related deaths as of August 28, 2021, based on autopsies of the victims and an underreporting factor of 41 derived from anaphylaxis rates pre- and post-vaccine. See Jessica Rose and Matthew Crawford, "Estimating the Number of COVID Vaccine Deaths in America," https://downloads.regulations.gov/CDC-2021-0089-0024/attach ment_1.pdf.

69. Pantazatos and Seligmann, "Covid Vaccination," 15.

70. Ibid., 12.

71. Steven Mosher, "Now It's Personal . . . Several of My Loved Ones Have Suffered Seriously from the So-Called 'Vaccines,'" LifeSiteNews, January 3, 2022, https://www .lifesitenews.com/blogs/now-its-personal-several-of-my-loved-ones-have-suffered-se riously-from-the-so-called-vaccines/.

72. Pantazatos and Seligmann, "Covid Vaccination," 13.

73. "A 5th Investigation of Scott Jensen's Medical License," Dr. Scott Jensen for Governor, https://drscottjensen.com/medical-license-jensen/.

74. Hannah Knowles, "After Doctor Derided Mask Wearing, His Medical License Has Been Suspended," *Seattle Times*, March 6, 2021, https://www.seattletimes.com /nation-world/after-oregon-doctor-derided-mask-wearing-his-medical-license-has-be en-suspended/. The attacks on such courageous truth-tellers were absolutely vicious, as articles from the time illustrate. Consider a CNN article by Rob Kuznia and colleagues in late 2021, "They Take an Oath to Do No Harm, but These Doctors Are Spreading Misinformation about the Covid Vaccine," CNN, October 20, 2021, https:// www.cnn.com/2021/10/19/us/doctors-covid-vaccine-misinformation-invs/index .html.

75. Carl Campanile, "Hochul Scraps Booster Mandate for Health Care Workers, Cites Staff Shortages," *New York Post*, February 18, 2022, https://nypost.com/2022/02/18 / hochul-scraps-booster-mandate-for-health-care-workers/.

76. Stanley Xu et al., "COVID-19 Vaccination and Non–COVID-19 Mortality Risk—Seven Integrated Health Care Organizations, United States, December 14, 2020–July 31, 2021," *Morbidity and Mortality Weekly Report* 70, no. 43 (October 29, 2021): 1520–24, https://www.cdc.gov/mmwr/volumes/70/wr/mm7043e2.htm.

77. Frank Kowalzik et al., "mRNA-Based Vaccines," National Center for Biotechnology Information, April 15, 2021, https://www.ncbi.nlm.nih.gov/pmc/articles/PMC8103 517/.

78. Dr. Malone is the discoverer of in-vitro and in-vivo RNA transfection and the inventor of mRNA vaccines, accomplishments he made while he was at the Salk Institute in 1988. Big Tech has done its best to "disappear" those who have raised questions about the experimental gene therapy that the mRNA vaccines rely upon, but archived information on Malone's background may be found at https://web.arch ive.org/web/20210608101002/https://www.rwmalonemd.com/about-us. See also Joseph Mercola, "COVID-19 Injection Campaign Violates Bioethics Laws," Citizens Journal, August 18, 2021, https://www.citizensjournal.us/covid-19-injection-campai gn-violates-bioethics-laws-2/.

79. Kowalzik et al., "mRNA-Based Vaccines."

80. Ibid. The authors also note that "mRNA vaccines are currently being tested clinically for a number of viral diseases, including rabies virus, influenza virus, Zika virus, cytomegalovirus, respiratory syncytial virus, and novel coronavirus (SARS-CoV-2).

With the exception of SARS-CoV-2, however, none of these clinical trials has passed the early phase" [emphasis added].

81. "Understanding mRNA COVID-19 Vaccines," Centers for Disease Control and Prevention, November 3, 2021, https://www.cdc.gov/coronavirus/2019-ncov/vaccines/different-vaccines/mRNA.html?s_cid=11347:+mRNA%2520+vaccines:sem.b:p:RG:GM:gen:PTN:FY21.

82. Hui Jiang and Ya-Fang Mei, "SARS–CoV–2 Spike Impairs DNA Damage Repair and Inhibits V(D)J Recombination In Vitro," National Center for Biotechnology Information, October 13, 2021, https://www.ncbi.nlm.nih.gov/pmc/articles/PMC853 8446/. The authors concluded, "Our findings reveal a potential molecular mechanism by which the spike protein might impede adaptive immunity and underscore the potential side effects of full-length spike-based vaccines."

83. Alex Berenson, "Playing God (Badly)," Unreported Truths (Substack), October 29, 2021, https://alexberenson.substack.com/p/playing-god-badly/comments.

84. Maggie Fox and Jamie Gumbrecht, "Vaccine Protection against Covid-19 Wanes over Time, Especially for Older People, CDC says," CNN, September 23, 2021, https://www.cnn.com/2021/09/22/health/cdc-vaccine-advisers-booster-wane/index.html.

85. Jen Christensen, "Immunocompromised May Need a Fourth Covid-19 Shot, CDC Says," CNN, October 26, 2021, https://www.cnn.com/2021/10/26/health/covid-19-fourth-dose-for-the-immunocompromised/index.html.

86. See Table 1, "Scenario 5: Current Best Estimate" in "COVID-19 Pandemic Planning Scenarios," Centers for Disease Control and Prevention, March 19, 2021, https://www.cdc.gov/coronavirus/2019-ncov/hcp/planning-scenarios.html.

87. Landon Mion, "Fauci: Mandating Covid-19 Vaccines for School Children Is a 'Good Idea,'" Townhall, August 29, 2021, https://townhall.com/tipsheet/landonmion/2021/08/29/fauci-mandating-covid19-vaccines-for-school-children-is-a-good-idea-n259 4947. A Swedish report notes, "In the US, a peer-reviewed paper has been published suggesting that children might be the best group to target for Covid-19 immunization in order to reduce the spread of the virus also to other groups, comparing it with other respiratory infections like influenza and pneumococcal infections. This theory is not supported by the findings in our report." The article it was referring to is Carol M. Kao et al., "The Importance of Advancing Severe Acute Respiratory Syndrome Coronavirus 2 Vaccines in Children," *Clinical Infectious Diseases* 72, no. 3 (February 1, 2021): 515–18, https://pubmed.ncbi.nlm.nih.gov/33527122/. The Swedish report is Public Health Agency of Sweden, "Covid-19 in Schoolchildren: A Comparison between Finland and Sweden," *Folkhälsomyndigheten*, no. 20108-1 (2020), https://www.folkhalsomyndigheten.se/contentassets/c1b78bffbfde4a7899eb0d8ffdb57b09/covid-19-school-aged-children.pdf.

88. Levi Quackenboss, "A Letter to Parents Planning to Vaccinate Their Children for COVID," LifeSiteNews, July 8, 2021, https://www.lifesitenews.com/opinion/a-letter -to-parents-planning-to-vaccinate-their-children-for-covid/.

89. Ali Zhang et al., "Original Antigenic Sin: How First Exposure Shapes Lifelong Anti–Influenza Virus Immune Responses," *Journal of Immunology* 202, no. 2 (January 15, 2019): 335–40, doi: 10.4049/jimmunol.1801149. The authors conclude that "it seems clear that [Original Antigenic Sin] can also be detrimental when the boosting of memory responses to conserved, but nonprotective, epitopes comes at the expense of generating new responses against protective, but antigenically drifted, epitopes."

90. Paul-Henri Lambert, Margaret Liu, and Claire-Anne Siegrist, "Can Successful Vaccines Teach Us How to Induce Efficient Protective Immune Responses?," *Nature Medicine* 11 (April 5, 2005): S54–S62, https://www.nature.com/articles/nm1216.

91. S. V. Subramanian and Akhil Kumar, "Increases in COVID-19 Are Unrelated to Levels of Vaccination across 68 Countries and 2947 Counties in the United States," *European Journal of Epidemiology* 36 (September 2021): 1237–40, https://doi .org/10.1007/s10654-021-00808-7.

92. Claire M. Midgley et al, "An in-Depth Analysis of Original Antigenic Sin in Dengue Virus Infection," *Journal of Virology* 85, no. 1 (2011): 410–21, https://www.ncbi.nlm. nih.gov/pmc/articles/PMC3014204/#!po=1.56250/.

93. U.S. FDA (@US_FDA), "You are not a horse . . . ," Twitter, August 21, 2021, 7:57 a.m., https://twitter.com/US_FDA/status/1429050070243192839.

94. Richard G. Frank, Leslie Dach, and Nicole Lurie, "It Was the Government That Produced COVID-19 Vaccine Success," *Health Affairs*, May 14, 2021, https://www.he althaffairs.org/do/10.1377/hblog20210512.191448/full/. The authors note that estimates of direct public spending on the development and manufacturing of Covid-19 vaccines vary from $18 billion and $39.5 billion. But the article leaves a crucial question unanswered: If the vaccines were an unmitigated "success," why would the government need to indemnify their manufacturers against lawsuits?

95. As the FDA explains, "An Emergency Use Authorization (EUA) is a mechanism to facilitate the availability and use of medical countermeasures, including vaccines, during public health emergencies, such as the current COVID-19 pandemic. Under an EUA, FDA may allow the use of unapproved medical products, or unapproved uses of approved medical products in an emergency to diagnose, treat, or prevent serious or life-threatening diseases or conditions when certain statutory criteria have been met, *including that there are no adequate, approved, and available alternatives*" [emphasis added]. "Emergency Use Authorization for Vaccines Explained," U.S. Food and Drug Administration, November 20, 2020, https://www.fda.gov/vaccines-blood-biologics /vaccines/emergency-use-authorization-vaccines-explained.

96. Other potentially useful treatments were attacked as well, such as a nasal spray developed by the leading U.S. manufacturer of xylitol-based products. See Alice

Giordano, "Feds Seek to Block Promotion of a Nasal Spray against COVID-19," *Epoch Times*, November 7, 2021, https://www.theepochtimes.com/mkt_morningbrief/feds -seek-to-block-promotion-of-a-nasal-spray-against-covid-19_4088366.html?utm_sour ce=Morningbrief&utm_medium=email&utm_campaign=mb-2021-11-08&mktids=3c 5eaec8ad7f65fdefca9f9b55b03803&est=UKwgQmFmdJMe8LPpcgUSoNFxgIvGp+RkY CYCgJdwV8OXi7oeprDR0KU=.

97. Maggie Fox and Jamie Gumbrecht, "Vaccine Protection against Covid-19 Wanes over Time, Especially for Older People, CDC Says," CNN, September 23, 2021, https:// www.cnn.com/2021/09/22/health/cdc-vaccine-advisers-booster-wane/index.html.

98. DonkeyHotey, "Anthony Stephen Fauci, aka Anthony Fauci, is an American physician and immunologist who has served as the director of the National Institute of Allergy and Infectious Diseases since 1984," Wikimedia Commons, https://upload .wikimedia.org/wikipedia/commons/0/08/Anthony_Fauci_-_Caricature_%28497410 46401%29.jpg, printed under a Creative Commons license: https://creativecommons .org/licenses/by/2.0/deed.en.

99. Myocarditis is a type of heart inflammation that, in serious cases, can lead to heart failure and death. A related condition, pericarditis, is similarly an inflammation, but of the pericardium, the membrane that surrounds the heart.

100. Gerhard Peters and John T. Woolley, "Donald J. Trump, Tweets of March 21, 2020 Online," American Presidency Project, March 21, 2020, https://www.presidency .ucsb.edu/documents/tweets-march-21-2020.

101. Tamara Keith and Malaka Gharib, "A Timeline of Coronavirus Comments from President Trump and WHO," NPR, April 15, 2020, https://www.npr.org/sections/goat sandsoda/2020/04/15/835011346/a-timeline-of-coronavirus-comments-from-preside nt-trump-and-who.

102. John Bacon and Jorge L. Ortiz, "Coronavirus Live Updates: Medical Aid for 3 States as US Death Tolls Hits 417; Stimulus, Checks Hit Snag; Utah Rep. Ben McAdams Hospitalized," *USA Today*, March 22, 2020, https://www.usatoday.com/story/news /health/2020/03/22/coronavirus-updates-us-state-lockdowns-stimulus-package-cong ress-pence/2877552001/.

103. Prabhash K. Dutta, "Remember Donald Trump–Touted Hydroxychloroquine? Study in India Backs It as Covid-19 Cure," *India Today*, June 7, 2021, https://www.indiatod ay.in/coronavirus-outbreak/story/remember-donald-trump-touted-hydroxychloroqu ine-study-india-backs-as-covid-19-cure-1811892-2021-06-07.

104. The National Institute of Allergy and Infectious Diseases (NIAID) budget for FY2020 was $5.89 billion. See "Budget Appropriation for Fiscal Year 2020," National Institute of Allergy and Infectious Diseases, https://www.niaid.nih.gov/grants-contracts/bud get-appropriation-fiscal-year-2020. Some of that money went to fund dangerous gain- of-function research in China. Newt Gingrich, "It's Time for Dr. Fauci to Retire,"

Newsweek, August 2, 2021, https://www.newsweek.com/its-time-dr-fauci-retire-opinion-1614824.

105. "Coronavirus (COVID-19) Update: FDA Revokes Emergency Use Authorization for Chloroquine and Hydroxychloroquine" [news release], U.S. Food and Drug Administration, June 15, 2020, https://www.fda.gov/news-events/press-announcements/coronavirus-covid-19-update-fda-revokes-emergency-use-authorization-chloroquine-and.

106. Julia Taliesin, "'Don't Do It': Dr. Fauci Warns against Using Ivermectin to Treat or Prevent COVID-19," *Boston Globe*, August 29, 2021, https://www.boston.com/news/coronavirus/2021/08/29/ivermectin-warnings-anthony-fauci-megan-ranney-fda/. In an interview with Jake Tapper referenced in the article, the CNN host called ivermectim a "horse-dewormer," and Fauci did not object.

107. U.S. FDA (@US_FDA), "You are not a horse."

108. "Rapid Increase in Ivermectin Prescriptions and Reports of Severe Illness Associated with Use of Products Containing Ivermectin to Prevent or Treat COVID-19," Centers for Disease Control and Prevention, August 26, 2021, https://stacks.cdc.gov/view/cdc/109271.

109. Taliesin, "Don't Do It."

110. "The Nobel Prize in Physiology or Medicine 2015: Press Release," Nobel Prize, October 5, 2015, https://www.nobelprize.org/prizes/medicine/2015/press-release/.

111. Maulshree Seth, "Uttar Pradesh Government Says Early Use of Ivermectin Helped to Keep Positivity, Deaths Low," *Indian Express*, May 12, 2021, https://indianexpress.com/article/cities/lucknow/uttar-pradesh-government-says-ivermectin-helped-to-keep-deaths-low-7311786/.

112. Mordechai Sones, "5-Fold Increase in Sudden Cardiac and Unexplained Deaths among FIFA Athletes in 2021," America's Frontline Doctors, https://americasfrontlinedoctors.org/2/frontlinenews/500-increase-in-sudden-cardiac-and-unexplained-deaths-among-fifa-athletes-in-2021/.

113. Emily Anthes and Noah Weiland, "Heart Problems More Common after Vaccination than after Covid-19, Study Finds," *New York Times*, August 25, 2021, https://www.nytimes.com/2021/08/25/health/covid-myocarditis-vaccine.html.

114. Matthew Oster et al., "Myocarditis Cases Reported after mRNA-Based COVID-19 Vaccination in the US From December 2020 to August 2021," *Journal of the American Medical Association* 327, no. 4 (2022): 331–40, doi:10.1001/jama.2021.24110.

115. Public Health Agency of Sweden, "Covid-19 in Schoolchildren"; also see the Swedish researchers' summary of the report in the *New England Journal of Medicine*: J. F. Ludvigsson et al., "Open Schools, Covid-19, and Child and Teacher Morbidity in Sweden," *New England Journal of Medicine* 384, no. 7 (February 18, 2021): 669–71, https://www.nejm.org/doi/full/10.1056/NEJMc2026670.

116. Eugyppius, "More on Original Antigenic Sin and the Folly of Our Universal Vaccination Campaign," Eugyppius: A Plague Chronicle (Substack), October 26, 2021, https://eugyppius.substack.com/p/more-on-original-antigenic-sin-and?utm_source=substack&utm_campaign=post_embed&utm_medium=web.

117. "8 Things Health Experts Want You to Know about the Delta Variant," UC Davis Health, July 22, 2021, https://health.ucdavis.edu/coronavirus/news/headlines/8-things-health-experts-want-you-to-know-about-the-delta-variant/2021/07.

118. David Leonhardt, "Omicron Is Milder," *New York Times*, January 5, 2022, https://www.nytimes.com/2022/01/05/briefing/omicron-risk-milder-pandemic.html.

119. Vimal Patel, "How Omicron, the New Covid-19 Variant, Got Its Name," *New York Times*, November 27, 2021, https://www.nytimes.com/2021/11/27/world/africa/omicron-covid-greek-alphabet.html.

120. Martin Kulldorff and Jay Bhattacharya, "How Fauci Fooled America," *Newsweek*, November 1, 2021, https://www.newsweek.com/how-fauci-fooled-america-opinion-1643839.

121. Alex Berenson, "Vaccinated English Adults under 60 Are Dying at Twice the Rate of Unvaccinated People the Same Age," Unreported Truths (Substack), November 20, 2021, https://alexberenson.substack.com/p/vaccinated-english-adults-under-60.

122. Jonathan Rothwell and Sonal Desai, "How Misinformation Is Distorting COVID Policies and Behaviors," Brookings, December 22, 2020, https://www.brookings.edu/research/how-misinformation-is-distorting-covid-policies-and-behaviors/. Those surveyed also grossly overestimated the risk that the China Virus posed to those under sixty-five, and particularly to children and young adults.

123. David Zweig, "Our Most Reliable Pandemic Number Is Losing Meaning," *The Atlantic*, September 13, 2021, https://www.theatlantic.com/health/archive/2021/09/covid-hospitalization-numbers-can-be-misleading/620062/. Zweig noted a recent study showing "that roughly half of all the hospitalized patients showing up on COVID-data dashboards in 2021 may have been admitted for another reason entirely, or had only a mild presentation of disease."

124. Amanda Henwood and Paul Dolan, "Part Four—the Effects of Fear at a Time of Crisis," Collateral Global, June 1, 2021, https://collateralglobal.org/article/the-effects-of-fear-at-a-time-of-crisis/.

125. Debanjan Banerjee et al., "Biopsychosocial Intersections of Social/Affective Touch and Psychiatry: Implications of 'Touch Hunger' during COVID-19," *International Journal of Social Psychiatry* (2021): 1–15, https://journals.sagepub.com/doi/pdf/10.1177/0020764021997485. The authors concluded, "Human touch is essential for both short-term and long-term neuropsychological well-being and mental health. This is particularly critical during stress and period of elevated anxiety, as is happening because of the COVID-19 pandemic mandated social distancing. Human touch is also

important for our ability to recover from illnesses." Like many articles critical of the pandemic response, it has since been retracted by the authors. The forces of conformity were powerful.

126. By, for example, Hollywood has-been Robert de Niro on BBC in mid-May of 2020. Felix Allen, "Trump-Hater Robert De Niro Rants about 'Lunatic' President Who Doesn't Care 'How Many People Die from Coronavirus,'" *U.S. Sun*, May 13, 2020, https://www.the-sun.com/news/822338/robert-de-niro-rant-trump-lunatic-coronavirus/.

127. Alux, "15 Reasons Why the Biggest Wealth Transfer in History Is Happening Right Now," YouTube, November 15, 2020, https://youtu.be/ggIp2k1Z8Mg.

128. Gary Chapman, *The 5 Love Languages: The Secret to Love that Lasts* (Chicago: Northfield Publishing, 2015), 22.

129. Jon Miltimore and Dan Sanchez, "America's Small Business Owners Have Been Horribly Abused during These Riots and Lockdowns. That Will Have Consequences," Foundation for Economic Education, June 5, 2020, https://fee.org/articles/america-s-small-business-owners-have-been-horribly-abused-during-these-riots-and-lockdowns-that-will-have-consequences/.

130. The original article from the *Global Times* has been sent down the memory hole by CCP censors, but I quoted it in my article, "Did China's Leaders Deliberately 'Seed' Coronavirus around the World?," LifeSiteNews, April 20, 2020, https://www.lifesitenews.com/blogs/did-chinas-leaders-deliberately-seed-coronavirus-around-the-world/.

131. Mark Zuckerberg's metaverse follows naturally from the current lockdowns. He presumably sees a business opportunity in locking the minds of millions of impressionable young people, already suffering from social isolation, inside an alternate reality forever. Some of those who are freed from Covid lockdowns will undoubtedly refuse to leave their "cells," preferring to voluntarily imprison themselves in a comforting mirage rather than confront what they now perceive as the terrors of the real world.

132. Alex Berenson, *Pandemia: How Coronavirus Hysteria Took Over Our Government, Rights, and Lives* (Washington, D.C: Regnery, 2021), 156.

Chapter 10: Made in China: Thanks, Bat Lady (and Thank Your American Colleagues)

1. Ian Birrell, "China's FIRST Virus Cover-Up: Damning Research Reveals Beijing's Response to SARS Two Decades Ago Created the Template for Its Outrageous Deception over Covid, Writes Ian Birrell," *Daily Mail*, July 24, 2021, https://www.dailymail.co.uk/news/article-9821629/Research-reveals-Beijings-response-SARS-created-template-Covid-deception-writes-IAN-BIRRELL.html.

2. "WHO Finds No Evidence of Airborne Spread of SARS," Center for Infectious Disease Research and Policy, October 20, 2003, https://www.cidrap.umn.edu/news-perspec tive/2003/10/who-finds-no-evidence-airborne-spread-sars.

3. Moira Chan-Yeung and Rui-Heng Xu, "SARS: Epidemiology," *Respirology* 8, supplement 1 (2003): S9–S14, doi: 10.1046/j.1440-1843.2003.00518.x.

4. Tom Pyman and Mark Nicol, "China Was Preparing for a Third World War with Biological Weapons—including Coronavirus—Six Years Ago, according to Dossier Produced by the People's Liberation Army in 2015 and Uncovered by the US State Department," *Daily Mail*, May 8, 2021, https://www.dailymail.co.uk/news/article-95 56415/China-preparing-WW3-biological-weapons-six-years-investigators-say.html.

5. Sharon Lerner and Mara Hvistendahl, "NIH Officials Worked with EcoHealth Alliance to Evade Restrictions on Coronavirus Experiments," The Intercept, November 3, 2021, https://theintercept.com/2021/11/03/coronavirus-research-ecohea lth-nih-emails/; Paul D. Thacker, "Covid-19: Lancet Investigation into Origin of Pandemic Shuts Down over Bias Risk," *British Medical Journal*, October 1, 2021, https://www.bmj.com/content/375/bmj.n2414; Christopher White, "New Emails Reveal Fauci's Communication with Researcher Tied to Wuhan Lab under Scrutiny," Fox 45 News, June 3, 2021, https://foxbaltimore.com/news/nation-world/new-emails -reveal-faucis-communication-with-researcher-tied-to-wuhan-lab-under-scrutiny.

6. Ning Wang et al., "Serological Evidence of Bat SARS-Related Coronavirus Infection in Humans, China," *Virologica Sinica* 33 (March 2, 2018): 104–7, https://link.springer .com/article/10.1007%2Fs12250-018-0012-7. Note that this article was coauthored by Peter Daszak and Zheng-Li Shi, and that the funding for the research came in part from grants from the National Institute of Allergy and Infectious Diseases of the National Institutes of Health (Award Number R01AI110964) to Peter Daszak and Zheng-Li Shi, and from a United States Agency for International Development (USAID) Emerging Pandemic Threats PREDICT project grant (Cooperative Agreement No. AID-OAA-A-14-00102) to Peter Daszak.

7. Zachary Stieber, "WHO Now Says China Never Reported CCP Virus Outbreak," *Epoch Times*, July 3, 2020, https://www.theepochtimes.com/who-now-says-china-ne ver-reported-ccp-virus-outbreak_3411173.html. The WHO originally claimed that CCP officials had informed it of the outbreak, repeatedly praising the Communist authorities for their supposed transparency. See "Covid-19: China," World Health Organization, January 5, 2020, https://www.who.int/emergencies/disease-outbreak -news/item/2020-DON229. A U.S. congressional investigation concluded that the WHO "enabled the CCP cover-up by failing to investigate and publicize reports conflicting with the official CCP line, while at the same time praising the CCP's response." See House Foreign Affairs Committee Minority Staff Interim Report, "The Origins of the Covid-19 Global Pandemic, Including the Roles of the Chinese

Communist Party and the World Health Organization," House Foreign Affairs Committee Minority Staff Interim Report, June 12, 2020, https://gop-foreignaffairs .house.gov/wp-content/uploads/2020/08/Interim-Minority-Report-on-the-Origins-of -the-COVID-19-Global-Pandemic-Including-the-Roles-of-the-CCP-and-WHO-8.17.20 .pdf.

8. See "Disease Outbreak News: Pneumonia of Unknown Cause—China," World Health Organization, January 5, 2020, https://www.who.int/emergencies/disease-outbreak -news/item/2020-DON229.

9. "WHO, China Leaders Discuss Next Steps in Battle against Coronavirus Outbreak," World Health Organization, January 28, 2020, https://www.who.int/news/item/28-01 -2020-who-china-leaders-discuss-next-steps-in-battle-against-coronavirus-outbreak.

10. Steven Mosher, "You Can Thank the Chinese Communist Party for the Coronavirus Epidemic," LifeSiteNews, January 30, 2020, https://www.lifesitenews.com/blogs/you -can-thank-the-chinese-communist-party-for-the-coronavirus-epidemic/.

11. "WHO-Convened Global Study of Origins of SARS-CoV-2: China Part," World Health Organization, March 30, 2021, https://www.who.int/publications/i/item/who-con vened-global-study-of-origins-of-sars-cov-2-china-part.

12. Steven Nelson, "WHO Report Blaming Animals—Not Lab—for COVID Met with Bipartisan Criticism," New York Post, March 29, 2021, https://nypost.com/2021/03/29 /who-report-blaming-animals-for-covid-19-met-with-criticism/.

13. Steven Mosher, "Don't Buy China's Story: The Coronavirus May Have Leaked from a Lab," New York Post, February 22, 2020, https://nypost.com/2020/02/22/dont-buy-ch inas-story-the-coronavirus-may-have-leaked-from-a-lab/. In the article, I cite specifically the new directive of the Chinese Ministry of Science and Technology. "确保生物安全！科技部要求加强对实验室特别是对病毒的管理,"[Guarantee Biological Safely: The Ministry of Science and Technology Demands Increased Oversight of Research Labs, Especially Those Dealing with Viruses], ScienceNet News (Chinese), February 15, 2020, http://news.sciencenet.cn/htmlnews/2020/2/435780.shtm.

14. Ibid.; Miranda Devine, "What Is China Covering Up about the Coronavirus?: Devine," New York Post, May 6, 2020, https://nypost.com/2020/05/06/what-is-china-covering -up-about-the-coronavirus-devine/.

15. Facebook "fact-checkers" didn't wait for the evidence. They quickly moved to suppress my column as "False Information" (without, of course, being able to specify exactly what about it was false). Facebook refused to unblock my article until April 17, 2020, two months later. The mainstream media piled on, too, slamming the New York Post for publishing the writings of a "conspiracy theorist." Others who raised questions about the pandemic's origins were heavily censored as well—or "canceled" entirely. See Sohrab Ahmari, "Facebook Lab-Leak Censors Owe the Post, and America, an Apology," New York Post, May 27, 2021, https://nypost.com/2021/05/27

/facebook-and-its-censorious-fact-checkers-have-utterly-discredited-themselves/;
and Olafimihan Oshin, "Twitter Bans Conservative Author Alex Berenson," *The Hill*,
August 29, 2021, https://thehill.com/homenews/media/569908-twitter-bans-con
servative-author-Alex-Berenson.

16. Ibid.

17. David Cyranoski, "Did Pangolins Spread the China Coronavirus to People?" *Nature
Medicine*, February 7, 2020, https://www.nature.com/articles/d41586-020-00364-2/.

18. Jonathan Latham and Allison K. Wilson, "The Hunt for the Origins of COVID—
Where It Led and Why It Matters," The Defender, August 20, 2021, https://childrenshe
althdefense.org/defender/chinese-international-searches-origins-covid-zoonotic-lab
-leak/.

19. Associated Press, "Hunt for Virus's Origins Hindered," *Journal Gazette*, December 31,
2020, https://www.journalgazette.net/news/world/20201231/hunt-for-viruss-origins
-hindered.

20. Dake Kang, Maria Cheng, and Sam McNeil, "China Clamps Down in Hidden Hunt for
Coronavirus Origins," AP News, December 30, 2020, https://apnews.com/article/unit
ed-nations-coronavirus-pandemic-china-only-on-ap-bats-24fbadc58cee3a40bca2ddf
7a14d2955. See also Bill Bostock, "China Is Guarding Ancient Bat Caves against
Journalists and Scientists Seeking to Discover the Origins of the Coronavirus,"
Business Insider, December 30, 2020, https://www.businessinsider.in/science/news
/china-is-guarding-ancient-bat-caves-against-journalists-and-scientists-seeking-to
-discover-the-origins-of-the-coronavirus/articleshow/80031366.cms.

21. Lisa Winter, "Chinese Officials Blame US Army for Coronavirus," *The Scientist*,
March 13, 2020, https://www.the-scientist.com/news-opinion/chinese-officials-bla
me-us-army-for-coronavirus-67267.

22. Matthew Brown, "Fact Check: Coronavirus Originated in China, Not Elsewhere,
Researchers and Studies Say," *USA Today*, March 16, 2020, https://www.usatoday
.com/story/news/factcheck/2020/03/16/coronavirus-fact-check-where-did-covid-19
-start-experts-say-china/5053783002/.

23. Monika Chansoria, "Is China Producing Biological Weapons? Look at Its Capabilities
and International Compliance," Japan Forward, March 5, 2020, https://japan-forward
.com/is-china-producing-biological-weapons-look-at-its-capabilities-and-intern
ational-compliance/.

24. As I will detail in the next chapter, Dr. David Asher, who led the State Department's
investigation into the origins of the coronavirus, was convinced that it was a product
of the PLA's bioweapons program. "Former State Department Official: Probe into
COVID Found Almost No Evidence Supporting Natural Origin," Fox News, May 27,
2021, https://video.foxnews.com/v/6256307843001#sp=show-clips.

25. Interview of Yan Li-Meng by the author, July 29, 2020. See also Tucker Carlson, "Tucker Carlson: Coronavirus Was Enhanced during 'Reckless, Ghoulish, Very Dangerous Experiments,'" Fox News, May 21, 2021, https://www.foxnews.com/opinion/tucker-carlson-coronavirus-enhanced-dangerous-experiments.

26. Sharri Markson, "US Paid Chinese People's Liberation Army to Engineer Coronaviruses," *The Australian*, June 4, 2021, https://www.theaustralian.com.au/science/us-paid-chinese-peoples-liberation-army-to-engineer-coronavirus/news-story/4adee56c1433fad332a76ffe043390ea. I detail the involvement of the Wuhan Institute of Virology with the PLA's bioweapons program in the next chapter.

27. Bruno Coutard et al., "The Spike Glycoprotein of the New Coronavirus 2019-nCoV Contains a Furin-Like Cleavage Site Absent in CoV of the Same Clade," *Antiviral Research* 176 (2020): 104742, doi: 10.1016/j.antiviral.2020.104742. Aside from the supercharged site found by Coutard and his team, Steven Quay and Richard Muller also note, "There is additional scientific evidence that points to CoV-2's gain-of-function origin. The most compelling is the dramatic differences in the genetic diversity of CoV-2, compared with the coronaviruses responsible for SARS and MERS." See Steven Quay and Richard Muller, "The Science Suggests a Wuhan Lab Leak," *Wall Street Journal*, June 6, 2021, https://www.wsj.com/articles/the-science-suggests-a-wuhan-lab-leak-11622995184.

28. Steven Mosher, "Here's All the Proof Biden Needs to Conclude COVID-19 Was Leaked from a Lab," *New York Post*, July 24, 2021, https://nypost.com/2021/07/24/heres-all-the-proof-biden-needs-to-conclude-covid-19-was-leaked-from-a-lab/.

29. Interview of Yan Li-Meng by the author.

30. Li-Meng Yan, Shu Kang, and Shanchang Hu, "Unusual Features of the SARS-CoV-2 Genome Suggesting Sophisticated Laboratory Modification Rather than Natural Evolution and Delineation of Its Probable Synthetic Route," ResearchGate, September 14, 2020, https://www.researchgate.net/profile/Limeng-Yan/publication/344240007.

31. Aksel Fridstrøm, "The Evidence Which Suggests That This Is No Naturally Evolved Virus," *Minerva*, July 2020, https://www.minervanett.no/angus-dalgleish-birger-sorensen-coronavirus/the-evidence-which-suggests-that-this-is-no-naturally-evolved-virus/362529.

32. Interview of Nikolai Petrokvsy by the author, August 4, 2020.

33. Bernardo Cervellera, "Prof Tritto: COVID-19 Was Created in the Wuhan Laboratory and Is Now in the Hands of the Chinese Military," Asia News, August 4, 2020, http://www.asianews.it/news-en/Prof-Tritto:-COVID-19-was-created-in-the-Wuhan-laboratory-and-is-now-in-the-hands-of-the-Chinese-military-50719.html. See my summary of Professor Tritto's book at Steven Mosher, "Renowned European Scientist: COVID-19 Was Engineered in China Lab, Effective Vaccine 'Unlikely,'" LifeSiteNews, August

10, 2020, https://www.lifesitenews.com/blogs/renowned-european-scientist-covid-19-was-engineered-in-china-lab-effective-vaccine-unlikely/.

34. Leslie Eastman, "Report: China Destroyed Evidence of Wuhan Coronavirus in December," Legal Insurrection, March 19, 2020, https://legalinsurrection.com/2020/03/report-china-destroyed-evidence-of-wuhan-coronavirus-in-december/.

35. Sharri Markson, "US Paid Chinese People's Liberation Army to Engineer Coronaviruses," *The Australian*, June 4, 2021, https://www.theaustralian.com.au/science/us-paid-chinese-peoples-liberation-army-to-engineer-coronavirus/news-story/4adee56c1433fad332a76ffe043390ea. Markson reports that "American money was funding risky research on coronaviruses with People's Liberation Army scientists—including decorated military scientist Zhou Yusen and the Wuhan Institute of Virology's 'Bat Woman,' Shi Zhengli. . . . National security sources said the ties between Zhou and Dr Shi supported claims by US intelligence that the Wuhan Institute of Virology was engaged in 'secret military activity.'" See also Adam Shaw, "Pompeo Says Wuhan Lab Was Engaged in Military Activity alongside Civilian Research," Fox News, May 29, 2021, https://www.foxnews.com/politics/pompeo-wuhan-lab-military-activity-alongside-civilian-research.

36. Steven Mosher, "Did China's Leaders Deliberately 'Seed' Coronavirus around the World?," LifeSiteNews, April 20, 2020, https://www.lifesitenews.com/blogs/did-chinas-leaders-deliberately-seed-coronavirus-around-the-world/.

37. Gianluca Veneziani, "Coronavirus, il professor Joseph Tritto: 'Nato in laboratorio. Tracce di Hiv nel genoma, perché è la prova definitive,'" *Libero Quotidiano*, July 27, 2020, https://www.sabinopaciolla.com/cina-covid-19-la-chimera-che-ha-cambiato-il-mondo/.

38. Steven Mosher, "Was the Coronavirus Created by Chinese Scientists?"

39. Nectar Gan, Caitlin Hu, and Ivan Watson, "Beijing Tightens Grip over Coronavirus Research, amid US-China Row on Virus Origin," CNN, April 16, 2020, https://www.cnn.com/2020/04/12/asia/china-coronavirus-research-restrictions-intl-hnk/index.html.

40. Mosher, "Was the Coronavirus Created by Chinese Scientists?"

41. Interview of Jonathan Latham by the author, August 6, 2020. See also Jonathan Latham and Allison Wilson, "A Proposed Origin for SARS-CoV-2 and the COVID-19 Pandemic," Independent Science News, July 15, 2020, https://www.independentsciencenews.org/commentaries/a-proposed-origin-for-sars-cov-2-and-the-covid-19-pandemic/.

42. Dr. Yan convincingly rebutted Latham and Ebright, pointing out that the arguments of both are based on the belated and unconvincing claim by Dr. Shi Zhengli that way back in 2013 she had "found a close relative to the China Virus in nature." Steven Mosher, "Chinese Scientist Who Defected to US: COVID-19 Not from Nature but

Created in Lab," LifeSiteNews, September 15, 2020, https://www.lifesitenews.com/bl ogs/chinese-scientist-who-defected-to-us-covid-19-not-from-nature-but-created-in -lab/.

43. "RaTG13—the Undeniable Evidence That the Wuhan Coronavirus Is Man-Made," *Nerd Has Power* (blog), May 2, 2020, https://nerdhaspower.weebly.com/ratg13-is-fake .html.

44. Lawrence Sellin, "Is China Lying about the Science of COVID-19?," WION, May 6, 2020, https://www.wionews.com/opinions-blogs/is-china-lying-about-the-science-of -covid-19-297002.

45. Mosher, "Was the Coronavirus Created by Chinese Scientists?"

46. Shi Zhengli's Wuhan Institute of Virology bio reads: Title: Principal Investigator E-mail: zlshi@wh.iov.cn **Education** 1987, B.S. Genetics, Department of Biology, Wuhan University 1990 M.Sc. Virology, Wuhan Institute of Virology, Chinese Academy of Sciences 2000, Ph.D. Virology, University Montpellier II **Research Interests** For more than a decade, Prof. Shi has been working on epidemiology and interspecies mechanism of emerging viruses of wildlife origin, especially bats and rodents. She has gained rich research experiences in discovery and characterization of viruses from bats. In the past twelve years, her research group has discovered a wild range of novel viruses or viral antibodies in bats, included coronaviruses, adenoviruses, orthoreoviruses, circoviruses, paramyxoviruses, filoviruses, hepatitis viruses, etc. Her group has highlighted findings on the animal origin of SARS-CoV. Their long-term surveillance of SARS-like coronaviruses in bat populations in China led to the new recognition of genetically diverse SARS-like coronaviruses, including strains not only sharing very high sequence similarity to SARS-CoV but also able to use the human ACE2 as an entry receptor. Their findings provide unequivocal evidence that bats are natural reservoir of SARS-CoV and reveal the origin of pandemic SARS-CoV from these bat CoVs. "Zhengli Shi," Wuhan Institute of Virology, http://www.whiov.cas.cn/sourcedb_whiov_cas/yw/rck/200907/t20090718 _2100074.html. Rather remarkably, under the circumstances, she is still listed as a member of the American Society of Microbiology as of February 22, 2022. See "Zhengli Shi, Ph.D.," American Society for Microbiology, https://asm.org/Biographi es/Zhengli-Shi,-Ph-D.

47. Xing-Yi Ge et al., "Isolation and Characterization of a Bat SARS-like Coronavirus That Uses the ACE2 Receptor," *Nature Medicine*, October 30, 2013, https://www.natu re.com/articles/nature12711.

48. Ibid.; Katherine Eban, "The Lab-Leak Theory: Inside the Fight to Uncover COVID-19's Origins," *Vanity Fair*, June 3, 2021, https://www.vanityfair.com/news/2021/06/the -lab-leak-theory-inside-the-fight-to-uncover-covid-19s-origins. Shi Zhengli was well compensated for her collaboration with Peter Daszak and EcoHealth Alliance. On her

resume, Shi mentions receiving grant funding from U.S. government sources totaling more than $1.2 million, including $665,000 from the National Institutes of Health from 2014 to 2019, as well as $559,500 over the same period from the U.S. Agency for International Development. And as the Wuhan Institute of Virology proudly noted on August 3, 2019, "Prof. Shi Zhengli elected a fellow of the American Academy of Microbiology," http://english.whiov.cas.cn/ne/201903/t20190308_206697 .html.

49. Wuze Ren et al., "Difference in Receptor Usage between Severe Acute Respiratory Syndrome (SARS) Coronavirus and SARS-Like Coronavirus of Bat Origin," *Journal of Virology* 82, no. 4 (December 22, 2020), https://doi.org/10.1128/JVI.01085-07.

50. Cockrell et al., "Efficient Reverse Genetic Systems for Rapid Genetic Manipulation of Emergent and Preemergent Infectious Coronaviruses," Springer Link, May 16, 2017, https://link.springer.com/protocol/10.1007/978-1-4939-6964-7_5; Savio Rodrigues, "Covid-19 Secret Is with Baric, Daszak and Zhengli," Sunday Guardian Live, September 11, 2021, https://www.sundayguardianlive.com/news/covid-19-secret-ba ric-daszak-zhengli.

51. Steven Carl Quay, "A Bayesian Analysis Concludes beyond a Reasonable Doubt that SARS-CoV-2 Is Not a Natural Zoonosis but Instead Is Laboratory Derived (Version 3)," Zenodo, March 29, 2021, https://zenodo.org/record/4642956.

52. Adam S. Cockrell et al., "Efficient Reverse Genetic Systems."

53. Steven Mosher, "How COVID-19 May Have Been Deliberately Engineered in a China Biolab," LifeSiteNews, April 22, 2020, https://www.lifesitenews.com/blogs/ how-co vid-19-may-have-been-deliberately-engineered-in-a-china-biolab/.

54. Anjeanette Roberts et al., "A Mouse-Adapted SARS-Coronavirus Causes Disease and Mortality in BALB/c Mice," *PLOS Pathogens*, January 12, 2007, https://journals.plos .org/plospathogens/article?id=10.1371/journal.ppat.0030005.

55. Adam S. Cockrell et al., "Efficient Reverse Genetic Systems for Rapid Genetic Manipulation of Emergent and Preemergent Infectious Coronaviruses," National Center for Biotechnology Information, May 16, 2017, https://www.ncbi.nlm.nih.gov /pmc/articles/PMC7120940/.

56. Vineet D. Menachery et al., "A SARS-like Cluster of Circulating Bat Coronaviruses Shows Potential for Human Emergence," *Nature Medicine* 21 (November 9, 2015): 1508–13, https://www.nature.com/articles/nm.3985. Two notes were appended to this study after it was first published. The first disclosed that there was funding flowing from Peter Daszak's EcoHealth Alliance to Shi Zheng-Li and her lab as early as 2015. The second is an "Editor's Note" dated March 2020, which reads, "We are aware that this article is being used as the basis for unverified theories that the novel coronavirus causing COVID-19 was engineered. There is no evidence that this is true; scientists believe that an animal is the most likely source of the coronavirus." Since

the article describes the *exact procedure* that was later followed in Dr. Shi's lab to create a dangerous coronavirus capable of infecting human beings, *Nature Medicine*'s attempt to deny the obvious is an abandonment not only of science but of reason.

57. *U.S. Government Gain-of-Function Deliberative Process and Research Funding Pause on Selected Gain-of-Function Research Involving Influenza, MERS, and SARS Viruses*, Department of Health and Human Services, October 17, 2014, https://www .phe.gov/s3/dualuse/Documents/gain-of-function.pdf. The White House justified the pause as a response to "recent biosafety incidents." See "Doing Diligence to Assess the Risks and Benefits of Life Sciences Gain-of-Function Research," White House, October 17, 2014, https://obamawhitehouse.archives.gov/blog/2014/10/17/doing-dilig ence-assess-risks-and-benefits-life-sciences-gain-function-research.

58. The quotation is from *U.S. Government Gain-of-Function Deliberative Process.*

59. Francis S. Collins, "NIH Lifts Funding Pause on Gain-of-Function Research," National Institutes of Health, December 19, 2017, https://www.nih.gov/about-nih/who-we-are/nih-director/sta tements/nih-lifts-funding-pause-gain-function-research.

60. "Dr. Fauci and CDC Director Walensky Testify on Efforts to Combat COVID-19," C-SPAN, May 11, 2021, https://www.c-span.org/video/?511511-1/dr-fauci-cdc-director-walensky-testify-efforts -combat-covid-19.

61. Guy Reschenthaler and Anthony Bellotti, "The Time for Transparency about COVID-19 Origins Is Now," *Newsweek*, January 14, 2022, https://www.newsweek.com/time-transparency-about-co vid-19-origins-now-opinion-1668785.

62. Matthew Cullinan Hoffman, "Did Anthony Fauci's Promotion of Dangerous Research Help Create the COVID-19 Pandemic?," LifeSiteNews, June 15, 2020, https://www.lifesitenews.com/ne ws/did-anthony-faucis-promotion-of-dangerous-research-help-create-the-covid-19-pan demic/. Daszak had a very close working relationship with Shi. See Keoni Everington, "WHO Inspector Caught on Camera Revealing Coronavirus Manipulation in Wuhan before Pandemic," *Taiwan News*, January 18, 2021, https://www.taiwannews.com.tw/en/news/4104828.

63. Charles Creitz, "New House GOP Wuhan Lab Report Discredits Facebook 'Fact Checkers' That Censored Covid Origin Claims," Fox Business, May 24, 2020, https://www.foxbusiness.com /media/coronavirus-origin-wuhan-lab-gop-report-facebook-fact-check.

64. Peter Daszak (@PeterDaszak), "Not true—we've made great progress with bat SARS-related CoVs . . . ," Twitter, November 21, 2019, 4:42 p.m., https://twitter.com/peterdaszak/status/1197631383 470034951?lang=en.

65. Matthew Cullinan Hoffman, "Did Anthony Fauci's Promotion of Dangerous Research Help Create the COVID-19 Pandemic?," LifeSiteNews, June 15, 2020, https://www.lifesitenews.com/ne ws/did-anthony-faucis-promotion-of-dangerous-research-help-create-the-covid-19-pan demic/. Daszak's involvement with the Wuhan lab is ably summarized in Bruce Golding, "Who Is Peter Daszak, the Nonprofit Exec Who Sent Taxpayer Money to Wuhan Lab?," *New York Post*,

June 4, 2021, https://nypost.com/2021/06/04/who-is-peter-daszak-exec-who-sent-taxpayer-money
-to-wuhan-lab/.

66. Charles Callisher et al., "Statement in Support of the Scientists, Public Health Professionals, and Medical Professionals of China Combatting COVID-19," *The Lancet* 395, no. 10226 (March 7, 2020), https://www.thelancet.com/journals/lancet/article/PIIS0140-6736(20)30418-9/fulltext.

67. Kristian G. Andersen et al, "The Proximal Origins of SARS-CoV-19," *Nature Medicine* 26 (April 2020): 450–52, https://www.nature.com/articles/s41591-020-0820-9.

68. James Gorman and Julian E. Barnes, "The C.D.C.'s Ex-Director Offers No Evidence in Favoring Speculation That the Coronavirus Originated in a Lab," *New York Times*, March 29, 2021, https:// www.nytimes.com/2021/03/26/science/redfield-coronavirus-wuhan-lab.html; Adam Taylor, "Experts Debunk Fringe Theory Linking China's Coronavirus to Weapons Research," *Washington Post*, January 29, 2020, https://www.washingtonpost.com/world/2020/01/29/experts-debunk-frin ge-theory-linking-chinas-coronavirus-weapons-research/.

69. Rich Lowry, "Media, 'Experts' Utterly Discredited Themselves by Suppressing the Lab-Leak Theory," *New York Post*, May 25, 2021, https://nypost.com/2021/05/25/media-experts-utterly-disc redited-themselves-by-suppressing-the-lab-leak-theory/.

70. Jesse D. Bloom et al., "Investigate the Origins of COVID-19," *Science* 372, no. 6543 (May 14, 2021), 694, https://www.science.org/doi/10.1126/science.abj0016.

71. Cristiano Lima, "Facebook No Longer Treating 'Man-Made' Covid as a Crackpot Idea," *Politico*, May 26, 2021, https://www.politico.com/news/2021/05/26/facebook-ban-covid-man-made-49 1053.

72. Mark Moore, "Fauci 'Not Convinced' COVID Developed Naturally, Backs Investigation," *New York Post*, May 23, 2021, https://nypost.com/2021/05/23/fauci-not-convinced-covid-19-developed -naturally/.

73. Chris Jewers, "Revealed: 26 out of the 27 Lancet Scientists Who Trashed Theory that Covid Leaked from a Chinese Lab Have Links to Wuhan Researchers," *Daily Mail*, September 11, 2021, https://www.dailymail.co.uk/news/article-9980015/26-Lancet-scientists-trashed-theory-Covid-le aked-Chinese-lab-links-Wuhan.html.

74. Jacques van Helden et al., "An Appeal for an Objective, Open, and Transparent Scientific Debate about the Origin of SARS-CoV-2," *The Lancet* 398, no. 10309 (October 16, 2021), https://www.the lancet.com/journals/lancet/article/PIIS0140-6736(21)02019-5/fulltext.

75. "TWiV 615: Peter Daszak of EcoHealth Alliance," This Week in Virology, May 19, 2020, https:// www.microbe.tv/twiv/twiv-615/. A partial transcript can be found at Everington, "WHO Inspector Caught on Camera Revealing Coronavirus Manipulation." See also Tucker Carlson, "Tucker Carlson: Anthony Fauci Let the Coronavirus Pandemic Happen, Why Isn't There a Criminal Investigation?," Fox News, May 11, 2021, https://www.foxnews.com/opinion/tucker-carl son-anthony-fauci-let-the-coronavirus-pandemic-happen-why-isnt-there-a-criminal-investi gation.

76. Peter Daszak (@PeterDaszak), "Not true. . . ."

77. Daszak's naivety where China is concerned comes through in statements such as this: "It's all collaborative science. People love to interact in collaborative science. What I've found is, especially in places like China, where increasingly there's a paranoia about collaboration, science collaboration is open and transparent because of the nature of what you are trying to do. You are trying to discover stuff quickly, understand what it means, and publish it in a high-impact journal. And that drives openness and transparency. That's been great for us around the world, it's also great for the U.S." ("TWiV 615: Peter Daszak.") That quotation didn't age well.

78. Sharon Lerner, Mara Hvistendahl, and Maia Hibbett, "NIH Documents Provide New Evidence U.S. Funded Gain-of-Function Research in Wuhan," The Intercept, September 10, 2021, https://theintercept.com/2021/09/09/covid-origins-gain-of-function-research/.

79. Ibid.

80. Ibid.

Chapter 11: Bio War Games: How the Chinese People's Liberation Army Released a Bioweapon on the World

1. "Military-Civil Fusion and the People's Republic of China," U.S. State Department, May 2020, https://www.state.gov/wp-content/uploads/2020/05/What-is-MCF-One-Pager.pdf.

2. Keoni Everington, "PLA Experimented in Wuhan Lab, Covered Up Outbreak," Taiwan News, February 22, 2021, https://www.taiwannews.com.tw/en/news/4133486.

3. Peter Wade, "'Molecularly Impossible': Fauci Blasts Rand Paul for Covid Lab Theory," Rolling Stone, October 24, 2021, https://www.rollingstone.com/politics/politics-news/fauci-blasts-rand-paul-covid-lab-theory-1247137/.

4. Jocelyn Kaiser, "NIH Says Grantee Failed to Report Experiment in Wuhan That Created a Bat Virus That Made Mice Sicker," Science, October 21, 2021, https://www.science.org/content/article/nih-says-grantee-failed-report-experiment-wuhan-created-bat-virus-made-mice-sicker.

5. "Transcript: Bioweapons Expert Dr. Francis Boyle on Coronavirus," Great Game India, February 5, 2020, https://greatgameindia.com/transcript-bioweapons-expert-dr-francis-boyle-on-coronavirus/. Boyle is a professor of international law at the University of Illinois College of Law. He drafted the U.S. domestic implementing legislation for the Biological Weapons Convention, known as the Biological Weapons Anti-Terrorism Act of 1989, which was approved unanimously by both Houses of the U.S. Congress and signed into law by President George H. W. Bush.

6. Li-Meng Yan, Shu Kang, and Shanchang Hu, "Unusual Features of the SARS-CoV-2 Genome Suggesting Sophisticated Laboratory Modification Rather than Natural

Evolution and Delineation of Its Probable Synthetic Route," Zenodo, September 14, 2020, https://zenodo.org/record/4028830#.YWw9MS-cZ5t.

7. Dr. Yan Li-Meng, personal communication to the author, July 29, 2020.

8. "More Reason to Think Beijing's to Blame for the Pandemic," *New York Post*, March 16, 2021, https://nypost.com/2021/03/16/more-reason-to-think-beijings-to-blame-for-the-pandemic/.

9. "Biological Weapons Convention," United Nations Office for Disarmament Affairs, https://www.un.org/disarmament/biological-weapons/.

10. David Asher and Miles Yu, "Transcript: The Origins of COVID-19: Policy Implications and Lessons for the Future," Hudson Institute, March 17, 2021, https://www.hudson.org/research/16762-transcript-the-origins-of-covid-19-policy-implications-and-lessons-for-the-future.

11. Mike Pompeo and Miles Yu, "China's Reckless Labs Put the World at Risk," *Wall Street Journal*, February 23, 2021, https://www.wsj.com/articles/chinas-reckless-labs-put-the-world-at-risk-11614102828.

12. Elsa B. Kania and Wilson VornDick, "Weaponizing Biotech: How China's Military Is Preparing for a 'New Domain of Warfare,'" Defense One, August 14, 2019, https://www.defenseone.com/ideas/2019/08/chinas-military-pursuing-biotech/159167/.

13. "Former State Department Official: Probe into COVID Found Almost No Evidence Supporting Natural Origin," Fox News, May 27, 2021, https://video.foxnews.com/v/6256307843001# sp = show-clips.

14. Kylie Atwood, "Pompeo-Led Effort to Hunt Down Covid Lab Theory Shut Down by Biden Administration over Concerns about Quality of Evidence," CNN, May 26, 2021, https://edition.cnn.com/2021/05/25/politics/biden-shut-down-trump-effort-coronavirus-chinese-lab/index.html.

15. Brooke Singman and Jennifer Griffin, "Biden State Department Quietly Ended Team's Work Probing COVID Origin," Fox News, May 26, 2021, https://www.foxnews.com /politics/biden-state-department-shut-down-team-covid-origin-investigation. See also Mark Lungariello, "Biden Team Shut Down State Dept. Inquiry Probing Possible Lab Link to COVID: Report," *New York Post*, May 25, 2021, https://nypost.com/2021/05/25/biden-team-shut-down-inquiry-to-prove-lab-link-to-covid-report/?utm_source=NYPTwitter&utm_campaign=SocialFlow&utm_medium=SocialFlow.

16. "Statement by President Joe Biden on the Investigation into the Origins of COVID-19," The White House, May 26, 2021, https://www.whitehouse.gov/briefing-room/statements-releases/2021/05/26/statement-by-president-joe-biden-on-the-investigation-into-the-origins-of-covid-19/.

17. "Biden's Intelligence Agencies Bow to Beijing and Claim They Can't Make a Conclusion on COVID," *New York Post*, August 25, 2021, https://nypost.com/2021/08/25/bidens-intelligence-agencies-bow-to-beijing-claim-no-conclusion-on-covid/.

18. Steven Nelson, "WH Doesn't Have 'Anything to Preview' on Getting COVID Answers from China," *New York Post*, August 25, 2021, https://nypost.com/2021/08/25/wh-doesnt-have-anything-to-preview-on-china-covid-transparency/.

19. Steven W. Mosher, "Here's All the Proof Biden Needs to Conclude COVID-19 Was Leaked from a Lab," *New York Post*, July 24, 2021, https://nypost.com/2021/07/24/heres-all-the-proof-biden-needs-to-conclude-covid-19-was-leaked-from-a-lab/.

20. "Transcript: Matt Pottinger on 'Face the Nation,'" CBS News, February 21, 2021, https://www.cbsnews.com/news/transcript-matt-pottinger-on-face-the-nation-february-21-2021/.

21. Everington, "PLA Experimented in Wuhan Lab."

22. Asher and Yu, "Transcript: The Origins of COVID-19."

23. "Documents Reveal Chinese Scientists Discussed Weaponising Coronavirus 5 Years before Pandemic," MSN, September 5, 2021, https://www.msn.com/en-in/news/world/documents-reveal-chinese-scientists-discussed-weaponising-coronavirus-in-2015/ar-BB1gxluD.

24. Riah Matthews, "Leaked Chinese Document Reveals a Sinister Plan to 'Unleash' Coronaviruses," News.com.au, May 8, 2021, https://www.news.com.au/world/coronavirus/leaked-chinese-document-reveals-a-sinister-plan-to-unleash-coronaviruses/news-story/53674e8108ad5a655e07e990daa85465. See also Tom Pyman and Mark Nicol, "China Was Preparing for a Third World War with Biological Weapons—including Coronavirus—Six Years Ago, according to Dossier Produced by the People's Liberation Army in 2015 and Uncovered by the US State Department," *Daily Mail*, May 8, 2021, https://www.dailymail.co.uk/news/article-9556415/China-preparing-WW3-biological-weapons-six-years-investigators-say.html.

25. Matthews, "Leaked Chinese Document Reveals."

26. Ibid.; Kania and VornDick, "Weaponizing Biotech."

27. Steven Mosher, "The Coronavirus Is a Bioweapon, China Expert Steven Mosher Argues," LifeSiteNews, April 6, 2021, https://www.lifesitenews.com/blogs/the-coronavirus-is-a-bioweapon-china-expert-steven-mosher-argues/.

28. Balamurali K. Ambati et al., "MSH3 Homology and Potential Recombination Link to SARS-CoV-2 Furin Cleavage Site," *Frontiers in Virology* (February 21, 2022), https://www.frontiersin.org/articles/10.3389/fviro.2022.834808/full.

29. Jennifer Griffin, "Former US investigator: COVID-19 May Have Come from Bioweapons Research Accident," *New York Post*, March 12, 2021, https://nypost.com/2021/03/12/former-us-investigator-covid-19-may-have-come-from-bioweapons-research-accident/.

30. Peter Wade, "'Molecularly Impossible': Fauci Blasts Rand Paul for Covid Lab Theory," *Rolling Stone*, October 24, 2021, https://www.rollingstone.com/politics/politics-news/fauci-blasts-rand-paul-covid-lab-theory-1247137/.

31. Mosher, "The Coronavirus Is a Bioweapon."

32. Sharon Lerner and Mara Hvistendahl, "NIH Officials Worked with EcoHealth Alliance to Evade Restrictions on Coronavirus Experiments," The Intercept, November 3, 2021, https://theintercept.com/2021/11/03/coronavirus-research-ecohealth-nih-emails/; Paul D. Thacker, "Covid-19: *Lancet* Investigation into Origin of Pandemic Shuts Down over Bias Risk," *British Medical Journal*, October 1, 2021, https://www.bmj.com/content/375/bmj.n2414; Christopher White, "New Emails Reveal Fauci's Communication with Researcher Tied to Wuhan Lab under Scrutiny," Fox 45 News, June 3, 2021, https://foxbaltimore.com/news/nation-world/new-emails-reveal-faucis-communication-with-researcher-tied-to-wuhan-lab-under-scrutiny.

33. Yan Li-Meng, Shu Kang, and Hu Shanchang, "SARS-CoV-2 Is an Unrestricted Bioweapon: A Truth Revealed through Uncovering a Large-Scale, Organized Scientific Fraud," Zenodo, October 2, 2020, https://zenodo.org/record/4073131#.Yf2xl_hOlPY.

34. "Lawrence C. Sellin, Ph.D." Rutgers Graduate School of Biomedical Sciences, 2006, http://gsbs.rutgers.edu/alumni/sellin2006.html. Lawrence Sellin earned his Ph.D. in physiology from the University of Medicine and Dentistry of New Jersey (now the Rutgers Graduate School of Biomedical Sciences), and Rutgers awarded Dr. Sellin its Distinguished Leadership Award in 2006. Dr. Sellin, who is also a retired U.S. Army colonel, spent much of 2020–2021 investigating the origins of the Covid virus, detailing the PLA's bioweapons program, and investigating the backgrounds of the PLA scientists involved. He was one of the first to point out that the China Virus contains a unique furin cleavage site on its spike protein.

35. Joe Hoft, "Exclusive: More Evidence Leaked from China on the Deliberate Release of COVID-19 by the Chinese Military," Gateway Pundit, July 23, 2021, https://www.thegatewaypundit.com/2021/07/report-deliberate-release-covid-19-chinese-military/.

36. Ibid.

37. "WHO SARS Risk Assessment and Preparedness Framework," World Health Organization, October 2004, https://www.who.int/csr/resources/publications/CDS_CSR_ARO_2004_2.pdf?ua=1. The WHO reported, "Since July 2003, there have been four occasions when SARS has reappeared. Three of these incidents were attributed to breaches in laboratory biosafety and resulted in one or more cases of SARS. . . . The most recent laboratory incident [in Beijing] resulted in 9 cases, 7 of which were associated with one chain of transmission and with hospital spread. Two additional cases at the same laboratory [in Beijing] with a history of illness compatible with SARS in February 2004 were detected as part of a serosurvey of contacts at the

facility." See also Robert Walgate, "SARS Escaped Beijing Lab Twice," *The Scientist*, April 24, 2004, https://www.the-scientist.com/news-analysis/sars-escaped-beijing-lab-twice-50137.

38. Dr. Yan Li-Meng, personal communication to the author, July 29, 2020.

39. "Fact Sheet: Activity at the Wuhan Institute of Virology," U.S. Department of State, January 15, 2021, https://2017-2021.state.gov/fact-sheet-activity-at-the-wuhan-institute-of-virology/index.html. See also Michael R. Gordon, Warren P. Strobel, and Drew Hinshaw, "Intelligence on Sick Staff at Wuhan Lab Fuels Debate on Covid-19 Origin," *Wall Street Journal*, May 23, 2021, https://www.wsj.com/articles/intelligence-on-sick-staff-at-wuhan-lab-fuels-debate-on-covid-19-origin-11621796228.

40. Atossa Therapeutics Inc. (Nasdaq: ATOS) is a clinical-stage biopharmaceutical company developing novel therapeutics for treating breast cancer and Covid-19. Dr. Quay is also the author of the bestselling book on surviving the pandemic, *Stay Safe: A Physician's Guide to Survive Coronavirus* (Seattle, Washington: Ensisheim Partners, 2020).

41. Steven Carl Quay, "A Bayesian Analysis Concludes beyond a Reasonable Doubt That SARS-CoV-2 Is Not a Natural Zoonosis but Instead Is Laboratory Derived," Zenodo, March 29, 2021, https://zenodo.org/record/4642956.

42. Steven Carl Quay et al., "Contamination or Vaccine Research? RNA Sequencing Data of Early COVID-19 Patient Samples Show Abnormal Presence of Vectorized H7N9 Hemagglutinin Segment," Zenodo, July 3, 2021, https://zenodo.org/record/5067706.

43. Zhuang Pinghui, "Coronavirus: WHO Backed China's Emergency Use of Experimental Vaccines, Health Official Says," *South China Morning Post*, September 26, 2020, https://www.scmp.com/news/china/society/article/3103121/coronavirus-who-backed-chinas-emergency-use-experimental.

44. Lawrence Sellin (@LawrenceSellin), "In 2017, Maj Gen Wei Chen[,] CCP's presumed biowarfare chief . . . ," Twitter, April 10, 2021, 6:09 a.m., https://twitter.com/lawrencesellin/status/1380825202137956355. The translation of the Chinese phrase is mine.

45. Ibid; Hoft, "Exclusive: More Evidence Leaked from China."

46. Charlie Coë and Levi Parsons, "Chinese Whistleblower Claims First COVID Outbreak Was Intentional and Happened in October 2019 at Military World Games in Wuhan—Two Months before China Notified the World about Virus," *Daily Mail*, September 21, 2021, https://www.dailymail.co.uk/news/article-10014895/Ex-Chinese-Communist-Party-insider-Wei-Jingsheng-speaks-Wuhan-theory-relating-Covid-19.html.

47. Sam Cooper, "The Virus Cover-up: How China Stockpiled the World's Supply of PPEs," Sunday Guardian, July 31, 2021, https://www.sundayguardianlive.com/news/virus-cover-china-stockpiled-worlds-supply-ppes.

48. Michael Houston, "More Athletes Claim They Contracted COVID-19 at Military World Games in Wuhan," Inside the Games, May 17, 2020, https://www.insidethegames.biz/articles/1094347/world-military-games-illness-covid-19.

49. Nectar Gan and Steve George, "China Doubles Down on Baseless 'US Origins' Covid Conspiracy as Delta Outbreak Worsens," CNN, August 6, 2021, https://www.cnn.com/2021/08/06/china/china-covid-origin-mic-intl-hnk/index.html. Gan and George wrote, "At a news conference last week, Chinese Foreign Ministry spokesman Zhao Lijian called for WHO to investigate both the Fort Detrick lab and a laboratory at the University of North Carolina, helmed by leading US coronavirus expert Ralph Baric. Zhao also suggested American military athletes who attended the World Military Games in Wuhan in October 2019 could have brought the coronavirus into China—reiterating a baseless claim he made on Twitter in March 2020."

50. Hoft, "Exclusive: More Evidence Leaked from China."

Conclusion: The Once and Future Bioweapon

1. See Steven Mosher, *A Mother's Ordeal: One Woman's Fight against China's One-Child Policy* (New York: HarperCollins, 1993), especially chapter 2, "Famine and Death."

2. Population density is a key factor in the spread of plagues. Chinese cities have been among the largest and most densely populated human settlements on the planet for thousands of years, and rural population densities were—and still are today—also quite high. "In simulated epidemics involving less dense rural communities, epidemics went extinct 94.5 to 99.6 percent of the time." Jonathan Pekar et al., "Timing the SARS-CoV-2 Index Case in Hubei Province," *Science* 372, no. 6540 (April 23, 2021): 412–17, https://www.science.org/doi/full/10.1126/science.abf8003.

3. Wan Lin, "China Passes First Biosafety Law following COVID-19 Epidemic, Raises Level to National Security," *Global Times*, October 18, 2020, https://www.globaltimes.cn/page/202010/1203840.shtml.

4. Bi Chunli, president of the Chinese Academy of the Sciences, had said earlier in 2021 that two new P4 labs and eighty-one new P3 labs were already in operation. Press Trust of India, "China to Build More Bio Labs amid Scrutiny over Wuhan Facility on Covid," NDTV, April 16, 2021, https://www.ndtv.com/world-news/china-to-build-more-bio-labs-amid-scrutiny-over-wuhan-facility-on-covid-2415488; Bruce Golding, "China Building More Facilities Similar to Suspected COVID Leak Lab, Book Claims," *New York Post*, July 12, 2021, https://nypost.com/2021/07/23/china-building-more-facilities-similar-to-suspected-covid-leak-lab-book-claims/.

5. Golding, "China Building More Facilities."

6. Dr. Yan Li-Meng, personal communication to the author, July 29, 2020.

7. Liu Caiyu, "New Law Fortifies China's Legal Shield on Biosecurity Labs against Future Infectious Diseases," *Global Times*, April 15, 2021, https://www.globaltimes.cn/page/202104/1221202.shtml.

8. "Military-Civil Fusion and the People's Republic of China," U.S. State Department, May 2020, https://www.state.gov/wp-content/uploads/2020/05/What-is-MCF-One-Pager.pdf; Elsa B. Kania and Wilson VornDick,"Weaponizing Biotech: How China's Military Is Preparing for a 'New Domain of Warfare," Defense One, August 14, 2019, https://www.defenseone.com/ideas/2019/08/chinas-military-pursuing-biotech/159167/; Adam Shaw, "Pompeo Says Wuhan Lab Was Engaged in Military Activity alongside Civilian research," Fox News, May 29, 2021, https://www.foxnews.com/politics/pompeo-wuhan-lab-military-activity-alongside-civilian-research.

9. Jasper Becker, "China's Mutant Monkeys: These Are Just Two of the Countless Animals Used in Secret Genetic Engineering Tests in Labs—Many with Appalling Biosecurity. No Wonder So Many Experts Say Covid Did Leak from Wuhan Research Center," *Daily Mail*, June 5, 2021, https://www.dailymail.co.uk/news/article-9655357/JASPER-BECKER-No-wonder-experts-say-Covid-DID-leak-Wuhan-research-centre.html.

10. Sabrina Tavernise, "A 'Zero Covid' Olympics," *The Daily* (*New York Times* podcast), February 4, 2022, https://www.nytimes.com/2022/02/04/podcasts/the-daily/a-zero-covid-olympics.html?.

11. Golding, "China Building More Facilities."

12. Daniel Case, "Empty paper towel shelves at Hannaford supermarket, Walden, NY, during coronavirus pandemic," Wikimedia Commons, March 13, 2020, https://commons.wikimedia.org/w/index.php?search=new+york+empty+shelves+2020&title=Special:MediaSearch&go=Go&type=image.

13. See, for example, Marlene Lenthang, "Texas Doctor Who Promoted Ivermectin Suspended by Hospital," NBC News, November 15, 2021, https://www.nbcnews.com/news/us-news/texas-doctor-touted-ivermectin-covid-treatment-suspended-rcna5588.

14. Jack Kelly, "In A Dramatic Turn, the Once-Heralded Nurses and Healthcare Workers Are Being Fired for Not Getting Their Vaccination Shots," *Forbes*, September 30, 2021, https://www.forbes.com/sites/jackkelly/2021/09/30/in-a-dramatic-turn-the-once-herald-nurses-and-healthcare-workers-are-being-fired-for-not-getting-their-vaccination-shots/?sh=3489609f2b62; Deon J. Hampton, "U.S. Vaccine Mandate on Freight Drivers Coming from Canada May Worsen Auto Supply Chain Shortage," NBC News, January 19, 2022, https://www.nbcnews.com/news/us-news/us-vaccine-mandate-freight-drivers-coming-canada-may-exacerbate-auto-s-rcna12649.

15. James Bovard, "COVID-Positive Nurses Are in Our Hospitals. But Biden's Mandate Forbids Unvaccinated Ones," *USA Today*, January 7, 2022, https://www.usatoday.com /story/opinion/2022/01/07/biden-vaccine-mandate-nurses/9093551002/?gnt-cfr=1.

16. Katelyn Caralle, "'The Experts Say We Know That This Virus Is, in Fact, Uh, Um, Uh, It's Going to Be, or Excuse Me': Biden Loses His Thoughts on Vaccines, Flubs Answer on His Foreign Policy Work and Falsely Tells Town Hall You Won't Get Covid If You Have the Shot," *Daily Mail*, July 22, 2021, https://www.dailymail.co.uk/news/article -9814723/Biden-flubs-answer-foreign-policy-work-falsely-says-WONT-COVID-shot .html.

17. Kaylee McGhee White, "Covid Vaccines Aren't Working the Way We Were Told They Would," *Washington Examiner*, December 27, 2021, https://www.washingtonexamin er.com/opinion/the-covid-vaccines-arent-working-the-way-we-were-told-they-would.

18. Eric Sykes, "CDC Director: Covid Vaccines Can't Prevent Transmission Anymore," KMOX News Radio St. Louis, January 10, 2022, https://www.msn.com/en-us/health /medical/cdc-director-covid-vaccines-cant-prevent-transmission-anymore/ar-AAS Dndg.

19. It would take a book, and the services of a professional statistician, to document all the ways in which the public health data from many countries that should be readily available has been rendered opaque, misinterpreted to suit the pandemic narrative, or obscured from public view entirely.

20. Apoorva Mandavilli, "The C.D.C. Isn't Publishing Large Portions of the Covid Data It Collects," *New York Times*, February 20, 2022, https://www.nytimes.com/2022/02/20 /health/covid-cdc-data.html.

21. Lauren Brownlie, "Covid Data Will Not Be Published over Concerns It's Misrepresented by Anti-Vaxxers," *Glasgow Times*, February 17, 2022, https://www.gl asgowtimes.co.uk/news/19931641.covid-data-will-not-published-concerns-misrepre sented-anti-vaxxers/.

22. Alex Berenson, "Data about the Vaccines Is Disappearing," Unreported Truths (Substack), February 17, 2022, https://alexberenson.substack.com/p/data-about-the -vaccines-is-disappearing/comments?r=x1alp.

23. See Alex Berenson, "Whistling Past the mRNA Graveyard," Unreported Truths (Substack), February 25, 2022, https://alexberenson.substack.com/p/whistling-past- the-mrna-vaccine-graveyard/comments?s=r.

24. "Breakdown of Science Funding in 2021 Appropriations Request," American Society for Microbiology, https://asm.org/Articles/Policy/2020/Breakdown-of-Science-Fun ding-in-the-President-s-20.

25. As I noted earlier, I was among those wrongly censored. My article for the *New York Post* on the lab origins of the China Virus was posted by the *Post* on its Facebook page. It was wrongly declared to be misinformation and taken down.

26. Chris Ka Pun Mok et al., "Comparison of the Immunogenicity of BNT162b2 and CoronaVac Covid-18 Vaccines in Hong Kong," *Respirology* (November 24, 2021), https://onlinelibrary.wiley.com/doi/10.1111/resp.14191.

27. "Great Barrington Declaration," https://gbdeclaration.org/.

28. "Fauci Criticizes 'Herd Immunity'; Suggests People Rethink Thanksgiving Travel," NBC Bay Area, October 15, 2020, https://www.nbcbayarea.com/news/coronavirus/fauci-criticizes-herd-immunity-suggests-people-rethink-thanksgiving-travel/2381019/.

29. Users found that Googling "Great Barrington Declaration" produced a spate of articles critical of the declaration, rather than the declaration itself. See, for instance, Dr. Delbert Meyer, "Why Has Google Censored the Great Barrington Declaration?" DelMeyer.net, January 20, 2021, http://delmeyer.net/the-great-barrington-declaration/.

30. Spencerbdavis, "COVID-19 Vaccine Vial Prop—mRNA," Wikimedia Commons, April 8, 2021, https://commons.wikimedia.org/wiki/File:Solo-mrna-vaccine-2.jpg.

31. "Exclusive: Former Harvard Prof. Martin Kulldorff: 'Science and Public Health Are Broken,'" *Epoch Times*, February 16, 2022, https://www.theepochtimes.com/mkt_app/exclusive-former-harvard-prof-martin-kulldorff-science-and-public-health-are-broken_4270247.html. Professor Kulldorff and Harvard University parted company after he grew increasingly critical of the failed pandemic response. He is now happily ensconced at Hillsdale College's Brownstone Institute.

32. Johan Ahlander, "Sweden Declare[s] Pandemic Over, despite Warnings from Scientists," Euronews, February 10, 2022, https://www.euronews.com/2022/02/10/uk-health-coronavirus-sweden-restrictions.

33. "Covid-19: Lifting of All Domestic Restrictions and Restrictions at the Border," Government of Iceland Ministry of Health, February 23, 2022, https://www.government.is/news/article/2022/02/23/COVID-19-Lifting-of-all-domestic-restrictions-and-restrictions-at-the-border/.

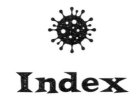

Index

Y

Z